Breast Pathology

Editor

KIMBERLY H. ALLISON

SURGICAL PATHOLOGY CLINICS

www.surgpath.theclinics.com

Consulting Editor

JASON L. HORNICK

March 2022 • Volume 15 • Number 1

ELSEVIER

1600 John F. Kennedy Boulevard • Suite 1800 • Philadelphia, Pennsylvania, 19103-2899

http://www.theclinics.com

SURGICAL PATHOLOGY CLINICS Volume 15, Number 1
March 2022 ISSN 1875-9181, ISBN-13: 978-0-323-89684-9

Editor: Katerina Heidhausen
Developmental Editor: Diana Grace Ang

Surgical Pathology Clinics (ISSN 1875-9181) is published quarterly by Elsevier Inc., 360 Park Avenue South, New York, NY 10010. Months of issue are March, June, September, and December. Business and Editorial Office: Elsevier Inc., 1600 John F. Kennedy Blvd., Ste. 1800, Philadelphia, PA 19103-2899. Accounting and Circulation Offices: Elsevier Inc., 3251 Riverport Lane, Maryland Heights, MO 63043. Periodicals postage paid at New York, NY and at additional mailing offices. Subscription prices are $237.00 per year (US individuals), $376.00 per year (US institutions), $100.00 per year (US students/residents), $283.00 per year (Canadian individuals), $395.00 per year (Canadian Institutions), $284.00 per year (foreign individuals), $395.00 per year (foreign institutions), and $120.00 per year (international students/residents), $100.00 per year (Canadian students/residents). Foreign air speed delivery is included in all *Clinics'* subscription prices. All prices are subject to change without notice. **POSTMASTER:** Send address changes to *Surgical Pathology Clinics*, Elsevier, 3251 Riverport Lane, Maryland Heights, MO 63043. **Customer Service: 1-800-654-2452 (US). From outside the United States, call 1-314-447-8871. Fax: 1-314-447-8029. E-mail:** JournalsCustomerServiceusa@elsevier.com **(for print support)** and JournalsOnlineSupport-usa@elsevier.com **(for online support).**

Reprints. For copies of 100 or more, of articles in this publication, please contact the Commercial Reprints Department, Elsevier Inc., 360 Park Avenue South, New York, NY 10010-1710. Tel. 212-633-3874; Fax: 212-633-3820; E-mail: reprints@elsevier.com.

Surgical Pathology Clinics of North America is covered in *MEDLINE/PubMed (Index Medicus).*

Contributors

CONSULTING EDITOR

JASON L. HORNICK, MD, PhD
Director of Surgical Pathology and
Immunohistochemistry, Brigham and Women's
Hospital, Professor of Pathology, Harvard
Medical School, Boston, Massachusetts, USA

EDITOR

KIMBERLY H. ALLISON, MD
Professor of Pathology, Vice Chair of
Education, Director of Breast Pathology and
Breast Pathology Fellowship, Director of
Pathology Residency Training, Department of
Pathology, Stanford University School of
Medicine, Stanford, California, USA

AUTHORS

EMILY B. AMBINDER, MD
Assistant Professor, Breast Imaging Division,
The Russell H. Morgan Department of
Radiology and Radiological Science, Johns
Hopkins Medicine, Baltimore, Maryland, USA

AGNES BALLA, MD, MHS
Assistant Professor of Pathology, Department
of Pathology and Laboratory Medicine, Larner
College of Medicine, University of Vermont,
UVM Medical Center, Burlington, Vermont,
USA

BENJAMIN C. CALHOUN, MD, PhD
Associate Professor, Director of Anatomic
Pathology, Director of Breast Pathology,
Department of Pathology and Laboratory
Medicine, The University of North Carolina at
Chapel Hill, Chapel Hill, North Carolina, USA

ASHLEY CIMINO-MATHEWS, MD
Associate Professor, Departments of
Pathology and Oncology, Johns Hopkins
School of Medicine, Baltimore, Maryland, USA

ALLISON S. CLEARY, MD, PhD
Assistant Professor, Department of Pathology,
University of Utah School of Medicine,
Huntsman Cancer Hospital, Salt Lake City,
Utah, USA

TIMOTHY M. D'ALFONSO, MD
Associate Attending Pathologist, Memorial
Sloan Kettering Cancer Center, New York, New
York, USA

QINGQING DING, MD, PhD
Department of Anatomical Pathology, The
University of Texas MD Anderson Cancer
Center, Houston, Texas, USA

LEISHA A. EMENS, MD, PhD
Professor, Department of Oncology, UPMC
Hillman Cancer Center/Magee Women's
Hospital, Pittsburgh, Pennsylvania, USA

MEGHAN R. FLANAGAN, MD, MPH
Assistant Professor, Department of Surgery,
University of Washington, Seattle, Washington,
USA

TANYA GUPTA, MD
Clinical Assistant Professor, Department of
Medicine, Division of Oncology, Stanford
University School of Medicine, Palo Alto,
California, USA

KELLY HUNT, MD
Department of Breast Surgical Oncology, The
University of Texas MD Anderson Cancer
Center, Houston, Texas, USA

GEETHA JAGANNATHAN, MBBS
Surgical Pathology Assistant, Department of
Pathology, Johns Hopkins School of Medicine,
Baltimore, Maryland, USA

THAER KHOURY, MD
Professor of Oncology, Pathology Department,
Roswell Park Comprehensive Cancer Center,
Buffalo, New York, USA

MARK R. KILGORE, MD
Director of Breast Pathology and Assistant
Professor, Department of Laboratory Medicine
and Pathology, University of Washington,
University of Washington Medical Center,
Seattle, Washington, USA

SUSAN C. LESTER, MD, PhD
Associate Pathologist, Department of
Pathology, Brigham and Women's Hospital,
Assistant Professor, Harvard Medical School,
Boston, Massachusetts, USA

**ELAINE HSUEN LIM, MBBCh (Cantab),
MRCP (UK), PhD (Cantab)**
Senior Consultant, Division of Medical
Oncology, National Cancer Centre, Singapore

KATHRYN P. LOWRY, MD
Assistant Professor, Department of Radiology,
University of Washington, Seattle Cancer Care
Alliance, Seattle, Washington, USA

TIMOTHY ISAAC MILLER, MD, MA
Pathology Resident, Department of Laboratory
Medicine and Pathology, University of
Washington, University of Washington Medical
Center, Seattle, Washington, USA

MIRNA B. PODOLL, MD
Assistant Professor of Pathology,
Microbiology, and Immunology, Vanderbilt
University Medical Center, Nashville,
Tennessee, USA

DARA S. ROSS, MD
Associate Attending Pathologist, Memorial
Sloan Kettering Cancer Center, New York, New
York, USA

AYSEGUL SAHIN, MD
Department of Anatomical Pathology, The
University of Texas MD Anderson Cancer
Center, Houston, Texas, USA

MELINDA E. SANDERS, MD
Professor of Pathology, Microbiology, and
Immunology, Vanderbilt University Medical
Center, Nashville, Tennessee, USA

**BENJAMIN YONGCHENG TAN, MBBS,
FRCPath**
Consultant, Department of Anatomical
Pathology, Singapore General Hospital,
Singapore

PUAY HOON TAN, MBBS, FRCPA
Chairman and Senior Consultant, Division of
Pathology, Singapore General Hospital,
Singapore, Singapore

MEGAN L. TROXELL, MD, PhD
Professor, Department of Pathology, Stanford
University School of Medicine, Stanford
Pathology, Stanford, California, USA

DONALD L. WEAVER, MD
Professor of Pathology, Department of
Pathology and Laboratory Medicine, Larner
College of Medicine, University of Vermont,
UVM Cancer Center, UVM Medical Center,
Burlington, Vermont, USA

MARISSA J. WHITE, MD
Assistant Professor, Department of Pathology,
Johns Hopkins School of Medicine, Baltimore,
Maryland, USA

RENA R. XIAN, MD
Assistant Professor, Departments of Pathology
and Oncology, Johns Hopkins School of
Medicine, Baltimore, Maryland, USA

ESTHER YOON, MD
Department of Anatomical Pathology, The
University of Texas MD Anderson Cancer
Center, Houston, Texas, USA

Contents

Errors in anatomic pathology can result in patients receiving inappropriate treatment and poor patient outcomes. Policies and procedures are necessary to decrease error and improve diagnostic concordance. Breast pathology may be more prone to diagnostic errors than other surgical pathology subspecialties due to inherit borderline diagnostic categories such as atypical ductal hyperplasia and low-grade ductal carcinoma in situ. Mandatory secondary review of internal and outside referral cases before treatment is effective in reducing diagnostic errors and improving concordance. Assessment of error through amendment/addendum tracking, implementing an incident reporting system, and multidisciplinary tumor boards can establish procedures to prevent future error.

The presence of detected metastases in locoregional lymph nodes of women with breast cancer is an important prognostic variable for cancer staging, prognosis, and treatment planning. Standardized and systematic lymph node evaluation with gross and microscopic protocols designed to detect all macrometastases larger than 2.0 mm is the appropriate objective based on clinical outcomes evidence. By random chance, pathology sections will either detect or miss smaller micrometastases and isolated tumor cell clusters (ITCs) depending on their location in the paraffin block. Although these smaller metastases have prognostic significance, they are not predictive of recurrence for chemotherapy naïve patients. Thus, protocols to reliably detect metastases smaller than 2.0 mm are not required or recommended by guidelines. Women with T1-T2 breast cancer with a clinically negative axilla but with 1 or 2 pathologically positive sentinel nodes now have alternative options including observation and axillary irradiation and do not necessarily require completion axillary dissection.

Breast cancer is the most common malignant tumor in females. While most carcinomas are categorized as invasive carcinoma, no special type (NST), a diverse group of tumors with distinct pathologic and clinical features is also recognized, ranging in incidence from relatively more common to rare. So-called "special histologic type" tumors display more than 90% of a specific, distinctive histologic pattern, while a spectrum of tumors more often encountered in the salivary gland may also arise in the breast. Metaplastic carcinomas can present diagnostic challenges. Some uncommon tumors harbor pathognomonic genetic alterations. This article provides an overview of the key diagnostic points and differential diagnoses for this group of disparate lesions, as well as the salient clinical characteristics of each entity.

Cytotoxic or endocrine therapy before surgery (neoadjuvant) for breast cancer has become standard of care, affording the opportunity to assess and quantify response in the subsequent resection specimen. Correlation with radiology, cassette mapping, and histologic review with a semi-quantitative reporting system such as residual cancer burden (RCB) provides important prognostic data that may guide further therapy. The tumor bed should be identified histologically, often as a collagenized zone devoid of normal breast epithelium, with increased vasculature. Identification of residual treated carcinoma may require careful high power examination, as residual tumor cells may be small and dyscohesive; features are widely variable and include hyperchromatic small, large, or multiple nuclei with clear, foamy, or eosinophilic cytoplasm. Calculation of RCB requires residual carcinoma span in 2 dimensions, estimated carcinoma cellularity (% area), number of involved lymph nodes, and span of largest nodal carcinoma. These RCB parameters may differ from AJCC staging measurements, which depend on only contiguous carcinoma in breast and lymph nodes.

Most of the high-grade spindle cell lesions of the breast are malignant phyllodes tumors (MPTs), spindle cell carcinomas (SpCCs), and matrix-producing metaplastic breast carcinomas (MP-MBCs). MPTs have neoplastic spindle stromal cells and a classic leaf-like architecture with subepithelial stromal condensation. MPTs are often positive for CD34, CD117, and bcl-2 and are associated with MED12, TERT, and RARA mutations. SpCCs and MP-MBCs are high-grade metaplastic carcinomas, whereas neoplastic epithelial cells become spindled or show heterologous mesenchymal differentiation, respectively. The expression of epithelial markers must be evaluated to make a diagnosis. SAS, or rare metastatic spindle cell tumors, are seen in the breast, and clinical history is the best supporting evidence. Surgical resection is the standard of care.

As the first node in treatment algorithms for breast disease, pathologists have the potential to play a critical role in refining appropriate therapy for lesions in the atypical ducal hyperplasia-ductal carcinoma in situ (ADH-DCIS) spectrum by conservatively approaching diagnosis of lesions limited in size on core needle biopsy. Appropriate efforts to downgrade the diagnosis of lesions at the borderline of ADH and DCIS will certainly lead to more breast conservation and avoid the common morbidities of mastectomy, sentinel node biopsy, and radiation therapy. Whether results of clinical trials of active surveillance will successfully identify a subset of women who may successfully forgo even limited breast-conserving surgery is eagerly anticipated. Given the increasing concern that a significant number of women with DCIS are overtreated, identification of patients at very low risk for progression who may forgo surgery and radiation therapy safely is of significant interest.

Geetha Jagannathan, Marissa J. White, Rena R. Xian, Leisha A. Emens, and Ashley Cimino-Mathews

Predictive biomarker testing on metastatic breast cancer is essential for determining patient eligibility for targeted therapeutics. The National Comprehensive Cancer Network currently recommends assessment of specific biomarkers on metastatic tumor subtypes, including hormone receptors, HER2, and BRCA1/2 mutations, on all newly metastatic breast cancers subtypes; programmed death-ligand 1 on metastatic triple-negative carcinomas; and PIK3CA mutation status on estrogen receptor-positive carcinomas. In select circumstances mismatch repair protein deficiency and/or microsatellite insufficiency, tumor mutation burden, and NTRK translocation status are also testing options. Novel biomarker testing, such as detecting PIK3CA mutations in circulating tumor DNA, is expanding in this rapidly evolving arena.

Allison S. Cleary and Susan C. Lester

Video content accompanies this article at http://www.surgpath.theclinics.com

Gross examination is the foundation for the pathologic evaluation of all surgical specimens. The rapid identification of cancers is essential for intraoperative assessment and preservation of biomolecules for molecular assays. Additional key components of gross examination include the accurate identification of the lesions of interest, correlation with clinical and radiologic findings, assessment of lesion number and size, relationship of lesions to surgical margins, documenting the extent of disease spread to the skin and chest wall, and the identification of axillary lymph nodes. Although the importance of gross evaluation is undeniable, current challenges include the difficulty of teaching grossing well and its possible perceived undervaluation compared with microscopic and molecular studies. In the future, new rapid imaging techniques without the need for tissue processing may provide an ideal melding of gross and microscopic pathologic evaluation.

Dara S. Ross and Timothy M. D'Alfonso

Papillary neoplasms of the breast are a heterogeneous group of tumors characterized by fibrovascular cores lined by epithelium, with or without myoepithelial cells. Papillary neoplasms include benign, atypical, and malignant tumors that show varying histopathologic features and clinical outcomes. Appropriate pathologic classification is crucial to guide clinical treatment. Classification of papillary neoplasms is largely based on morphology, with immunohistochemistry playing an ancillary role to establish diagnoses. Recent molecular studies have provided insight into the genomics of these lesions. This review summarizes the histologic, immunohistochemical, and molecular features of papillary neoplasms of the breast that are important for diagnosis and treatment.

Image-guided core needle biopsies (CNBs) of the breast frequently result in a diagnosis of a benign or atypical lesion associated with breast cancer risk. The subsequent clinical management of these patients is variable, reflecting a lack of consensus on criteria for selecting patients for clinical and radiological follow-up versus immediate surgical excision. In this review, the evidence from prospective studies of breast CNB with radiologicalepathological correlation is evaluated and summarized. The data support an emerging consensus on the importance of radiologicalpathological correlation in standardizing the selection of patients for active surveillance versus surgery.

Metaplastic breast carcinoma (MpBC) is a heterogeneous group of tumors that clinically could be divided into low risk and high risk. It is important to recognize the different types of MpBC, as the high-risk subtypes have worse clinical outcomes than triple-negative breast cancer. It is important for the pathologist to be aware of the MpBC entities and use the proposed algorithms (morphology and immunohistochemistry) to assist in rendering the final diagnosis. Few pitfalls are discussed, including misinterpretation of immunohistochemistry and certain histomorphologies, particularly spindle lesions associated with complex sclerosing lesions.

SURGICAL PATHOLOGY CLINICS

SERIES OF RELATED INTEREST

Clinics in Laboratory Medicine
http://www.labmed.theclinics.com/
Medical Clinics
https://www.medical.theclinics.com/

THE CLINICS ARE AVAILABLE ONLINE!
Access your subscription at:
www.theclinics.com

Preface
The Importance of Addressing Diagnostic Challenges in Breast Pathology with an Understanding of Current Clinical Treatment Implications

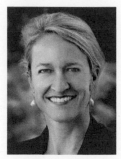

Kimberly H. Allison, MD
Editor

In this issue of *Surgical Pathology Clinics*, we present a collection of reviews focused on Breast Pathology, entitled "Diagnostic Challenges in Breast Pathology and Their Clinical Implications." The topics in this breast pathology issue have been selected because of their relevance to clinical treatment. These are often challenging areas for the practicing pathologist, where subtle diagnostic differences can have major clinical implications. In these articles, the invited breast pathology experts, often with their clinical colleagues as coauthors, not just explain diagnostic criteria and how to resolve differentials but also provide answers to the question of what difference it can make clinically.

Several of these reviews focus on key clinical questions and provide practical approaches to answering them with an emphasis on possible clinical treatment algorithms. Is the high-grade spindle cell lesion in the breast a sarcoma or a carcinoma, and how will the clinical team manage either diagnosis? If you diagnose a special histologic type of breast cancer, what specific differences in treatment pathways and options occur? Why does it matter that we identify, characterize, and quantify the amount of residual breast cancer after neoadjuvant treatment? How hard do we need to work to identify microscopic axillary lymph node spread of breast cancer, and what are actionable thresholds that make treatment differences? What tests in the metastatic breast cancer setting are recommended; how are they performed, and what therapies do they make a patient a candidate for?

In the era of deescalation of treatment and individualized risk management, the pathologist's

Surgical Pathology 15 (2022) xi–xii
https://doi.org/10.1016/j.path.2021.11.012
1875-9181/22/© 2021 Published by Elsevier Inc.

approach to diagnosing risk lesions on core biopsy, including the spectrum of atypical ductal hyperplasia to low-grade ductal carcinoma in situ (DCIS), has also become a critical component of the multidisciplinary conversation. A deeper molecular understanding of the spectrum of papillary neoplasms of the breast is also presented with their associated diagnostic challenges and clinical implications. And importantly, methods to ensure accurate gross tissue sampling, to reduce errors and increase diagnostic concordance, are emphasized in novel ways, including with a QR code link to a video on grossing techniques.

Thank you to all the experts who contributed to this multifaceted issue and helped to provide such a valuable resource!

Kimberly H. Allison, MD
Department of Pathology
Stanford University School of Medicine
300 Pasteur Drive
Lane Room 235
Stanford, CA 94305-5324, USA

E-mail address:
allisonk@stanford.edu

Error Reduction and Diagnostic Concordance in Breast Pathology

Timothy Isaac Miller, MD, MA[a],*,
Meghan R. Flanagan, MD, MPH[b], Kathryn P. Lowry, MD[c],
Mark R. Kilgore, MD[a]

KEYWORDS

• Breast • Error • Pathology • Anatomic • Accuracy • Review • Concordance

Key points

- Anatomic breast pathology may be more prone to error due to borderline diagnostic categories such as atypical ductal hyperplasia (ADH) versus low-grade ductal carcinoma in situ (lgDCIS).

- Mandatory second review of atypical ductal hyperplasia (ADH) and worse diagnoses may reduce diagnostic errors and improve concordance.

- Pathology review of outside referral cases before treatment can decrease error, improve concordance, and change patient management.

- Practical approaches to reduce error include inking biopsies, controlling cold ischemia (CIT) and formalin fixation time (FFT), assuring rad-path calcification concordance, surgeon intraoperative inking of lumpectomies, and standardized reporting.

- Ongoing assessment of error through amendment/addendum tracking, implementing an incident reporting system, and multidisciplinary tumor boards can help establish procedures to prevent future error.

ABSTRACT

A 2017 case report details the story of an 18-year-old female diagnosed with concurrent invasive ductal and tubulo-lobular carcinoma after undergoing excisional biopsy for a 4-cm periareolar breast mass[1]; this was in the context of no significant past medical history and no significant family oncologic history. The patient sought second opinion and treatment options at another institution, which upon mandatory pathology review identified dystrophic calcifications in the intima of medium-sized arteries. This uncommon finding in a patient of this age prompted the reviewing pathologist to suggest the possibility of a specimen mix-up at the outside institution. After an investigation, it was determined that the 18-year-old's specimen label had been swapped with that of an elderly woman. The correct diagnosis of the 18-year-old was mammary fibromatosis.[1] Thankfully, the young patient never underwent any type of oncologic treatment of invasive carcinoma, largely due to institutional policies for systematic and mandatory confirmation of outside diagnoses before initiation of treatment. Because of the astute pathology review, no patient harm occurred.

This case report is a chilling reminder that errors in pathology occur, but it also highlights that errors can be detected and prevented. In this case, the

[a] Department of Laboratory Medicine and Pathology, University of Washington, University of Washington Medical Center, 1959 Northeast Pacific Street, Box 357100, Seattle, WA 98195, USA; [b] Department of Surgery, University of Washington, 1100 Fairview Avenue, M4-B874, Seattle, WA 98109, USA; [c] Department of Radiology, University of Washington, Seattle Cancer Care Alliance, 1144 Eastlake Avenue East, LG-215, Seattle, WA 98109, USA
* Corresponding author.
E-mail address: timiller@uw.edu

Surgical Pathology 15 (2022) 1–13
https://doi.org/10.1016/j.path.2021.11.001
1875-9181/22/© 2021 Elsevier Inc. All rights reserved.

pathologist used clinical context to detect the error: if a diagnosis is highly unlikely or does not make sense clinically or radiographically, it is prudent for the pathologist to investigate. Evidence suggests that breast pathology, specifically, may be more susceptible to errors than other surgical pathology subspecialties, making awareness and techniques to reduce it more essential. A blinded review of 8916 surgical pathology and nongynecologic cytology cases within an institution resulted in 69 (0.8%) amendments, and of these, breast core biopsies were overrepresented (4.4%).[2] A review of 335 pathology malpractice claims from 1998 to 2003 at one law firm reported that 12.5% were for breast biopsy specimens (20 cases of missed cancer diagnoses, 22 cases of false-positive cancer diagnoses). Only melanoma cases had a higher percentage of claims.[3]

This article, devoted to error and diagnostic concordance within breast pathology, will first define error and then discuss best practice recommendations (clinical care points) for error prevention, including the following: secondary review,

institutional review of outside cases, using breast subspecialty-trained surgical pathologists, inter (or multi) disciplinary approach, practical/technical workflow interventions, and leveraging ongoing assessment of error (**Box 1**).

HOW TO DEFINE ERROR

A 2005 College of American Pathologists (CAP) Q-probe study looked at self-reported data from 74 laboratories that resulted in a mean and median discrepancy rate of 6.7% and 5.1%, respectively.[4] The study broadly defined *discrepancy* as encompassing everything from a change in diagnosis to a change in patient information to a typographic error. Obviously, an insignificant typographical error likely has no impact on patient care, whereas change in a benign or malignant diagnosis may have life-altering consequences. Of the discrepancies in the study, 5.3% resulted in changes to patient care. Although minimizing all discrepancies is ideal, those that impact patient care may result in patient harm and are therefore the

---

Box 1
Summarized best practice recommendations (clinical care points) to reduce error within breast pathology

Clinical care points: best practice recommendations
- Secondary review by another pathologist
  - Diagnosis of atypia or higher
- Institutional review of outside cases
  - Required before treatment (surgery, chemoradiation)
- Using breast subspecialty-trained surgical pathologists (consultation)
  - In unclear diagnoses that may affect patient management
    - Benign versus atypia
    - Benign versus malignant
    - Atypical papillary lesions
    - DCIS with microinvasion
- Interdisciplinary approach
  - Multidisciplinary breast subspecialty clinics (tumor board)
- Practical/technical practices to reduce error
  - Catching specimen mislabeling and core biopsy inking
  - Controlling cold ischemia time and formalin fixation time.
  - Rad-path correlation of biopsies of calcifications
  - Surgeon intraoperative inking of lumpectomies
  - Standardized reporting
- Leveraging ongoing assessment of error

most important to prevent. This study highlights a major challenge when researching error—the definition matters, and the data obtained are largely based on what is included and excluded from the category of error.

Entire careers have focused on error in pathology and medicine. For the purposes of this article, error will be defined as inaccurate or incorrect information in the patient's surgical pathology report that results in inappropriate treatment decisions and/or prognostication of the patient's true disease.[5] Pathologists are well aware of preanalytical, analytical, and postanalytical subclassifications of error. A similar and expanded model of error by Zarbo and colleagues[6] describes error in the context of defective specimen, defective identification, defective interpretation, or defective report. This classification scheme may help pathologists identify the issues generating errors and target resolutions.[6]

ERROR VERSUS OPINION: IS THERE A DIFFERENCE?

A major underlying source of diagnostic error within pathology occurs at the level of *Defective Interpretation* and involves equivocating or "borderline" diagnostic categories. The inherent challenge with such cases occurs when the same microscopic/histologic entity is reviewed by different pathologists with varying interpretations. Oftentimes the practice, for lack of an alternative, is to defer to the more experienced/senior pathologist for the "correct" diagnosis or refer the case to an expert consultant. The unfortunate reality of these equivocal cases is that obtaining the ultimate truth is problematic. Whether treated or not, one may never know the alternative outcome. A lesion considered to have malignant potential is often treated, which for many patients results in overtreatment. Alternatively, undertreatment may result in progression of disease and poor patient outcomes. Borderline lesions in pathology exemplify this diagnostic and treatment dilemma. By definition, opinions will vary as to the best classification of such entities.

Some of the best examples of such equivocal lesions exist in breast pathology. The inherit equivocation within the diagnoses of atypical ductal hyperplasia (ADH) and low-grade ductal carcinoma in situ (lgDCIS) is well documented. One study compared the diagnoses of 115 practicing pathologists who interpret breast specimens with the diagnoses of an expert-derived breast consensus panel. The study concluded that there was 96% agreement for invasive carcinoma, but only 48% agreement for atypical hyperplasia and

a 13% underinterpretation rate for lgDCIS.[7] Another study looked at 122 amended breast pathology reports at an academic institution and reported that 28% were for misinterpretations, including ADH interpreted as lgDCIS.[8] One must consider if these types of disagreements are classified as errors or a matter of opinion.

Considering the previously mentioned definition of error, it is most important to consider how the interpretation of ADH and lgDCIS impacts patient care. If ADH or lgDCIS is identified on core biopsy, excision is recommended regardless. Although the surgical procedure for lgDCIS (lumpectomy/ partial mastectomy) attempts to obtain clear margins, which may result in a larger-volume specimen, both lesions require excision. Therefore, the distinction of ADH versus lgDCIS at the time of biopsy is not an error under this definition.[9,10] However, after excision, there is an opportunity for changes to patient care. Most notably, if the disease process is more obvious in the excisional specimen compared with the prior biopsy, ADH can be upgraded to lgDCIS and treated appropriately. However, lgDCIS cannot be reduced to ADH without amending the original biopsy report and overturning the diagnosis. Thus, a unique scenario for error is created in which the outcome for overinterpretation of ADH as lgDCIS on core biopsy may result in irreversible changes to patient care, whereas lgDCIS underinterpreted as ADH may have little consequence. It must be noted that treatment plans are evolving based on advances in literature, and practices also depend on the clinical context of an individual patient. Alternatively, the same paradigm exists in the opposite direction for ADH and usual ductal hyperplasia (UDH). Overinterpretation of UDH as ADH may result in unnecessary excision, whereas underinterpretation of ADH may result in inadequate care and the potential to miss advanced disease (DCIS and/or invasive carcinoma). Several ancillary tests and diagnostic criteria exist to help better define these 3 entities (UDH, ADH, and lgDCIS), which is discussed in the article Melinda E. Sanders and Mirna Podoll's article, "ADH-DCIS Spectrum: Diagnostic Considerations and Treatment Impact in the Era of De-escalation," in this issue. For the purposes of this article, these borderline lesions are discussed to highlight error versus opinion and introduce the first best practice recommendation (clinical care point): secondary review.

SECONDARY REVIEW

Common practice within many anatomic pathology (AP) departments includes secondary review—requiring a second in-house pathologist to agree with a diagnosis. A 2010 report of 45 pathology laboratories found that approximately 6.6% of cases underwent secondary review before sign-out.[11] Requirements for secondary review vary across practices and may be required only for new malignant diagnoses. Similarly, some groups require secondary review for diagnoses that result in significant patient care decisions (excision, additional testing, medical treatment, etc.). Essentially, any diagnosis in which a false-positive diagnosis may result in significant patient harm (surgical procedure, chemotherapy/radiation, etc.) may warrant review by another pathologist. The most stringent of practices require secondary reads on all negative biopsy cases as well, as a false-negative diagnosis may be as detrimental. Although not specific to breast pathology, one study of AP errors identified that false-negative diagnoses were the most common type of error, comprising 33% of identified errors.[12] Studies have demonstrated the utility of secondary review, showing that it reduces amendment rates.[13] A review of 3417 amendments (out of 1,667,547 specimens) from 359 laboratories identified that institutions with routine diagnostic slide review before case sign-out had an amendment rate of 1.2 per 1000 specimens and those without routine slide review had an amendment rate of 1.4 per 1000 specimens.[14] These studies support The CAP recommendation that AP groups have a defined system for secondary review of selected cases.[15] However, this recommendation does not specify which cases require secondary review, and ultimately the system is determined by each pathology group.

One option used by a minority of practices is review of every case. A 1993 study performed secondary review on all AP cases, which detected 14 instances (out of 5397 cases, 0.25%) of potentially clinically significant discrepancies.[16] However, this time-intensive technique is not feasible for most pathology groups in our current health care system. An alternative study investigated randomly generated cases that require secondary review before sign-out, which decreased amendment rates compared with no formal review system.[17] Intuitively, though, a system that picks specific cases for review, rather than at random, is superior for many reasons. At least one study has demonstrated that a focused system for selecting secondary review is better at detecting errors than a random system.[18]

If a focused system for secondary review is done for breast cases, what are the optimal criteria? Should review be performed on all cases, for atypia or worse diagnoses, for DCIS or worse diagnoses, or only for malignant/invasive neoplasms? Elmore and colleagues[19] evaluated the cutoff for secondary review of breast specimens. If secondary review was required only for malignant diagnoses, this did not result in significantly improved accuracy. However, when secondary review was required for all atypia, DCIS, and invasive carcinoma, or for only DCIS and invasive carcinoma, this did improve accuracy.[19] A 2014 survey of 252 pathologists who sign-out breast specimens found many institutions already require secondary review: 65% of pathologists surveyed reported mandatory secondary review for invasive diagnoses, 56% for DCIS, and 36% for ADH. In addition, 81% reported they often sought second opinion, even if there was not a policy.[20] As mentioned previously, many malignant diagnoses have relatively straightforward histology and high interobserver agreement, whereas atypia and DCIS are more challenging diagnoses with less concordance. With this in mind, it is interesting that many institutions do not require secondary review for an interpretation of atypia, when it is more often misinterpreted; this may be related to departmental policy, in which many groups have an overarching policy to review malignant diagnoses only. By definition, atypia is not malignant and, therefore, does not fall under the purview of mandatory review. However, unlike many other organ systems, a diagnosis of atypia in the breast typically results in surgical excision. ADH and lgDCIS are on a biologic spectrum, whereas other specimen types use the term "atypia" to describe benign processes that do not warrant additional treatment.

Even without an official policy, pathologists may be seeking secondary review of atypia diagnoses. One study showed 115 pathologists different breast cases to determine when they would request a second opinion, and in 67% to 78% of atypia cases, pathologists reported they would want a second opinion.[21] However, instituting a policy rather than relying on a pathologist's own intuition to seek a secondary review may be the best strategy. There is at least one study that found pathologists overestimated their actual diagnostic agreement for breast cases with an expert panel.[22] This finding suggests breast subspecialty services or specialists within pathology groups may need to implement their own policy to trigger secondary review of atypia or higher diagnoses.

This strategy does miss false-negative diagnoses because it requires the initial pathologist to recognize at least atypia to trigger mandatory secondary review. The ideal method to catch false-negative diagnoses is to require every single case undergo secondary review, but as previously discussed, this is not possible in all settings given the high case volume to breast pathologist ratio. Therefore, culture that encourages secondary review whenever the initial pathologist is not fully confident in their diagnosis, even if secondary review is not mandatory, is critical for success. Scheduling systems that ensure at least 2 breast-experienced pathologists are on service each day ensures easy and timely access to another breast-trained pathologist for secondary review. Depending on the size of an institution, these methods may not be feasible. Alternative strategies for timely secondary review of cases may be necessary. This discussion of secondary review for internal cases serves as a transition to the second best practice recommendation (clinical care point): institutional review of outside cases before treatment.

INSTITUTIONAL REVIEW OF OUTSIDE CASES

Like the case vignette at the start of the article demonstrated, many tertiary treatment centers also require pathology review of outside referral cases to their institution. This approach may also help satisfy Joint Commission on Accreditation of Healthcare Organization (JCAHO) standards. JCAHO requires hospitals collect data on significant discrepancies between preoperative and postoperative diagnoses, including pathology (see Joint Commission [JCHAO] Standards PI.01.01.01 EP5). Breast pathology-specific studies have looked retrospectively at how often these reviews result in clinically significant changes to the patient's treatment plan. Several of these are mentioned here, and when possible, whether or not the review resulted in a change in patient management.

Of 430 reviewed cases in one study, 43 (10%) resulted in a difference in interpretation that changed surgical management. Twelve cases with benign diagnoses changed to malignant interpretations, and 4 cases with malignant diagnoses changed to benign interpretations.[23] A study of 1970 referral cases reviewed over 1 year found that 11.5% had discrepancies that impacted patient care.[24] Another study evaluating review of all referred node-negative invasive carcinoma and DCIS cases over a 4-year period resulted in 6% of patients with significant changes in their care based on the reviews.[25] A study of 205 reviewed cases (when requested by the treating clinician rather than mandatory review) discovered that 52 cases (25.4%) had significant changes that altered patient care.[26] Another study of 502 mandatory reviews of needle core biopsies identified that 21% of cases were discordant (8%

deemed as major) with 3% of the cases resulting in actual changes to patient management. Most commonly, discordant cases were of premalignant lesions (16 cases) followed by prognostic markers (10 cases).[27] This study also highlights the importance of prognostic/predictive marker (ER/PR/HER2 status) review in addition to routine histologic sections. An additional study with mandatory review of prognostic/predictive markers (1139 cases) identified a difference in interpretation that resulted in alternative patient management (0.6% of cases).[28]

Overall, the findings of these referral studies demonstrate the importance of requiring interinstitutional breast pathology review before initiating treatment. This requires close working relationships between clinical care teams and reviewing pathologists. Strong administrative support and institutional policy are also necessary to support this type of systematic review. Our system requires that all newly referred patients have their pathology reviewed in-house before undergoing evaluation for treatment or surgery. Retrospective review in our system identifies major interpretative changes at the time of referral to be approximately 3% to 5%; this is significant for 2 reasons, the most notable being patient care. These data imply that 5 of 100 patients may require more or less treatment (ie, changes to surgical management, changes to chemotherapy and/or radiation) based on review alone. The second reason is cost savings. Reviewing outside pathology material generates decreased revenue when compared with internal cases (a cost to the system). However, this is more than accounted for when one considers decreased cost to the health care system by identifying inappropriate patient mement before it occurs. Reports estimate that up to 30% of annual health care spending in the United States ($750 billion) may be spent unnecessarily on services and other inefficiencies.[29] These are important considerations when discussing approaches for systematic reviews of outside pathology material with institutional leadership. Typically, review of outside cases at a tertiary treatment center involves advanced levels of care, which serves as a transition to the third best practice recommendation (clinical care point): using breast subspecialty-trained surgical pathologists.

BREAST-TRAINED PATHOLOGISTS

Large tertiary treatment centers often have subspecialized pathologists, including a team of specialty-trained and dedicated breast pathologists. The previously mentioned studies supporting mandatory pathology review of outside material are largely focused on this setting and illuminate the potential gap between pathologists with breast expertise and a general surgical pathology model. Notably, these studies did not specify with what frequency the outside pathology was interpreted by a breast-trained pathologist. Nonetheless, smaller community-based pathology groups without breast-specific trained pathologists (or those without extensive experience with breast cases) may require a lower threshold for sending out cases for consultation.

Although most breast cases can be appropriately managed by a well-trained general surgical pathologist, there are unique and diagnostically challenging cases that may warrant external consultation. One study looked at 281 papillary lesions with both a core biopsy and excisional specimen. The diagnostic correlation for the core biopsy and excision was compared for both breast-trained pathologists and non-breast-trained pathologists. The non-breast-trained pathologists had a higher rate (26%) of upgrade from benign papilloma (core biopsy) to atypical or malignant lesion (excision) when compared with breast-trained pathologists (16%).[30] Another study compared the agreement rates between general and breast-trained pathologists using the Kappa interrater reliability scale, finding poor agreement for pleomorphic lobular carcinoma in situ (pLCIS) and moderate agreement for ADH, low/intermediate-grade DCIS, and DCIS with microinvasion.[31] Although moderate agreement may seem reasonable, it indicates that only 41% to 60% of instances have actual agreement.[32] Of course, there is equivocation in components of diagnoses that ultimately would not affect patient care (ie, low vs intermediate-grade DCIS), whereas others may have profound impact (ie, benign diagnosis vs ADH). One study evaluated the most common reasons for outside pathology consultation to breast-trained pathologists at tertiary medical centers. Of 985 consultation cases at one institution, 33.3% were for atypia, 17.2% for papillary lesions, and 14% for subtyping carcinoma.[33]

A reasonable recommendation for pathology groups without significant breast experience or breast subspecialty-trained surgical pathologists is to consider obtaining consultation when the differential diagnosis will impact patient care and the diagnoses under consideration are known to be challenging; these include, but are not limited to, atypia versus benign, benign versus malignant, atypical papillary lesions, and DCIS with microinvasion. Before considering consultation, one must feel confident the lesion of interest has been sampled, which serves as a transition to the fourth best practice recommendation: inter (or multi) disciplinary approach.

INTERDISCIPLINARY APPROACH

A major source of error in breast pathology is pathology and radiology discordance. This discordance occurs when the pathologic diagnosis does not account for imaging features of the biopsied lesion, which may be due to inaccurate targeting or undersampling at the time of biopsy. This concept is briefly discussed here as it relates to error and is more fully discussed in the article Benjamin C. Calhoun and Emily B. Ambinder's article, "Risk-Associated Lesions of the Breast in Core Needle Biopsies: Current Approaches to Radiological-Pathological Correlation," in this issue.

Well-defined policies and procedures must exist for evaluating concordance. Documentation of imaging-pathology concordance and follow-up recommendations are standard components of image-guided biopsy reporting.[34] Clear communication and an integrated clinical relationship between pathology and radiology is likely as important as identification of discordance alone.[35] Pathologists must recognize potential discrepancies between the pathologic findings and the radiologic assessment and ensure that any concern for misdiagnosis is communicated clearly to prevent errors in diagnosis. Oftentimes, this involves direct communication between pathologists and radiologists to confirm that the histologic findings are representative of the imaging (eg, are there histologic findings that explain a mass or subtle distortion?). Formal interdepartmental collaboration to develop standard workflows ensure that both entities are aware of concordance and discordance and subsequent management recommendations.[35] It is worth noting that correlation often extends beyond pathology and radiology and includes clinical context as well.

Another tool to optimize care is a breast multidisciplinary tumor board. Studies indicate that multidisciplinary groups, including radiology, pathology, surgical oncology, medical oncology, and radiation oncology decrease error and improve patient outcomes. One retrospective study of 149 breast cases reviewed at a multidisciplinary breast tumor board found that review of pathology at the conference altered the surgical management plan for 9% of the patients.[36] Another study reported decreased time between diagnosis and treatment initiation (42.2 days vs 29.6 days; $P < .0008$) following implementation of a multidisciplinary breast cancer clinic.[37] As previously discussed, institutional review of outside cases is commonly performed in anticipation of tumor board presentation. Therefore, although not directly measured, the previously cited data with respect to discrepancy and change in diagnosis may further corroborate the benefit of multidisciplinary breast subspecialty practices. However, this requires accurate diagnoses using material that has been appropriately labeled and processed for the designated patient, which serves as a transition to the fifth best practice recommendation (clinical care point): practical/technical practices to reduce error.

PRACTICAL/TECHNICAL PRACTICES TO REDUCE ERROR

SPECIMEN MISLABELING AND CORE BIOPSY INKING

Specimen mislabeling is an overt error that can be missed without a policy or procedure for internal review. A 2011 study of 136 institutions identified 1811 mislabeling events, which subclassified the labeling errors into cases (27.1%), specimens (19.8%), blocks (25.5%), and slides (27.7%).[38] The errors (96.7%) were identified largely due to routine formal checks immediately after mislabeling occurred. Systematic review of patient name and specimen site in the gross description helped identify mislabeled specimen containers.[38] Best practice includes formal, routine label checks by every person involved with a specimen at each step in its workflow. A labeling error more specific to breast pathology is specimen laterality. An error in laterality designation (left vs right) can result in a catastrophic event, particularly if bilateral procedures were performed. A systematic review of imaging data to confirm the laterality of the abnormality at the time of sign out ensures laterality concordance because if the laterality is designated incorrectly on both the label and requisition form received by accessioning, this will otherwise pass formal internal checks for consistency.

In addition to standard accessioning and grossing techniques to reduce specimen misidentification, additional precautions can be taken to help identify errors. One method involves systematic inking of specimens when a series of similar biopsies are grossed sequentially (ie, breast needle core biopsies). As each breast core biopsy is grossed, it is inked a different color than the previous. Once all colors have been used, the pattern repeats itself. Confirming the ink color on the slide matches the ink color in the gross description decreases the likelihood of a specimen mix-up. This

additional safeguard helps ensure that the correct patient is receiving the appropriate diagnosis. Studies have demonstrated the utility of core biopsy inking in both prostate and breast core biopsies.[39,40] Of note, certain colors and ink types can autofluoresce and interfere with fluorescence in situ hybridization (FISH) results; this is problematic with breast core biopsies because they are commonly evaluated by ancillary FISH studies, which routinely use red/orange and green fluorescent signals.[41]

COLD ISCHEMIA AND FORMALIN FIXATION TIME

The status of prognostic/predictive markers (ER, PR, and HER2) in breast pathology changes patient management. Therefore, it is imperative that they be performed and interpreted in a controlled and systematic manner to ensure accuracy and prevent error. Current American Society of Clinical Oncology/CAP recommendations are that cold ischemia time (CIT) be as short as possible, ideally less than 1 hour, and that formalin fixation time (FFT) be within 6 to 72 hours.[42–44] Several studies have demonstrated that increased CIT negatively impacts the quality of breast biomarkers.[45–49] Many breast core biopsies are immediately placed in formalin at biopsy, making CIT irrelevant. However, for larger excisional specimens, reducing CIT can be more problematic. Under ideal circumstances, neoplastic tissue (tumor) is in close contact with formalin, which requires incision of the specimen; this is an operational challenge that increases with the complexity of a health care system. Maintaining standards for CIT and FFT requires clear expectations, communication, and coordination between the operating room and gross room laboratory staff. Uniquely, more complex systems with satellite sites and centralized laboratories (large tertiary centers) are more prone to challenges regarding CIT and FFT than smaller self-contained institutions (community practice). These scenarios necessitate resource allocation from the hospital to ensure current recommendations are met for optimal patient care and outcome.

One single-institution study assessed the effectiveness of a rapid triage protocol to obtain CIT and was able to achieve a CIT of less than 1 hour in 78% of excisional breast specimens. This study also emphasized the importance of treating every excision the same, regardless of the anticipated need for biomarker testing.[50] Otherwise, incidental malignant diagnoses and unexpected metastases may fail to meet current recommendations. One such rapid triage method includes the following: after excision, the specimen is appropriately prepared (oriented, inked, imaged, labeled) by the surgeon and immediately sent to the gross room. There is clear documentation of when the specimen was removed from the patient (start of CIT). Accessioning staff immediately deliver the specimen directly to the responsible gross examiner (pathology assistant, trainee, technician, or pathologist). The specimen is prepared, incised, and appropriately placed in formalin with the time documented (end of CIT, start of FFT). After hours, the operating room staff pages an assigned person on call directly to pick up the specimen, who follows the same procedure. The end of FFT is documented when the specimen is completely grossed, submitted in cassettes, and embedded in paraffin wax (formalin-fixed paraffin-embedded tissue). Such well-defined policies/procedures for controlling and documenting CIT and FFT are essential in modern-day pathology practices to account for current guidelines and prevent inaccurate biomarker results.

BIOPSIES OF CALCIFICATIONS

Documenting adequate sampling in breast biopsies performed for calcifications at times requires additional measures. Calcifications are commonly associated with malignancy; therefore, it is essential to identify the presence or absence of calcifications within the biopsy.[51] Oftentimes, calcifications are present and obviously identified as aggregates of deep purple (basophilic) calcium phosphate crystals (type II) on hematoxylin and eosin (H&E)-stained slides[52,53] (**Fig. 1**). Occasionally, calcifications are not identified on the initial levels. A common approach is to first polarize the light to see if this demonstrates less common calcium oxalate crystals (type I), which are often clear and refractile[52,53] (**Fig. 2**). If this fails to reveal calcifications, further evaluation through deeper histologic sections (additional levels) can be considered. At least one study has demonstrated that calcifications not identified in the initial levels are often present in deeper sections.[54] If additional levels do not reveal calcification the tissue block can be imaged by radiograph; this can be helpful when multiple blocks are present to avoid unnecessary leveling of material unlikely to have calcifications.

It is important that biopsies targeting calcifications are thoroughly evaluated before interpreted as benign when calcifications are absent. At minimum, communication to radiology (whether via report comment or directly) about the presence or absence of calcifications is necessary for

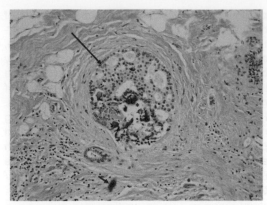

Fig. 1. Calcium phosphate crystals (*asterisk*) associated with lgDCIS (*long arrow*) and benign stroma (*short arrow*). The crystals are basophilic and nonbirefringent and may be more associated with neoplastic disease; original magnification ×200, H&E, nonpolarized.[52,53] (*Data from* Scott R, Stone N, Kendall C, et al. Relationships between pathology and crystal structure in breast calcifications: an in situ X-ray diffraction study in histological sections. NPJ breast cancer. 2016;2(1):1–6; and Radi MJ. Calcium oxalate crystals in breast biopsies. An overlooked form of microcalcification associated with benign breast disease. Arch Pathol Lab Med. 1989;113(12):1367–9.)

adequate radiology-pathology concordance and avoidance of sampling error. Although many practices follow similar approaches, there is no consensus guideline for how to proceed in

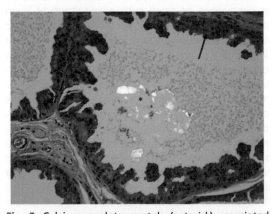

Fig. 2. Calcium oxalate crystals (*asterisk*) associated with apocrine metaplasia (*arrow*). The crystals are birefringent and colorless and may be more associated with benign findings; original magnification, ×200, H&E, polarized.[52,53] (*Data from* Scott R, Stone N, Kendall C, et al. Relationships between pathology and crystal structure in breast calcifications: an in situ X-ray diffraction study in histological sections. NPJ breast cancer. 2016;2(1):1–6; and Radi MJ. Calcium oxalate crystals in breast biopsies. An overlooked form of microcalcification associated with benign breast disease. Arch Path Lab Med. 1989;113(12):1367–9.)

evaluating breast biopsies performed for calcifications. In the absence of national guidelines, it is important for institutions to have standardized procedures to ensure a consistent approach across pathologists.

SURGEON INTRAOPERATIVE INKING OF LUMPECTOMIES

Proper orientation of a lumpectomy specimen is essential for accurately reporting margin status. Studies suggest that intraoperative inking/orientation results in decreased reexcision rates. One study reported 17% in cost savings for invasive carcinoma and 5% in cost savings for DCIS after implementing intraoperative inking.[55] Another study reported a decreased reexcision rate from 38% to 19% after implementation of intraoperative inking.[56] Thus, intraoperative inking by the surgeon is an immediate and simple way to improve patient care if surgeons and their institution are amenable to its implementation. Despite widespread implementation of such techniques, some institutions still rely on gross room personnel to ink previously oriented specimens.

STANDARDIZED REPORTING

Standardized synoptic cancer pathology reports increase physician and patient satisfaction and ensure complete reporting.[57,58] The Commission on Cancer of the American College of Surgeons requires 90% of cancer pathology reports have the required CAP elements to be designated a cancer center[59]; it is also a requirement by CAP, The Joint Commission, and the National Accreditation for Breast Centers.[60] Therefore, it is essential to adhere to CAP cancer reporting protocol templates when reporting results for invasive carcinoma and DCIS of the breast,[61] which ensures pertinent information is not excluded from the report and that standardized terminology is present in a reproducible manner across institutions.[62] One method to ensure compliance with standardized reporting practices is to use CAP electronic Cancer Checklists (eCC) directly within the laboratory information system (LIS). CAP eCC are available as modules for most AP LIS vendors (Cerner CoPathPlus, Dolbey, Epic Beaker, mTuitive, Novopath, Psyche Systems, Sunquest Powerpath, Voicebrook). A major benefit of this method is updates to the eCC modules coincide with changes to CAP Cancer Protocols.

Although not required, CAP breast biopsy templates for invasive carcinoma and DCIS are available in addition to templates for prognostic/predictive markers. Similar to synoptic reporting practices for excisional specimens, standardized reporting for biopsies and prognostic markers ensures complete reports and reproducibility. A well-organized reporting system also allows for systematic review of finalized reports, which serves as a transition to the sixth best practice recommendation (clinical care point): leveraging ongoing assessment of error.

LEVERAGING ONGOING ASSESSMENT OF ERROR

The ability to audit amendments presents a powerful tool that pathology groups can use to assess sources of error. A formal process to track amendments and develop interventions to address underlying reasons can decrease amendments long term.[63] Errors identified that result in an amendment can be further subclassified as type of error, discovery method, and patient impact.[64] This information can inform appropriate institution-specific interventions that decrease future errors. An intradepartmental partnership between information technology and breast pathology can develop a system to track errors occurring within their institution.

A confounding variable in this type of review is the delineation of addendum and amendment reports. A survey of AP directors documents wide variation in designation. Although most agree that change in malignant diagnosis (benign to malignant, malignant to benign) warrants an amendment, there is variable practice patterns for other report changes.[65,66] Therefore, individual pathology groups need an internal system for evaluation of both amendment and addendum reports to thoroughly evaluate report error.

Besides a periodic systematic review of addenda and amendments, groups could consider implementing an incident reporting system that any personnel can use; this allows capture of near-miss events and provides an avenue for all employees in a specimen's lifespan, from receipt in the laboratory to the final report, to be able to raise any concerns that could have resulted in error (**Fig. 3**for an example). Once the report is submitted, there is a systematic review process with the appropriate leadership personnel and potential escalation. If needed, policy or workflow changes can be implemented. A necessary component of this process is an official policy that prevents retaliation against any employee for submitting a report; otherwise, employees may be hesitant to report out of fear for punishment.

An additional tool to reduce future errors is to leverage the power of breast tumor boards. If

The Laboratory Event Management System (LEMS) is for documenting non-conforming laboratory events. If the issue you are reporting is time sensitive, please contact the section supervisor or section lead.

For "Type of Request", please change from "General Request" to select one of the following:

- **Pre-analytic** events occur prior to testing, processing, interpretation or diagnosis.
- **Analytic** events occur during testing, processing, interpretation or diagnosis.
- **Post-analytic** events occur after testing, processing, interpretation or diagnosis.

Please document the problem fully, any suggestions for solutions, and help us by suggesting who else needs to be involved in further communications.

Your Name:　　　　　　　　　　　　　Change your default information in the Settings
CC:
Email:
Building
Room Number:
Division:
Phone:
Target Date (YYYY-MM-DD):　　　　　High Priority Request: ☐
Division:
Site:
Type of request:　　　General Request
Description of Problem/Request:

Fig. 3. Example of an incident reporting form. A link to this form is present on the desktop of work computers, and all personnel involved in a specimen's life cycle are capable of submitting a report.

one works within a system in which all new malignant diagnoses and excisions are presented to a multidisciplinary care team, this is an opportunity for review, and to correct an error before it reaches patient care. Detailed quality assurance records of cases presented at tumor board allows for easy data collection (**Fig. 4**). This method also presents an opportunity to review prognostic/predictive markers and obtain consensus across pathologists (CAP accreditation requires 95% concordance). Last, it can evaluate if more than 90% of required cases contain the necessary CAP elements for accreditation as previously mentioned.[59,60]

SUMMARY

Error is challenging to define, and there is no universally accepted definition. From a clinical standpoint, identifying error that affects patient management and outcome is most important. This article highlights 6 techniques that can decrease error and improve diagnostic concordance in breast pathology. These techniques

*Conference Presenters: PLEASE **return** completed forms to the mailbox labeled: **Conference QA forms**

Date of Conference:		Conference Case Quality Assessment					
Pathologist*:		Cancer Conference:	**Breast Tumor Board**				
Trainee*:		Required Data Elements (RDEs) Synoptic Reporting Format *CAP Cancer Protocols revised 1/4, based on AJCC/UICC TNM, 8th Edition*					
Patient Initials	**Case #**	**Resection specimen** (CAP Cancer Protocols apply)	**RDEs present in synoptic reporting format** (CAP Cancer Protocols)	**Sign Out Pathologist Name**	**Diagnosis discrepancy code** (see legend)		**Comments**
		Y / N	Y / N / NA				
		Y / N	Y / N / NA				
		Y / N	Y / N / NA				
		Y / N	Y / N / NA				

Legend – Diagnosis Discrepancy Codes	
A = No discrepancy on review	D = Interpretive error with potential for or actual minor adverse clinical consequences
B = Gross or microscopic sampling error	E = Major interpretive error with potential for serious adverse clinical consequences
C = Minor interpretive error with no significant potential for adverse clinical outcome	F1 = Deferred appropriate
	F2 = Deferred inappropriate

Fig. 4. Example of a conference quality assurance (QA) form. Discrete data elements can be entered in electronic databases for director review; they record if the required data elements (RDE) in synoptic reporting format are present for accreditation. In addition, discrepancy codes are tabulated with designation of "A" indicating complete concordance (including prognostic/predictive marker review). Data retrieved from these forms have been successfully used to satisfy CAP accreditation checklist requirements.

include secondary review, institutional review of outside cases, using breast subspecialty-trained surgical pathologists, interdisciplinary approach, practical/technical workflow interventions, and leveraging ongoing assessment of error. These techniques are summarized as best practice recommendations (clinical care points) (**Box 1**).

DISCLOSURE

K.P. Lowry reports a research grant from GE Healthcare to her institution outside the submitted work. All other authors have nothing to disclose.

REFERENCES

1. Tozbikian G, Gemignani ML, Brogi E. Specimen Identification Errors in Breast Biopsies: Age Matters. Report of Two Near-Miss Events and Review of the Literature. Breast J 2017;23(5):583–8.
2. Renshaw AA, Gould EW. Comparison of disagreement and amendment rates by tissue type and diagnosis: identifying cases for directed blinded review. Am J Clin Pathol 2006;126(5):736–9.
3. Troxel DB. Medicolegal aspects of error in pathology. Arch Pathol Lab Med 2006;130(5):617–9.
4. Raab SS, Nakhleh RE, Ruby SG. Patient safety in anatomic pathology: measuring discrepancy frequencies and causes. Arch Pathol Lab Med 2005; 129(4):459–66.
5. Sirota RL. Defining error in anatomic pathology. Arch Pathol Lab Med 2006;130(5):604–6.
6. Zarbo RJ, Meier FA, Raab SS. Error detection in anatomic pathology. Arch Pathol Lab Med 2005; 129(10):1237–45.
7. Elmore JG, Longton GM, Carney PA, et al. Diagnostic concordance among pathologists interpreting breast biopsy specimens. Jama 2015;313(11): 1122–32.
8. Harrison BT, Dillon DA, Richardson AL, et al. Quality Assurance in Breast Pathology: Lessons Learned From a Review of Amended Reports. Arch Pathol Lab Med 2017;141(2):260–6.
9. Gradishar WJ, Anderson BO, Balassanian R, et al. Breast Cancer, Version 4.2017, NCCN Clinical Practice Guidelines in Oncology. J Natl Compr Canc Netw 2018;16(3):310–20.
10. Consensus guidelines on concordance assessment of image-guided breast biopsies and management of borderline or high-risk lesions. The American Society of Breast Surgeons. Available at: https://www.breastsurgeons.org/docs/statements/Consensus--Guideline-on-Concordance-Assessment-of-Image--Guided-Breast-Biopsies.pdf. Accessed April 27 2021.
11. Nakhleh RE, Bekeris LG, Souers RJ, et al. Surgical pathology case reviews before sign-out: a College of American Pathologists Q-Probes study of 45 laboratories. Arch Pathol Lab Med 2010;134(5):740–3.
12. Renshaw AA, Gould EW. Measuring errors in surgical pathology in real-life practice: defining what does and does not matter. Am J Clin Pathol 2007; 127(1):144–52.
13. Renshaw AA, Gould EW. Measuring the value of review of pathology material by a second pathologist. Am J Clin Pathol 2006;125(5):737–9.
14. Nakhleh RE, Zarbo RJ. Amended reports in surgical pathology and implications for diagnostic error detection and avoidance: a College of American Pathologists Q-probes study of 1,667,547 accessioned cases in 359 laboratories. Arch Pathol Lab Med 1998;122(4):303–9.
15. Nakhleh RE, Nosé V, Colasacco C, et al. Interpretive Diagnostic Error Reduction in Surgical Pathology and Cytology: Guideline From the College of American Pathologists Pathology and Laboratory Quality Center and the Association of Directors of Anatomic and Surgical Pathology. Arch Pathol Lab Med 2016;140(1):29–40.
16. Safrin RE, Bark CJ. Surgical pathology sign-out. Routine review of every case by a second pathologist. Am J Surg Pathol 1993;17(11):1190–2.
17. Owens SR, Wiehagen LT, Kelly SM, et al. Initial experience with a novel pre-sign-out quality assurance tool for review of random surgical pathology diagnoses in a subspecialty-based university practice. Am J Surg Pathol 2010;34(9):1319–23.
18. Raab SS, Grzybicki DM, Mahood LK, et al. Effectiveness of random and focused review in detecting surgical pathology error. Am J Clin Pathol 2008;130(6): 905–12.
19. Elmore JG, Tosteson AN, Pepe MS, et al. Evaluation of 12 strategies for obtaining second opinions to improve interpretation of breast histopathology: simulation study. BMJ 2016;i3069.
20. Geller BM, Nelson HD, Carney PA, et al. Second opinion in breast pathology: policy, practice and perception. J Clin Pathol 2014;67(11):955–60.
21. Geller BM, Nelson HD, Weaver DL, et al. Characteristics associated with requests by pathologists for second opinions on breast biopsies. J Clin Pathol 2017;70(11):947–53.
22. Carney PA, Allison KH, Oster NV, et al. Identifying and processing the gap between perceived and actual agreement in breast pathology interpretation. Mod Pathol 2016;29(7):717–26.
23. Romanoff AM, Cohen A, Schmidt H, et al. Breast pathology review: does it make a difference? Ann Surg Oncol 2014;21(11):3504–8.
24. Khazai L, Middleton LP, Goktepe N, et al. Breast pathology second review identifies clinically significant discrepancies in over 10% of patients. J Surg Oncol 2015;111(2):192–7.
25. Kennecke HF, Speers CH, Ennis CA, et al. Impact of routine pathology review on treatment for node-

negative breast cancer. J Clin Oncol 2012;30(18):
2227–31.

26. Marco V, Muntal T, García-Hernandez F, et al. Changes in breast cancer reports after pathology second opinion. Breast J 2014;20(3):295–301.

27. Soofi Y, Khoury T. Inter-Institutional Pathology Consultation: The Importance of Breast Pathology Subspecialization in a Setting of Tertiary Cancer Center. Breast J 2015;21(4):337–44.

28. Jorns JM, Healy P, Zhao L. Review of estrogen receptor, progesterone receptor, and HER-2/neu immunohistochemistry impacts on treatment for a small subset of breast cancer patients transferring care to another institution. Arch Pathol Lab Med 2013;137(11):1660–3.

29. Medicine Io. Best care at lower cost: the path to Continuously Learning health care in America. Washington, DC: The National Academies Press; 2013. p. 436.

30. Jakate K, De Brot M, Goldberg F, et al. Papillary lesions of the breast: impact of breast pathology subspecialization on core biopsy and excision diagnoses. Am J Surg Pathol 2012;36(4):544–51.

31. Gomes DS, Porto SS, Balabram D, et al. Interobserver variability between general pathologists and a specialist in breast pathology in the diagnosis of lobular neoplasia, columnar cell lesions, atypical ductal hyperplasia and ductal carcinoma in situ of the breast. Diagn Pathol 2014;9:121.

32. Viera AJ, Garrett JM. Understanding interobserver agreement: the kappa statistic. Fam Med 2005; 37(5):360–3.

33. East EG, Zhao L, Pang JC, et al. Characteristics of a Breast Pathology Consultation Practice. Arch Pathol Lab Med 2017;141(4):578–84.

34. ACR practice parameter for the performance of ultrasound-guided percutaneous breast interventional procedures American College of Radiology Updated. 2016. Available at: https://www.acr.org/-/media/acr/files/practice-parameters/us-guided-breast.pdf. Accessed April 27th 2021.

35. Jörg I, Wieler J, Elfgen C, et al. Discrepancies between radiological and histological findings in preoperative core needle (CNB) and vacuum-assisted (VAB) breast biopsies. J Cancer Res Clin Oncol 2021;147(3):749–54.

36. Newman EA, Guest AB, Helvie MA, et al. Changes in surgical management resulting from case review at a breast cancer multidisciplinary tumor board. Cancer 2006;107(10):2346–51.

37. Gabel M, Hilton NE, Nathanson SD. Multidisciplinary breast cancer clinics: do they work? Cancer Interdiscip Int J Am Cancer Soc 1997;79(12):2380–4.

38. Nakhleh RE, Idowu MO, Souers RJ, et al. Mislabeling of cases, specimens, blocks, and slides: a college of american pathologists study of 136 institutions. Arch Pathol Lab Med 2011;135(8): 969–74.

39. Renshaw AA, Kish R, Gould EW. The value of inking breast cores to reduce specimen mix-up. Am J Clin Pathol 2007;127(2):271–2.

40. Raff LJ, Engel G, Beck KR, et al. The effectiveness of inking needle core prostate biopsies for preventing patient specimen identification errors: a technique to address Joint Commission patient safety goals in specialty laboratories. Arch Pathol Lab Med 2009;133(2):295–7.

41. Gulbahce HE, Coleman JF, Sirohi D. Interference of Tissue-Marking Dyes With Fluorescence In Situ Hybridization Assays. Arch Pathol Lab Med 2019; 143(11):1299.

42. Hammond ME, Hayes DF, Dowsett M, et al. American Society of Clinical Oncology/College of American Pathologists guideline recommendations for immunohistochemical testing of estrogen and progesterone receptors in breast cancer (unabridged version). Arch Pathol Lab Med 2010;134(7):e48–72.

43. Wolff AC, Hammond ME, Hicks DG, et al. Recommendations for human epidermal growth factor receptor 2 testing in breast cancer: American Society of Clinical Oncology/College of American Pathologists clinical practice guideline update. J Clin Oncol 2013;31(31):3997–4013.

44. Wolff AC, Hammond MEH, Allison KH, et al. Human Epidermal Growth Factor Receptor 2 Testing in Breast Cancer: American Society of Clinical Oncology/College of American Pathologists Clinical Practice Guideline Focused Update. Arch Pathol Lab Med 2018;142(11):1364–82.

45. Khoury T, Sait S, Hwang H, et al. Delay to formalin fixation effect on breast biomarkers. Mod Pathol 2009;22(11):1457–67.

46. Khoury T. Delay to formalin fixation alters morphology and immunohistochemistry for breast carcinoma. Appl Immunohistochem Mol Morphol 2012;20(6):531–42.

47. Khoury T, Liu Q, Liu S. Delay to formalin fixation effect on HER2 test in breast cancer by dual-color silver-enhanced in situ hybridization (Dual-ISH). Appl Immunohistochem Mol Morphol 2014;22(9):688–95.

48. Khoury T. Delay to Formalin Fixation (Cold Ischemia Time) Effect on Breast Cancer Molecules. Am J Clin Pathol 2018;149(4):275–92.

49. Li X, Deavers MT, Guo M, et al. The effect of prolonged cold ischemia time on estrogen receptor immunohistochemistry in breast cancer. Mod Pathol 2013;26(1):71–8.

50. East EG, Gabbeart M, Roberts E, et al. A rapid triage protocol to optimize cold ischemic time for breast resection specimens. Ann Diagn Pathol 2018;34:94–7.

51. O'Grady S, Morgan MP. Microcalcifications in breast cancer: From pathophysiology to diagnosis and prognosis. Biochim Biophys Acta Rev Cancer 2018;1869(2):310–20.

52. Scott R, Stone N, Kendall C, et al. Relationships between pathology and crystal structure in breast calcifications: an in situ X-ray diffraction study in histological sections. NPJ breast cancer 2016;2(1):1–6.

53. Radi MJ. Calcium oxalate crystals in breast biopsies. An overlooked form of microcalcification associated with benign breast disease. Arch Pathol Lab Med 1989;113(12):1367–9.

54. Gallagher R, Schafer G, Redick M, et al. Microcalcifications of the breast: a mammographic-histologic correlation study using a newly designed Path/Rad Tissue Tray. Ann Diagn Pathol 2012;16(3):196–201.

55. Van Den Bruele AB, Jasra B, Smotherman C, et al. Cost-effectiveness of surgeon performed intraoperative specimen ink in breast conservation surgery. J Surg Res 2018;231:441–7.

56. Singh M, Singh G, Hogan KT, et al. The effect of intraoperative specimen inking on lumpectomy re-excision rates. World J Surg Oncol 2010;8:4. https://doi.org/10.1186/1477-7819-8-4.

57. Sluijter CE, van Lonkhuijzen LR, van Slooten H-J, et al. The effects of implementing synoptic pathology reporting in cancer diagnosis: a systematic review. Virchows Archiv 2016;468(6):639–49.

58. Torous VF, Simpson HW, Balani JP, et al. College of American Pathologists Cancer Protocols: From Optimizing Cancer Patient Care to Facilitating Interoperable Reporting and Downstream Data Use. JCO Clin Cancer Inform 2021;(5):47–55.

59. Optimal resources for cancer care (2020 standards). American College of Surgeons. Available at: https://www.facs.org/-/media/files/quality-programs/cancer/coc/optimal_resources_for_cancer_care_2020_standards.ashx. Accessed April 30 2021.

60. Cancer protocol and electronic cancer checklist: Frequently asked questions. College of American Pathologists. Available at: https://www.cap.org/protocols-and-guidelines/cancer-reporting-tools/cancer-protocol-templates/cancer-protocol-and-ecc--faqs. Accessed April 27 2021.

61. Cancer Protocol Templates College of American Pathologists. Available at: https://www.cap.org/protocols-and-guidelines/cancer-reporting-tools/cancer--protocol-templates. Accessed April 5 2021.

62. Kleer CG. Pathology re-review as an essential component of breast cancer management. Curr Oncol 2010;17(1):2–3.

63. Meier FA, Varney RC, Zarbo RJ. Study of amended reports to evaluate and improve surgical pathology processes. Adv Anat Pathol 2011;18(5):406–13.

64. Roy JE, Hunt JL. Detection and classification of diagnostic discrepancies (errors) in surgical pathology. Adv Anat Pathol 2010;17(5):359–65.

65. Parkash V, Fadare O, Dewar R, et al. Can the Misinterpretation Amendment Rate Be Used as a Measure of Interpretive Error in Anatomic Pathology?: Implications of a Survey of the Directors of Anatomic and Surgical Pathology. Adv Anat Pathol 2017;24(2):82–7.

66. Cooper K. Errors and error rates in surgical pathology: an Association of Directors of Anatomic and Surgical Pathology survey. Arch Pathol Lab Med 2006;130(5):607–9.

Pathologic Evaluation of Lymph Nodes in Breast Cancer
Contemporary Approaches and Clinical Implications

Agnes Balla, MD, MHS[a],*, Donald L. Weaver, MD[b]

KEYWORDS

- Breast cancer • Breast pathology • Sentinel lymph node biopsy • Macrometastasis
- Micrometastasis • Prognostic factors • Metastatic cancer

Key points

- Breast cancer screening has effectively reduced tumor size at diagnosis and secondarily decreased the prevalence of axillary lymph node metastases allowing limited axillary sampling for staging and prognosis.
- Sentinel lymph node biopsy has replaced axillary dissection as the standard procedure worldwide for evaluating lymph nodes in early-stage breast cancer presenting with a clinically negative axilla.
- The objective of the pathology evaluation of lymph nodes in breast cancer is the detection of all macrometastases larger than 2.0 mm using systematic gross and microscopic evaluation protocols.
- Metastases smaller than 2.0 mm will be detected or missed by chance; evidence-based outcome studies indicate these smaller metastases are not clinically significant in the prechemotherapy setting.
- When systemic therapy is planned, women with T1-T2 breast cancers and 1 or 2 positive sentinel nodes may elect to omit completion axillary dissection; observation or axillary irradiation are contemporary alternatives.

ABSTRACT

The presence of detected metastases in locoregional lymph nodes of women with breast cancer is an important prognostic variable for cancer staging, prognosis, and treatment planning. Systematic and standardized lymph node evaluation with gross and microscopic protocols designed to detect all macrometastases larger than 2.0 mm is the appropriate objective based on clinical outcomes evidence. Pathologists will detect smaller micrometastases and isolated tumor cell clusters (ITCs) by random chance but will also leave similar sized metastases undetected in paraffin blocks. Although these smaller metastases have prognostic significance, they are not predictive of recurrence for chemotherapy naïve patients. Thus, protocols to reliably detect metastases smaller than 2.0 mm are not required or recommended by guidelines. Women with T1-T2 breast cancer with a clinically negative axilla but with 1 or 2 pathologically positive sentinel nodes now have alternative options including observation and axillary irradiation and do not require completion axillary dissection.

[a] Department of Pathology and Laboratory Medicine, Larner College of Medicine, University of Vermont and UVM Medical Center, 111 Colchester Avenue, Burlington, VT 05401, USA; [b] Department of Pathology and Laboratory Medicine, Larner College of Medicine, University of Vermont, UVM Cancer Center, UVM Medical Center, Given Courtyard South, 89 Beaumont Avenue, Burlington, VT 05405-0068, USA
* Corresponding author.
E-mail addresses: Agnes.Balla@uvmhealth.org; donald.weaver@uvmhealth.org

Surgical Pathology 15 (2022) 15–27
https://doi.org/10.1016/j.path.2021.11.002
1875-9181/22/© 2022 Elsevier Inc. All rights reserved.

Abbreviations	
AJCC	American Joint Committe on Cancer
ALND	axillary lymph node dissection
DCIS	ductal carcinoma in situ
ITCs	isolated tumor cell clusters
SLNB	sentinel lymph node biopsy
UICC	International Union Against Cancer

INTRODUCTION

The presence, or absence, and the quantitative burden of metastatic disease in the regional lymph nodes remains a critical variable in understanding the prognosis and deciding appropriate adjuvant treatment for patients with breast cancer. Technical improvements in breast mammography and widespread adoption of breast cancer screening programs have led to the detection of smaller tumors and lower rates of positive lymph nodes. Although geographic and demographic disparities still exist today, most of the mammographically screened patients are diagnosed with early clinical stage I breast cancer. This shift to earlier detection combined with data from recent clinical trials showing axillary lymph node dissection (ALND) may be omitted in select patients with a limited number of positive sentinel nodes, necessitates a reexamination of how pathologists evaluate lymph nodes and report their findings. In this article, we present the evolutionary changes in breast cancer axillary staging, including intraoperative and permanent section evaluation strategy, significance of metastasis volume and size, and the basic principles for reporting lymph nodes containing metastatic disease. Special considerations for patients treated with neoadjuvant therapy are also discussed.

THE EVOLUTION OF AXILLARY STAGING

ALND generally involves removing all level I and II lymph nodes. Level III nodes are palpated intraoperatively and removed only if clinically suspicious; however, in some countries, additional removal of level III nodes is still a standard part of this procedure. Four decades ago, the seminal trials comparing simple mastectomy with and without axillary dissection and simple mastectomy with and without axillary irradiation demonstrated that axillary lymph node surgery does not improve overall survival and the addition of axillary irradiation can reduce and control axillary recurrence.[1,2] These trials established the basis for the TNM staging system and set the stage for subsequent trials that demonstrated improved outcomes in patients with positive nodes who received systemic chemotherapy. Despite the absence of a survival benefit from axillary dissection, the importance of the information gained from knowing whether positive nodes were present was so compelling that ALND was adopted as the standard surgical procedure performed on all patients with breast cancer for stratification into treatment groups based on the presence of axillary disease. The intent of ALND was to provide prognostic information and loco-regional control of disease at a time when most patients were presenting with locally advanced or node-positive disease.

The widespread adoption of screening mammography led to a major epidemiologic shift in the pathologic stage of breast cancer at diagnosis; smaller tumor sizes are associated with lower numbers of positive axillary nodes.[3,4] Data from the Breast Cancer Surveillance Consortium indicates less than 25% of women undergoing screening are expected to have positive nodes at diagnosis.[5] In addition, mammographically detected tumors have a statistically significant disease-free advantage over patients with clinically detected tumors.[6] This difference in survival is likely due to a combination of earlier detection, advancements in radiation and oncologic management, and a difference in the inherent biology and metastatic potential of screen-detected tumors. Host factors including genetic background, immune status, and social factors including environment, lifestyle choices, and access to medical care are also responsible.

Conservative breast surgery was widely adopted when foundational clinical trials initiated in the 1980s demonstrated equivalent long-term outcomes in patients undergoing partial mastectomy followed by radiation therapy compared with total mastectomy in early-stage breast cancer.[7] The trends toward increased screening, lower node-positive rates, smaller tumor size, and more conservative surgery prompted clinical trials to study whether more limited axillary staging approaches could lower morbidity while providing equivalent survival and regional control.[8] The sentinel lymph node biopsy (SLNB) concept emerged from the hypotheses that lymphatic drainage from an anatomic site follows a predictable pattern and that injection of a tracer could be used to map nodes and identify the most likely sites of lymphatic drainage from a tumor. For small breast cancers less than 5 cm (cT1-T2), lymphatic spread within the axilla is more likely to occur along predictable drainage pathways which is why the sentinel node technique for axillary staging is reliable and specifically indicated in this patient population. The information gained from pathologic examination of these select nodes can then be used to make informed adjuvant therapy decisions while sparing an unnecessary complete ALND for approximately 75% of women who will ultimately have negative sentinel lymph nodes.[5,9] Today, various guidelines recommend SLNB for patients with cT1-2 invasive breast cancer with a clinically negative axilla, patients with ductal carcinoma in situ (DCIS) sufficient to require mastectomy (or DCIS with suspected or diagnosed microinvasion) or patients with clinically negative axillary nodes following neoadjuvant chemotherapy.[10,11]

SENTINEL NODE SURGICAL PROCEDURE

Several methods exist for the detection of sentinel lymph nodes including direct visualization using blue dye, the radioisotope method, and newer methodologies involving optimal imaging-guided sentinel lymph node detection and magnetic tracer guided detection. The most widely used method in the United States is the radioisotope method for which the surgeon typically localizes the breast tumor and injects Tc99 sulfur colloid with or without vital blue dye circumferentially around the tumor, in the overlying dermis or into the subareolar plexus.[12] A handheld gamma detector is used before incising skin to locate the lymph nodes first receiving drainage from the tumor and then also used to guide the surgical dissection of the labeled "sentinel" node(s). Lymph nodes are removed as single nodes or small clusters of nodes until the radioactive counts decrease to less than 10% of the starting counts. These nodes are sent to the pathology laboratory labeled as sentinel nodes with accompanying radiotracer counts.

At this point in the operative procedure, the surgeon palpates the axillary tissue within the incision and removes any firm or suspicious nodes. These nodes may be labeled nonsentinel nodes, palpable axillary nodes, or nonradioactive sentinel nodes and should be submitted separately.

Importantly, nodes that are completely replaced by tumor may not have radiotracer uptake which is why palpation and removal of clinically enlarged lymph nodes is critical. Adding this final step to the sentinel node biopsy procedure reduces the procedural false-negative rate. It is important to know that the radiotracer only maps the lymphatic drainage from the breast. The 10-s counts obtained in the operating room are to verify a node is radiolabeled and receiving drainage from the tumor site but do not indicate nodal involvement. The relative difference in counts is more important than the absolute value of the counts as the absolute counts are related to the size of the colloid particles and the time since injection. If metastases are detected, they are more likely to be in the 3 nodes with the highest radioactivity counts. The optimal number of sentinel lymph nodes to excise is debated and may depend on tumor characteristics including size, location, histology, and even host factors including race.[13–15]

CONTEMPORARY INTRAOPERATIVE ASSESSMENT OF SENTINEL NODES

One of the more controversial procedural topics in breast pathology is the intraoperative assessment of sentinel nodes. The primary actionable intraoperative decision is whether to perform an immediate completion axillary dissection. Clinical trials comparing SLNB to axillary dissection used intraoperative frozen section or cytologic scrape/smear evaluation to make this decision. In the past, the conservative approach was an immediate axillary dissection for any detectable metastatic disease in a sentinel lymph node(s) at the time of intraoperative evaluation, regardless of the size and number of metastases. Detecting any malignant cells intraoperatively was of paramount importance and of huge clinical consequence. Today, axillary clearance is less likely to be performed in the context of intraoperative node positivity when few nodes or small metastases are identified.

Analysis of the US Surveillance, Epidemiology, and End Results (SEER) national cancer database first indicated that the inflection point for worse outcomes occurs between 2 and 3 nodes positive and not at the positive versus negative threshold.[16] Perhaps more convincing are the findings from the ACOSOG Z-0011 trial. Data from this trial demonstrated that ALND could be omitted in selected patients with tumors no larger than 5 cm (cT1-2) and with 1 or 2 positive sentinel lymph nodes if patients followed recommended guidelines for medical and radiation oncologic management. Outcomes at 10 years for women in the observation group were no worse than for women in the axillary dissection group.[17] Recent 10-year follow-up data from the AMAROS trial substantiate these findings and have shown comparable 10-year recurrence and survival rates following either axillary radiotherapy or ALND in patients with early-stage breast cancer with micro- or macrometastases detected in sentinel lymph nodes.[18] For this reason, some surgeons may elect to forego intraoperative assessment of sentinel lymph nodes in patients who meet the Z-0011 selection criteria.

Frozen section and cytologic evaluation each have their benefits and drawbacks for identifying metastatic disease in the intraoperative setting. Benefits of entirely freezing the tissue include increased ability to identify small metastases that may not be grossly appreciable and the ability to quantify the extent of metastatic disease in real-time. Cutting and freezing all the nodal tissue, however, increases operative times and time under anesthesia. Beyond being time-intensive, freeze artifact can make identification of some morphologic subtypes such as lobular carcinoma difficult. Further, getting a full face section can be challenging and tissue is sacrificed in this process ending up unexamined in the bottom of the cryostat. In contrast, cytologic evaluation has the benefit of preserving tissue for permanent sections while targeting suspicious areas for scrape prep examination. Some surgical pathologists may not be as comfortable interpreting cytologic smears and certain morphologies such as lobular carcinoma and carcinoma with histiocytoid features can be more challenging to identify on cytologic smears. Determining the exact size of a metastasis is problematic and micrometastases can be missed with this selective sampling methodology. In the era of more conservative axillary management, the identification of micrometastases and isolated tumor cell clusters (ITCs) intraoperatively is less critical than in the past.

Recognizing the importance of shared decision making with the patient, our breast care multidisciplinary team at the University of Vermont Medical Center has implemented an intraoperative policy and procedural change that reflects the dynamic changes we have witnessed in the surgical management of positive sentinel lymph nodes. Our focus in the intraoperative setting has evolved to detection of macrometastases. Our standard procedure involves intraoperative gross evaluation of sentinel nodes on a selective basis determined by the surgeon's assessment of the clinical risk for metastatic disease. Sentinel nodes are grossly sliced into 2 mm sections and each section is evaluated by a pathologist with a dissecting microscope. An inverted ocular lens can also be used. The pathologist then decides whether the nodes are reported to the surgeon as having no suspicious findings on macroscopic evaluation or the pathologist performs a cytologic evaluation of grossly or macroscopically suspicious areas and reports the result of the cytologic examination.. By only examining nodes that are grossly suspicious using scrape prep cytology, we avoid axillary clearance surgery for ITCs and micrometastases incidentally detected that may no longer be present on permanent sections or may not have clinical relevance. In cases that are false negative, with metastases later identified on permanent sections, our multi-disciplinary team is able to use clinical trial outcome data, primary tumor characteristics, patient demographics, and patient preference to make an informed decision about subsequent management. Following an investigational chart review at our institution, we discovered that when given treatment options, only 28% of women with false-negative intraoperative examinations and positive nodes on permanent sections chose any further axillary surgery. Further, when they declined completion axillary dissection, one-third chose axillary irradiation, and the remainder elected observation.[19] The false-negative cases included a spectrum of detected sizes on permanent section including macrometastases up to 3 mm in greatest dimension.

PERMANENT SECTION PATHOLOGIC EVALUATION OF LYMPH NODES

PREDICTING TUMOR VOLUME FROM GLASS SLIDES

Once the sentinel nodes leave the operating room, surgical pathologists are responsible for determining whether the nodes are "positive" or "negative" in a semiquantitative classification. The challenge is that tumor volume is the ideal variable but is difficult to measure in pathology specimens and is particularly elusive to estimate from 2-dimensional microscopic slides. For the purposes of T-classification and N-classification in the AJCC and UICC staging systems, we use a maximum dimension of tumor foci as a reasonable surrogate for tumor volume. Recognizing that we can't examine all tissue in a block, it is more scientifically accurate to consider metastases as "detected" or "not detected." *Our professional task is to identify lymph node metastases that are clinically significant.* Another challenge in breast pathology is how to classify multiple foci of tumor. It can be helpful to consider theoretic metastasis volumes.

Fig. 1. Relationship of tumor volume and lymph node metastasis size. (*A*) One 2.0 mm micrometastasis has a volume of 4.2 mm³ which is equivalent to the volume of 1000 isolated tumor cell clusters (ITCs) each measuring 0.2 mm and the volume of 1,000,000 single tumor cells measuring 20 uM (not shown). (*B*) One 5.0 mm round macrometastasis has a volume of 65 mm³ which is equivalent to 16 micrometastases each measuring 2.0 mm or one 8.0 × 4.0 mm oval macrometastasis.

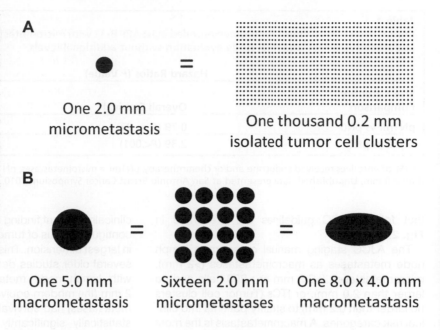

A

One 2.0 mm micrometastasis = One thousand 0.2 mm isolated tumor cell clusters

B

One 5.0 mm macrometastasis = Sixteen 2.0 mm micrometastases = One 8.0 x 4.0 mm macrometastasis

For example, the volume of a 2 mm micrometastasis is equivalent to 1000 ITCs each measuring 0.2 mm and one million single tumor cells. It takes a lot of small metastases to attain a volume equivalent to a single micrometastasis at the upper 2 mm threshold. For this reason, distinct tumor cell clusters seen on a slide should not be added together to attain a total linear dimension as this will inflate the volume of disease in the node. For additional examples see **Fig. 1**. These volumetric principles underscore why we should not overestimate the size of a nodal metastasis or inappropriately nudge a nodal metastasis into the next category because it is at a categorical size threshold. Examples of measuring metastases

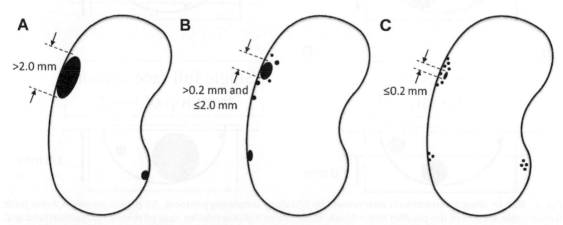

A >2.0 mm

B >0.2 mm and ≤2.0 mm

C ≤0.2 mm

Fig. 2. Measuring and categorizing metastases in individual lymph nodes. Examples of 3 node cross-sections with different categorical assessments. When a lymph node is submitted in multiple slices and/or in multiple cassettes, the nodal cross-section with the largest metastasis is used to categorize the lymph node. Each lymph node should be categorized separately and all positive nodes should be tabulated in the report. (*A*) Macrometastasis; At least one contiguous tumor deposit must be larger than 2.0 mm. (*B*) Micrometastasis; At least one contiguous tumor deposit must be larger than 0.2 mm and the largest contiguous tumor deposit must be no larger than 2.0 mm. Noncontiguous adjacent tumor deposits are not added. Multiple micrometastases may be present in a single lymph node. (*C*) Isolated tumor cell clusters (ITCs); The largest contiguous tumor deposit must be no larger than 0.2 mm. Multiple ITCs are often clustered and multiple foci are frequently present in a single node. Noncontiguous adjacent ITCs are not added. When more than 200 single tumor cells are present in a single lymph node cross-section, the node is classified as a micrometastasis.

Table 1
Comparison of outcomes[a] for women enrolled in NSABP B-32 with micrometastases, macrometastases and negative nodes on initial node evaluation without additional levels

| | Hazard Ratios (P Value) | |
Size Category Comparison	Overall Survival	Disease-Free Survival
pN1mi vs pN0	0.79 (P = .27)	0.99 (P = .99)
pN1a vs pN0	2.39 (P<.001)	1.78 (P<.001)

[a] 97% of enrollees received endocrine and/or chemotherapy. pN1mi = micrometastases; pN1a = macrometastases larger than 2.0 mm. Unpublished data presented at San Antonio Breast Cancer Symposium 2010, (Julian T, Abstract 851,740).

that follow AJCC guidelines are presented in **Fig. 2.**

The AJCC staging manual categorizes lymph node metastases as macrometastases (>2 mm), micrometastases (>0.2 mm or >200 cells and no larger than 2.0 mm), or ITCs (Tumor cell clusters no larger than 0.2 mm) to stratify patients into clinical risk categories. A macrometastasis is the most clinically relevant finding and is strictly defined as a contiguous focus of tumor cells greater than 2 mm in largest dimension. This cut off value comes from several older studies demonstrating that patients with lymph node metastases all smaller than 2 mm (the modern equivalent of pN1mi, or micrometastases) had survival outcomes that were not statistically significantly different from patients

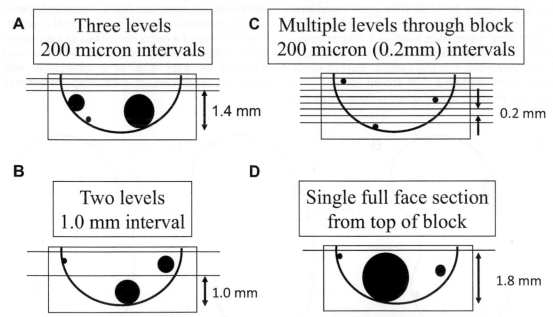

Fig. 3. Size of missed metastases is determined by histology sectioning protocol. All panels assume a 2 mm thick lymph node section in the paraffin tissue block; black circles indicate relative sizes of missed micrometastases and ITCs. (*A*) Typical 3 level protocol with generous 0.2 mm (200 uM) spacing between sections; 1.4 mm of unexamined tissue remains. Typical spacing between levels is often 20 to 50uM. (*B*) Systematic 2 level protocol with 1.0 mm between histologic sections; 1.0 mm of tissue unexamined between levels and 1.0 mm of tissue remains in the block. This theoretic protocol can be achieved with an automated microtome set at 0.005 mm (5 uM) and removing 200 sections before mounting on glass. (*C*) Systematic multi-level protocol with 0.2 mm between histologic sections. This protocol is designed to detect virtually all micrometastases, is labor-intensive, and will miss isolated tumor cell clusters present in unexamined tissue between histologic sections. (*D*) Guideline recommended protocol with single full-face section from the top of the block. The systematic approach for this protocol relies on careful gross sectioning of the lymph node before embedding in paraffin. It is accepted that micrometastases and ITCs will be detected or missed by chance but that virtually all macrometastases will be detected. The largest dimension of any detected metastasis may not be represented on the glass slide.

with "negative" nodes and that patients with metastases larger than 2 mm had statistically significantly worse outcomes.[20,21] An evaluation of initial node status used for clinical management on the B-32 trial provides sentinel node era data comparing macrometastases or micrometastases to "negative" nodes that also verifies this observation (**Table 1**).

MANAGING LYMPH NODES AT THE GROSS BENCH

The probability of missing (or detecting) a metastasis in a lymph node is directly correlated with the size of the metastasis and the thickness of any unexamined paraffin-embedded tissue (**Fig. 3**). Several mathematical models have explored this principle in theory.[22–24] The modeling clearly demonstrates that a sampling strategy must be designed to reliably detect metastases of a predetermined size and anything detected smaller than this targeted size is a random event. We know from the B-32 study that nodes sliced at 2 mm gross intervals evaluated with a single full-face surface histologic section have a low likelihood (0.04%) of containing a missed macrometastasis.[25] Traditional "levels" from the surface of the block do not significantly improve detection of macrometastases over a single full-face section from the paraffin block.[26] If the node was grossly sliced thicker than 2 mm before embedding, deeper levels may help compensate for this deficiency but only if the nodal tissue remaining in the block following levels is no thicker than 2 mm. For this principle reason, *one of the most important pathology procedural advances in evaluating breast cancer lymph nodes is to assure that the lymph node is sectioned into slices no thicker than 2 mm*. Further, all slices should be systematically placed in the cassette with non-opposing faces evaluated on glass slides (**Fig. 4**). The well-informed and fastidious pathologist will gain more satisfaction from knowing they attended to achieving 2 mm intervals than deriving any satisfaction from detecting ITCs with immunohistochemistry. With a single full-face section from the 2 mm thick node blocks, the likelihood of missing any metastasis larger than 2 mm, or a clinically significant metastasis, is very low.

ESTABLISHING THE NUMBER OF NODES EVALUATED

The total number of sentinel nodes should be based on the total number of nodes identified grossly, then subtract any candidate nodes that are not anatomically encapsulated lymph nodes;

lymphoid aggregates should not be added to the microscopic node count. When a sentinel node biopsy is performed and less than 6 total nodes are examined, the "(sn)" designation is appended to the N-classification. For example, if 3 nodes are examined and one contains a macrometastasis, the node evaluation is classified as pN1a(sn). The "(sn)" acknowledges the 5% to 9% inherent false-negative rate for SLNB. If 6 or more nodes are evaluated, whether all sentinel or a combination of sentinel and nonsentinel, the "(sn)" designation is omitted because the evaluation is then considered equivalent to a low axillary dissection. Thus, it is important to not inflate the number of nodes examined and infer a more extensive evaluation.

DOCUMENTING EXTRACAPSULAR EXTENSION

Accurately documenting the presence or absence of extracapsular extension in pathology reports is important for multidisciplinary discussions as it may impact decisions for axillary irradiation or more extensive axillary surgery even in the setting of pN1 disease. Extracapsular extension is defined as tumor cells extending beyond the lymph node capsule to involve pericapsular adipose or soft tissue. Although several studies have shown that the presence of extranodal extension in sentinel lymph nodes is associated with overall nodal tumor burden and may be a predictor for nonsentinel lymph node metastasis, the prognostic value of this information is still under investigation and debated.[27–30] Regardless of whether additional surgery or axillary irradiation is added following SLNB, these treatment approaches further disturb axillary lymphatics and increase the risk of lymphedema.

THE CLINICAL IMPACT OF UNDETECTED METASTASES

Many "node negative" cases have nodes with undetected (occult) metastases. From the discussion above, it should be evident that some metastases are systematically detected based on the sectioning protocol and smaller metastases are randomly detected or missed. On B-32, the initial "node positive" rate was 26% and "initially negative" nodes had metastases detected in 25% of cases using a comprehensive strategy of sections every 180 uM through the block, a protocol designed to systematically detect micrometastases.[26] Using the equally strategic but simpler strategy of 2 additional sections 0.5 mm and 1 mm from the top of the block detected additional

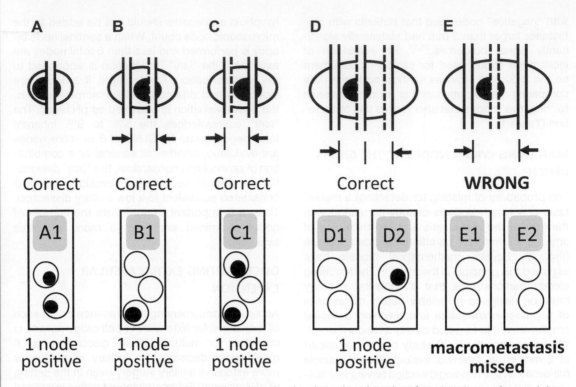

Fig. 4. Slicing, embedding, and sectioning lymph nodes. (*A–E*) Five lymph nodes of varying size, each containing a macrometastasis. Nodes are cut with each slice no thicker than 2 mm. Solid lines indicate the surface placed down in cassette, down in paraffin block and examined on glass slide. Dotted lines indicate the unexamined surface of tissue. The goal is to detect all macrometastases larger than 2.0 mm. (*A*) Opposing cut surfaces of bisected node placed down and sectioned with macrometastasis detected. (*B* and *C*) Cut ends of trisected node are sectioned; either surface of center slice is sectioned; by random chance, slides will have either 1 (*B*) or 2 (*C*) node cross-sections with macrometastasis detected. (*D*) Cut ends of quadrisected node are sectioned; care must be exercised to place center slices in cassette sequentially with surfaces to section no more than 2 mm apart to detect macro-metastasis on node cross-sections. (*E*) Note that in this node the center slices were incorrectly placed in the cassette with 4 mm of unexamined tissue between sections leading to a missed macrometastasis despite 2 mm thick slices. When a node is cut into 4 or more slices, consider the center slices as a deck of cards that must be stacked correctly so that all macrometastases are detected.

micrometastases and isolated tumor cells in 15.9% of initially node-negative cases.[25] Thus, groups of patients with "negative nodes" on initial evaluation comprise a mixed population of true node-negative cases and cases with undetected (occult) micrometastases and ITCs with detection dependent on the histology cutting protocol; this includes the older studies discussed above. These studies are indicating that it is clinically reasonable to miss (leave undetected) metastases that are smaller than 2 mm. In other words, our clinical goal in pathology is to detect all metastases that are greater than 2 mm using strategies that use systematic sectioning of lymph nodes with appro-priate evaluation of the resulting paraffin blocks.

Because small metastases are essentially randomly distributed within the lymph node paraffin blocks, there is a random chance that ITCs and micrometastases will be detected even

when the over-arching strategic goal is to identify all macrometases greater than 2 mm. This raises an important practical question: *Is there any clin-ical value of identifying and reporting these smaller metastases?* The B-32 and Z-0010 clinical trials evaluated this issue. Both studies were of similar size with almost 4000 patients. The B-32 correla-tive science study used a two-level strategy and identified additional metastases in 16% of cases; the Z-0010 study used a single level strategy and identified additional metastases in 11% of cases. Both studies demonstrated outcomes of similar magnitude (**Table 2**); however, the B-32 study demonstrated statistical significance due to the greater absolute number of occult metastases detected. This does not automatically support clinical significance but underscores how large datasets can detect small differences in outcome with statistical confidence. Importantly, the B-32

Table 2
Comparison of the effect of metastases detected on additional levels of initially negative sentinel nodes on survival in the B-32 and Z-0010 clinical studies

| | Occult Metastases | | | |
	Detected	Not Detected	Difference	P-Value
Overall survival				
B-32[a]	95.8%	94.6%	1.2%	.03
Z-0010[b]	95.7%	95.1%	0.6%	.64
Disease-free survival				
B-32[a]	89.2%	86.4%	2.8%	.02
Z-0010[b]	92.2%	90.4%	1.8%	.82

Abbreviation: IHC, cytokeratin immunohistochemical stain.
[a] Median follow-up 7.9 y; prevalence of occult metastases 15.9%; 2 additional levels plus IHC 0.5 and 1.0 mm deeper into block; detected occult metastases have prognostic significance but are not predictive of recurrence.
[b] Median follow-up 6.3 y; prevalence of occult metastases 10.5%; one additional level plus IHC from the surface of block; detected occult metastases do not have prognostic significance.

study demonstrated that the presence of micro-metastases and ITCs in sentinel nodes did not predict who would develop regional or distant recurrence.[25] Stated differently, this means micro-metastases and ITCs when aggregated into large groups of patients has some small prognostic value but there is no predictive value for the individual patient. From a pathology reporting perspective, we should carefully document the presence of even minute amounts of metastatic disease for future aggregate data analysis; however, we do not need to systematically look for micrometastases with additional levels/sections or use special techniques such as immunohisto-chemistry to identify micrometastases or ITCs.

EVALUATION OF SENTINEL LYMPH NODES FOLLOWING NEOADJUVANT CHEMOTHERAPY

Pathologists should consider SLNB in patients treated with neoadjuvant chemotherapy unique and distinctly different than in chemotherapy naïve patients. Following neoadjuvant chemotherapy, the technical success rate of the procedure may be lower and the implications for any detected residual metastatic disease are different. Studies have shown that SLNB is an appropriate initial axillary staging approach in patients who present with a clinically negative axilla at the time of primary breast surgery following neoadjuvant chemotherapy. In patients with biopsy-proven axillary nodal metastases before systemic therapy, the decision to pursue ALND or SLNB following a good clinical response can be difficult. This is an active area of study and management of these

patients varies. This decision is often left to the discretion of the surgeon and patient taking into account tumor and patient characteristics. Data from recent and ongoing prospective clinical trials including ACOSOG-Z1071 (ClinicalTrials.gov identifier: NCT00881361), SENTINA (Eudra Clinical Trial No: 2006–005,834–19), and SN-FNAC (ClinicalTrials.gov identifier: NCT00909441) may influence future clinical recommendations.

If SLNB is pursued, additional clinical effort should be made to minimize false-negative cases by using techniques such as the removal of 3 or more sentinel lymph nodes and using a dual tracer approach.[31] If a pretreatment lymph node was biopsied and pathologically positive, removal of this lymph node and all sentinel lymph nodes should be attempted following neoadjuvant chemotherapy. Although debate exists about whether nodes biopsied pretreatment should be marked with a clip during the biopsy, the presence of a clip may make it easier to identify the node clinically and pathologically following therapy. Knowledge of the patient's clinical axillary status is imperative and special care should be taken to note the presence or absence of a clip or marker grossly and/or biopsy site microscopically. Neoadjuvant-treated lymph nodes are processed in our laboratory in the same manner as treatment naïve cases and should be cut at 2 mm intervals and completely submitted for microscopic examination.

The aim of intraoperative evaluation of lymph nodes following chemotherapy is to identify any residual disease in the lymph nodes. Though the same limitations exist for freezing and cytologic evaluation, intraoperative evaluation of nodes is complicated by the fact that treatment effect and scarring can give the false impression of grossly positive disease. Further, fibrous scarring and histiocytes can make the interpretation of frozen and cytologic smears even more challenging. Extreme caution should be exercised in this setting and challenging cases should be deferred to permanent sections. Clinical trials are ongoing evaluating the use of ALND and axillary irradiation in the setting of residual nodal disease following chemotherapy; however, there are currently no data to support the safety of omitting axillary dissection in the setting of residual axillary disease, irrespective of the size of the sentinel lymph node metastasis.[32] For this reason, the approach described previously for treatment naïve patients whereby the focus is on the identification of macrometastases intraoperatively may not be appropriate in this setting. As always, the purpose and limitations of intraoperative evaluation should be clearly communicated and discussed with the breast surgeon up front.

Treatment response in lymph nodes can have a variable histologic appearance ranging from no obvious response with extensive residual tumor, to mild fibrous scarring, all the way to extensive necrotizing granulomatous inflammation. The use of immunohistochemistry to identify any residual disease following chemotherapy is indicated for any histologically suspicious areas because residual cancer cells in axillary nodes after neoadjuvant chemotherapy are a strong risk factor for locoregional relapse.[33] Some institutions prefer to document the presence of residual disease following chemotherapy using the MD Anderson residual tumor burden calculator.[34] However, AJCC classification should always be reported.

The most widely accepted definition of the pathologic complete response requires the absence of residual invasive disease in the breast (ypT0 or ypTis(DCIS)) and the absence of disease in any sampled axillary nodes (ypN0). In patients with a complete pathologic response in the lymph nodes, the report should include the number of lymph nodes that show characteristics of treatment effect and indicate whether or not a biopsy site or clip was identified.

INCIDENTAL FINDINGS IN BREAST AXILLARY LYMPH NODES

Although pathologists are primarily looking for metastatic carcinoma in sentinel or axillary lymph nodes, important and clinically relevant incidental diagnoses should not be overlooked. Occasionally, low-grade lymphomas can be identified in patients without a previous diagnosis of a hematologic malignancy. A wide range of benign incidental findings that mimic malignancy can also be found during axillary staging including findings such as the vascular transformation of lymph node sinuses, extensive pigment deposition from a dermal tattoo on the arm or back, or benign nevus cell aggregates. Even benign breast epithelium can be present in lymph nodes as incidental inclusions or as a result of mechanical transport from prior biopsy or surgical procedure. Benign epithelial cells, like tissue in the breast, can be hormonally responsive and undergo fibrocystic changes. Fortunately, morphology is typically classic and does not create diagnostic issues.

REPORTING LYMPH NODE FINDINGS

In light of the discussion presented above, statistical principles and good clinical judgment dictate the pathologic evaluation of lymph nodes in breast cancer. The available outcome data support an approach that optimizes detection of virtually all metastases larger than 2.0 mm (macrometastases) and recognizes that smaller metastases (micrometastases and ITCs) will be detected or missed by chance. Even though micrometastases and ITCs do not have the power to predict recurrence for the individual patient with breast cancer, at least for chemotherapy naïve patients, these 2 categories have prognostic significance when patients are aggregated into large outcomes analysis groups. This indicates that metastatic tumor burden is a continuous prognostic variable that should be accurately documented by pathologists for further study and entry into large cancer databases such as State Cancer Registries, the National Cancer Institute's SEER registry, or the American College of Surgeons' National Breast Cancer Database. The pathology report should include the total number of lymph nodes evaluated, the total number of sentinel lymph nodes evaluated, and the total number of positive nodes. If nodes are positive, a tabulation should be included that indicates the total number of positive nodes in each of the 3 metastasis categories (macrometastasis, micrometastasis, ITCs). The sum of the positive nodes in each category equals the total number of nodes reported as positive. When all positive nodes have ITCs only without micro or macrometastases detected in any nodes, the nodes are classified as pN0(i+). When no individual metastasis is larger than 2.0 mm, but at least one node has a metastasis larger than 0.2 mm or one node cross-section contains more than 200 single cells, the nodes are classified as pN1mi. Although the scientific evidence indicates the presence of micrometastases is not statistically significantly different from "node negative," clinicians may often consider pN1mi disease different from pN0 when advising on adjuvant therapy. The classification rules are more complex when macrometastases are detected; however, when nodes with macrometastases and micrometastases are considered, 1 to 3 positive nodes are generally classified as pN1a and 4 to 9 positive nodes are generally classified as pN2a. When macrometastases or micrometastases are present, nodes with ITCs only do not impact the N-classification because they add minimal additional volume to tumor burden. In countries following AJCC guidelines, nodes with ITCs should be tabulated and reported as positive nodes. These reporting guidelines are aligned with the AJCC manual for staging cancer[35] and the College of American Pathologists Protocols for reporting breast cancer.[36] In other countries and jurisdictions, reporting nodes with ITCs only may be optional when other nodes contain micrometastases or macrometastases.[37]

CLINICS CARE POINTS

- Clinical outcomes, including overall survival and disease-free survival, depend on the presence or absence of sentinel lymph node metastases and the size of those metastases.

- While survival is statistically significantly different for patients with metastases greater than 2 mm compared to patients without metastases detected, patients with smaller metastases less than or equal to 2 mm have survival that is not statistically significantly different from node negative patients.

- Macrometastases are reliably detected when sentinel lymph nodes are carefully sectioned at 2 mm intervals, all node sections are systematically embedded, and full-face microscopic sections are examined from each resulting lymph node cross section. Histology and grossing room personnel, including pathology resident trainees, should be continually reminded of the importance of 2 mm node sectioning.

- Special effort, including reflexively examining deeper sections from paraffin embedded lymph node blocks or universally performing immunohistochemical stains is not required for patients treated with adjuvant endocrine or chemotherapy following surgery. The presence of micrometastases or isolated tumor cell clusters does not predict distant recurrence or survival for these cases.

- In the neoadjuvant setting, the presence of any metastatic disease in the post treatment nodes is associated with higher locoregional recurrence risk. Conveying clinical data including history of neoadjuvant therapy, pre-treatment lymph node core biopsy result, and presence of a biopsy localizing clip is of paramount importance at the time post-chemotherapy nodes are submitted to pathology.

DISCLOSURE

The views expressed in this article are solely those of the authors and do not necessarily represent the official views of the National Cancer Institute or the U.S. government. Supported by grants (UO1-CA65121, U01-CA74137, R01CA74137) from the Public Health Service of the National Cancer Institute.

REFERENCES

1. Fisher B, Jeong J-H, Anderson S, et al. Twenty-five-year follow-up of a randomized trial comparing radical mastectomy, total mastectomy, and total mastectomy followed by irradiation. N Engl J Med 2002;347:567–75.
2. Elston CW, Gresham GA, Rao GS, et al. The cancer research campaign (King's/Cambridge) trial for early breast cancer: clinico-pathological aspects. Br J Cancer 1982;45:655–69.
3. Carter CL, Allen C, Henson DE. Relation of tumor size, lymph node status, and survival in 24,740 breast cancer cases. Cancer 1989;63:181–7.
4. Tubiana M, Koscielny S. The natural history of breast cancer: implications for a screening strategy. Int J Radiat Oncol Biol Phys 1990;19:1117–20.
5. Weaver DL, Rosenberg RD, Barlow WE, et al. Pathologic findings from the Breast Cancer Surveillance Consortium: population-based outcomes in women undergoing biopsy after screening mammography. Cancer 2006;106:732–42.
6. Salama JK, Heimann R, Lin F, et al. Does the number of lymph nodes examined in patients with lymph node-negative breast carcinoma have prognostic significance? Cancer 2005;103:664–71.
7. Fisher B, Anderson S, Bryant J, et al. Twenty-year follow-up of a randomized trial comparing total mastectomy, lumpectomy, and lumpectomy plus irradiation for the treatment of invasive breast cancer. N Engl J Med 2002;347:1233–41.

8. Krag DN, Julian TB, Harlow SP, et al. NSABP-32: phase III, randomized trial comparing axillary resection with sentinal lymph node dissection: a description of the trial. Ann Surg Oncol 2004;11(3 Suppl): 208S–10S.

9. Krag DN, Anderson SJ, Julian TB, et al. Sentinel-lymph-node-resection compared with conventional axillary-lymph-node-dissection in clinically node negative patients with breast cancer: overall survival findings from NSABP B-32 randomised phase 3 trial. Lancet Oncol 2010;11:927–33.

10. Performance and practice guidelines for sentinel lymph node biopsy in breast cancer patients. American Society of Breast Surgeons. Available at: https://www.breastsurgeons.org/docs/statements/Performance-and-Practice-Guidelines-for-Sentinel-Lymph-Node-Biopsy-in-Breast-Cancer-Patients.pdf. Accessed May 6, 2021.

11. Lyman GH, Somerfield MR, Bosserman LD, et al. Sentinel lymph node biopsy for patients with early-stage breast cancer: American Society of Clinical Oncology clinical practice guideline update. J Clin Oncol 2017;35:561–4. Available at: https://www.asco.org/research-guidelines/quality-guidelines/gu-idelines/breast-cancer#/9801. Accessed May 6, 2021.

12. Harlow SP. Sentinel lymph node biopsy in breast cancer: techniques. Available at: https://www.uptodate.com/contents/sentinel-lymph-node-biopsy-in-breast-cancer-techniques. Accessed May 6, 2021.

13. Yi M, Meric-Bernstam F, Ross MI, et al. How many sentinel lymph nodes are enough during sentinel lymph node dissection for breast cancer? Cancer 2008;113:30–7.

14. Bonneau C, Bendifallah S, Reyal F, et al. Association of the number of sentinel lymph nodes harvested with survival in breast cancer. Eur J Surg Oncol 2015;41:52–8.

15. Woznick A, Franco M, Bendick P, et al. Sentinel lymph node dissection for breast cancer: how many nodes are enough and which technique is optimal? Am J Surg 2006;191:330–3.

16. Michaelson JS, Silverstein M, Sgroi D, et al. The effect of tumor size and lymph node status on breast carcinoma lethality. Cancer 2003;98:2133–43.

17. Giuliano AE, Ballman KV, McCall L, et al. Overall survival among women with invasive breast cancer and sentinel node metastasis: the ACOSOG Z0011 (Alliance) randomized clinical trial. JAMA 2017;318:918–26.

18. Rutgers EJ, Donker M, Poncet C, et al. Radiotherapy or surgery of the axilla after a positive sentinel node in breast cancer patients: 10 year follow up results of the EORTC AMAROS trial (EORTC 10981/22023). San Antonio Breast Cancer Symposium 2018. Available at: https://www.abstracts2view.com/sabcs18/view.php?nu=SABCS18L_852&terms. Accessed May 6, 2021.

19. Ambaye AB, Ciampa A, Naud A, et al. Intraoperative sentinel lymph node evaluation leads to disparity in treatment of breast cancer patients (Abstract 83). United States and Canadian Academy of Pathology 96th Annual Meeting. Mod Pathol 2007;20(Suppl 2):23A.

20. Huvos AG, Hutter RVP, Berg JW. Significance of axillary macrometastases and micrometastases in mammary cancer. Ann Surg 1971;173:44–6.

21. Fisher E, Palekar A, Rockette H, et al. Pathologic findings from the national surgical adjuvant breast project (Protocol No. 4): V. Significance of axillary nodal micro- and macrometastases. Cancer 1978;42:2032–8.

22. Wilkinson EJ, Hause L. Probability in lymph node sectioning. Cancer 1974;33:1269–74.

23. Farshid G, Pradhan M, Kollias J, et al. Computer simulations of lymph node metastases for optimizing the pathologic examination of sentinel lymph nodes in patients with breast carcinoma. Cancer 2000;89:2527–37.

24. Cserni G. A model for determining the optimum histology of sentinel lymph nodes in breast cancer. J Clin Pathol 2004;57:467–71.

25. Weaver DL, Ashikaga T, Krag DN, et al. Effect of occult metastases on survival in node-negative breast cancer. N Engl J Med 2011;364:412–21.

26. Weaver DL, Le UP, Dupuis SL, et al. Metastasis detection in sentinel lymph nodes: comparison of a limited widely spaced (NSABP protocol B-32) and a comprehensive narrowly spaced paraffin block sectioning strategy. Am J Surg Pathol 2009;33:1583–9.

27. Joseph KA, El-Tamer M, Komenaka I, et al. Predictors of nonsentinel node metastasis in patients with breast cancer after sentinel node metastasis. Arch Surg 2004;139:648–51.

28. Changsri C, Prakash S, Sandweiss L, et al. Prediction of additional axillary metastasis of breast cancer following sentinel lymph node surgery. Breast J 2004;10:392–7.

29. Fujii T, Yanagita Y, Fujisawa T, et al. Implication of extracapsular invasion of sentinel lymph nodes in breast cancer: prediction of nonsentinel lymph node metastasis. World J Surg 2010;34:544–8.

30. Yang X, Ma X, Yang W, et al. Clinical significance of extranodal extension in sentinel lymph node positive breast cancer. Sci Rep 2020;10:14684.

31. Sutton TL, Johnson N, Garreau JR. Adequate sentinel node harvest is associated with low false negative rate in breast cancer managed with neoadjuvant chemotherapy and targeted axillary dissection. Am J Surg 2020;219:851–4.

32. Cavalcante FP, Millen EC, Zerwes FP, et al. Role of axillary surgery after neoadjuvant chemotherapy. JCO Glob Oncol 2020;6:238–41.

33. Mamounas EP, Anderson SJ, Dignam JJ, et al. Predictors of locoregional recurrence after neoadjuvant chemotherapy: results from combined analysis of National Surgical Adjuvant Breast and Bowel Project B-18 and B-27. J Clin Oncol 2012;30:3960–6.

34. Residual cancer burden calculator. Available at: http://www3.mdanderson.org/app/medcalc/index.cfm?pagename=jsconvert3. Accessed May 6, 2021.

35. AJCC Cancer Staging Manual, 8th edition, part XI, Breast. Available at: https://cancerstaging.org/references-tools/deskreferences/Documents/AJCC%208th%20Edition%20Breast%20Cancer%20Staging%20System.pdf. Accessed April 2, 2021.

36. College of American Pathologists. Protocol for the examination of resection specimens from patients with invasive carcinoma of the breast. https://documents.cap.org/protocols/cp-breast-invasive-resection-20-4400.pdf. Accessed April 2, 2021.

37. Cserni G, Brogi E, Cody HSIII, et al. Surgically Removed Lymph Nodes for Breast Tumours Histopathology Reporting Guide. Sydney, Australia: International Collaboration on Cancer Reporting; 2021.

Special Histologic Type and Rare Breast Tumors – Diagnostic Review and Clinico-Pathological Implications

Benjamin Yongcheng Tan, MBBS, FRCPath[c],
Elaine Hsuen Lim, MBBCh (Cantab), MRCP (UK), PhD (Cantab)[b],
Puay Hoon Tan, MBBS, FRCPA[a],*

KEYWORDS

- Breast • Carcinoma • Tumor • Special • Rare • Subtype

Key points

- Special histologic type and rare (such as metaplastic and salivary gland-type) breast carcinomas consist of morphologically heterogeneous tumors with distinct clinicopathological features.
- Accurate pathologic diagnosis of these tumors, many of which are uncommonly encountered, is key to appropriate management.
- A good working knowledge of the differential diagnoses for this diverse group of tumors aids in correct diagnosis.

ABSTRACT

Breast cancer is the most common malignant tumor in females. While most carcinomas are categorized as invasive carcinoma, no special type (NST), a diverse group of tumors with distinct pathologic and clinical features is also recognized, ranging in incidence from relatively more common to rare. So-called "special histologic type" tumors display more than 90% of a specific, distinctive histologic pattern, while a spectrum of tumors more often encountered in the salivary gland may also arise in the breast. Metaplastic carcinomas can present diagnostic challenges. Some uncommon tumors harbor pathognomonic genetic alterations. This article provides an overview of the key diagnostic points and differential diagnoses for this group of disparate lesions, as well as the salient clinical characteristics of each entity.

OVERVIEW

Breast cancer is the most common malignancy in women.[1] A breast carcinoma that displays a special histologic pattern in >90% of the tumor is by convention classified as a "pure special type" tumor.[2] Tumors that do not fulfill the preceding criterion fall into the category of invasive carcinoma, no special type (NST), which accounts for most diagnosed cases of breast carcinoma. Cases whereby a special subtype constitutes 10% to 90% of the tumor may be diagnosed as "mixed invasive breast carcinoma (NST) and (named) special subtype carcinoma", with a comment on the proportion constituted by the special subtype. As each

[a] Division of Pathology, Singapore General Hospital, Level 7, Diagnostics Tower, Academia, 20 College Road, Singapore 189856, Singapore; [b] Division of Medical Oncology, National Cancer Centre Singapore, 11 Hospital Crescent, Singapore 169610, Singapore; [c] Department of Anatomical Pathology, Singapore General Hospital, Level 10, Academia, 20 College Road, Singapore 169856, Singapore
* Corresponding author.
E-mail address: tan.puay.hoon@singhealth.com.sg

Surgical Pathology 15 (2022) 29–55
https://doi.org/10.1016/j.path.2021.11.003
1875-9181/22/© 2022 Elsevier Inc. All rights reserved.

tumor component may differ in grade and biomarker status, it may be of value to record these attributes independently.[2]

In the 5th edition of the WHO Classification of Breast Tumors (2019),[2] some unusual morphologic patterns are categorized under the histologic spectrum of invasive breast carcinoma (NST)—these include oncocytic, lipid-rich, glycogen-rich, clear cell, and sebaceous patterns, which, due to insufficiently robust data in support of their special distinction, are no longer regarded as special tumor subtypes. In addition, carcinomas with neuroendocrine differentiation, medullary, pleomorphic, choriocarcinomatous patterns, and melanocytic features do not currently warrant a special subtype designation. Regardless of the amount of such distinct patterns that may be observed in an individual tumor, the classification rule for special type carcinomas does not apply.

A variety of tumors more commonly identified in the salivary glands may be rarely encountered in the breast. Despite histologic and (sometimes) molecular similarities, site-specific clinical behavior is often distinct.

INVASIVE LOBULAR CARCINOMA

CLINICAL FINDINGS AND EPIDEMIOLOGY

Invasive lobular carcinoma constitutes approximately 5% to 15% of all invasive breast cancers,[3–6] with a mean age of 57 to 65 years, somewhat higher than that of patients with invasive carcinoma NST.[3,7,8] Bilateral tumors, including synchronous ones, seem to be more common.[9] Some studies have reported a higher incidence of multicentricity.[10–13]

Invasive lobular cancers are known for their surreptitious growth, more frequently being initially undetected on screening mammography until larger mass-forming lesions are present. Therefore, in certain series patients present with palpable breast masses. In some studies, ultrasonography demonstrates superior sensitivity to mammography in the detection of these tumors.[14–16] MRI may be helpful in defining multifocal lesions,[17] and is part of the radiological workup for these lesions in many centers.

Similar factors to other ER-positive cancers likely contribute to the etiology of invasive lobular carcinomas. But uniquely, patients harboring germline mutations in *CDH1* have a greatly increased risk for the development of diffuse-type gastric cancer and invasive lobular carcinoma of the breast.[18]

MACROSCOPIC FEATURES

While most invasive breast cancers are usually firm-to-hard tumors with irregular borders grossly, invasive lobular carcinomas may be grossly inconspicuous or diffusely involve large areas of the breast. Palpation rather than visual inspection may prove more helpful in delineating tumor margins, which feel firmer than surrounding parenchyma. Gross examination may substantially underestimate the microscopic extent of tumor.[19]

HISTOLOGY

The hallmark of invasive lobular carcinoma is the dyscohesion displayed by tumor cells, resulting most frequently in linear or individually-dispersed patterns of infiltration [**Fig. 1**A]. Classic features include small, rounded, or oval nuclei, a modest rim of cytoplasm, and occasional intracytoplasmic lumina containing mucoid material.

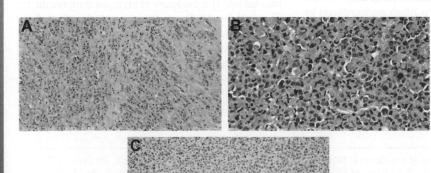

Fig. 1. (*A*) Linear strands of dyscohesive tumor cells are present in this classic invasive lobular carcinoma. (*B*) Marked nuclear pleomorphism characterizes invasive pleomorphic lobular carcinoma. (*C*) Invasive pleomorphic lobular carcinoma cells show loss of membranous E-cadherin immunohistochemical staining.

Variant patterns include the solid pattern with tumor arranged in cellular sheets; alveolar pattern characterized by rounded aggregates comprising at least 20 neoplastic cells; and tubulolobular pattern whereby a comingling of infiltrative tubules and linear files is seen, with membranous expression of E-cadherin.[20,21] Tumor cells may also display histiocytoid, apocrine or signet ring cytomorphological features.

Pleomorphic lobular carcinoma shows greater nuclear pleomorphism (more than 4x the size of normal lymphocytes), akin to the nuclei of high-grade ductal carcinoma-in-situ, and exhibits higher mitotic activity than classic invasive lobular carcinoma [Fig. 1B]. Admixed pleomorphic lobular carcinoma in situ may contain luminal necrotic material and harbor calcifications.

IMMUNOHISTOCHEMISTRY

Loss of membranous E-cadherin expression is a helpful immunohistochemical adjunct in the diagnosis of these tumors [Fig. 1C]; however, it is salient to note that approximately 15% of invasive lobular carcinomas (including most tubulolobular cancers) retain membranous E-cadherin staining,[22–24] while some invasive carcinomas NST may show loss of E-cadherin expression. In such cases, E-cadherin staining patterns should not be used to reclassify a tumor that would otherwise be placed in a definite diagnostic category. Aberrant (loss of distinct membranous) beta-catenin expression may also be seen in invasive lobular carcinomas, as well as a mis-localized (cytoplasmic, as opposed to membranous) staining pattern of p120-catenin.[25,26]

Most classic invasive lobular carcinomas are positive for ER (and, to a lesser extent, PR) and negative for ERBB2 (HER2) amplification; pleomorphic lobular carcinomas, on the other hand, can be ER-negative and may be ERBB2 (HER2) amplified.[27,28]

MOLECULAR TESTING

Not of current clinical relevance in the diagnosis of these tumors.

PROGNOSIS

Controversy exists over whether invasive lobular carcinoma has a more or less favorable outcome compared with invasive carcinoma NST.[29,30] Events in these tumors, such as distant metastases[31] and recurrences, may occur at a long interval, even decades, from initial diagnosis.

Grade relates to survival, as well as to histologic subtype.[32,33] Most grade 2 invasive lobular carcinomas are of the classic type, while variants, such as solid or pleomorphic cancers, are mostly grade 3. Conversely, tubulolobular and alveolar invasive lobular carcinomas are regarded as low-grade tumors. While patients with invasive lobular carcinoma have similar or even better outcomes than invasive carcinoma NST in the first decade following diagnosis, long-term events, such as recurrences, distant metastases, and mortality, appear more frequent.[34–36] Pleomorphic invasive lobular carcinoma has been found to be associated with a significantly worse recurrence-free survival, increased risk of distant metastases and decreased median survival time compared with classic invasive lobular carcinoma.[37–39]

Classic invasive lobular carcinomas (the majority being low-grade, ER-positive tumors) are typically sensitive to hormonal therapy[6,34,40,41]; however, they show an inferior response to neoadjuvant chemotherapy than invasive carcinoma NST, with poor rates of pathologic complete response.[41–43]

Difficulty in the accurate determination of tumor size can lead to challenges in achieving negative surgical margins.[44,45] The use of preoperative MRI has been reported to reduce reexcision rates in patients who undergo breast-conserving surgery.[46,47]

Of practical import is the challenge of diagnosing lobular carcinoma in metastatic sites. Lobular carcinoma involving the stomach may mimic a poorly cohesive (diffuse type, "linitis plastica") gastric carcinoma.[48,49] Osseous or splenic metastases can simulate hematopoeitic elements.[50–52] Cytokeratin immunohistochemistry may be helpful in the detection of obscure neoplastic cells.[51–53]

CLINICS CARE POINTS

- Dyscohesive tumor cells; often show loss of membranous E-cadherin expression and aberrantly localized p120 catenin staining
- Imaging and gross examination may substantially underestimate tumor extent
- Due to subtle, infiltrative growth pattern, surgical margins may be compromised
- Metastases can be difficult to detect
- Classic invasive lobular carcinoma is sensitive to hormonal therapy, but responds poorly to neoadjuvant chemotherapy
- The risk of recurrence persists for decades

TUBULAR CARCINOMA

CLINICAL FINDINGS AND EPIDEMIOLOGY

Tubular carcinomas most frequently occur in postmenopausal patients,[54,55] constituting 2% to 4%

of all breast carcinomas.[56–58] They may present as incidental "pick-ups" on mammographic screening due to their (relatively) smaller sizes at presentation.

MACROSCOPIC FEATURES

When mass-forming, tubular carcinoma forms a firm-to-hard mass with irregular, stellate borders and a grayish-white cut appearance. Many tubular carcinomas are quite small and may not be apparent grossly.

HISTOLOGY

The tumor forms haphazardly distributed, "open," rounded-to-angulated tubules and glands, lined by a single layer of relatively uniform neoplastic cells with small-to-intermediate sized nuclei, within a desmoplastic stroma [**Fig. 2**]. Luminal "snouts," secretions and calcifications may be present. By definition, more than 90% of the tumor should consist of the pattern described above, and the histologic grade is 1. Therefore, definitive classification should not occur on a core needle biopsy but instead in a surgical specimen whereby the entire cancer can be evaluated. When these features are present on a core biopsy, it can be appropriate to indicate that the cancer has features of this special histologic type ("tubular features"), and if on surgical excision it proves to have a similar uniformly tubular morphology it could be classified as a pure tubular carcinoma.

Common coexistent lesions include columnar cell lesions, flat epithelial atypia, lobular neoplasia, atypical ductal hyperplasia, and low-grade ductal carcinoma in situ,[59] which together with tubular carcinoma are lesions in the spectrum of a posited low-grade breast neoplasia pathway.[60–64]

IMMUNOHISTOCHEMISTRY

Tubular carcinoma is typically uniformly positive for ER, variably positive for PR, and negative for

ERBB2 (HER2).[55] Deviance from the expected expression pattern should provoke the consideration of alternative diagnoses,[65] such as low-grade adenosquamous carcinoma or adenoid cystic carcinoma, both being tumors with tubule formation.

MOLECULAR TESTING

Not of current clinical relevance in the diagnosis of these tumors.

DIFFERENTIAL DIAGNOSIS

Microglandular adenosis: The glands in MGA tend to be small and oval-to-rounded without angular contours, and contain dense, eosinophilic colloid-like secretions. Both tubular carcinoma and MGA lack myoepithelial rimming. Immunohistochemical interrogation shows strong S100 staining in MGA and negativity for ER and PR, in contradistinction to tubular carcinoma which is ER and PR positive.

Sclerosing adenosis and radial scar: Sclerosing adenosis is lobulocentric, compared with tubular carcinoma which shows infiltrative borders. The glandular epithelium of sclerosing adenosis and radial scars are invested by myoepithelium, which can be demonstrated by appropriate immunohistochemical markers, such as CK5/6, CK14, p63, and smooth muscle myosin-heavy chain; tubular carcinoma lacks myoepithelial participation.

PROGNOSIS

Patients with tubular carcinoma, in general, have excellent prognoses, and as such, tubular carcinoma is considered a "favorable histologic subtype."[55] It is notable that the NCCN breast cancer treatment guidelines have a separate treatment pathway for the pure favorable histologic types, including tubular carcinoma, with the avoidance of chemotherapy regardless of size (not considered unless lymph node positive) and there is therefore no need to test with ancillary tests such as OncotypeDX to predict benefit from chemotherapy (see https://www.nccn.org/guidelines/guidelines-detail?category=1&id=1419).

This is in contrast to the recommended use of this test in most ER-positive breast cancers larger than 0.5 cm to determine if chemotherapy should be added to endocrine therapy. Most patients with tubular carcinoma present with stage I disease[66]; and unifocal tubular carcinoma is, therefore, commonly treated with breast-conservation therapy followed by adjuvant radiotherapy and hormonal therapy.[67] Recurrence after adequate excision is a rare occurrence.

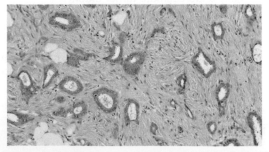

Fig. 2. Well-formed, "open" tubules and glands lined by tumor cells with low-to-intermediate grade nuclei are present in tubular carcinoma, associated with a desmoplastic stromal reaction.

CLINICS CARE POINTS

- "Open," round to angulated tubules lined by a single layer of tumor cells
- Grade 1
- ER positive, HER2 negative
- Favorable prognosis; genomic testing (OncotypeDX) is not required, and chemotherapy is not recommended

INVASIVE CRIBRIFORM CARCINOMA

CLINICAL FINDINGS AND EPIDEMIOLOGY

Pure invasive cribriform carcinoma is a rare entity, accounting for less than 0.5% of all breast carcinomas.[68–70] There are no specific distinguishing clinical features of significance. It is recommended that the "invasive" prefix is applied for these invasive cancers, to distinguish them from cribriform ductal carcinoma in situ.

MACROSCOPIC FEATURES

No specific characteristic gross morphologic features.

HISTOLOGY

Angulated and ovoid neoplastic nests of epithelium are seen within a desmoplastic stroma, displaying a well-defined cribriform, sieve-like architecture (architecturally akin to cribriform ductal carcinoma-in-situ), and lacking myoepithelial rimming. The neoplastic cells are relatively uniform and of low-to-intermediate nuclear grade [**Fig. 3**]. The Nottingham grade is usually 1 (with tubule score of 1 applied to the cribriform pattern). Mucinous secretions may be seen.[68] Admixed DCIS of a similar pattern is often present.

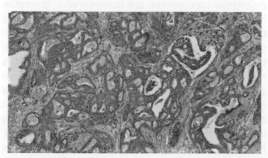

Fig. 3. Invasive cribriform carcinoma displays well-formed, "sieve-like" architecture and uniform tumor cell morphology.

IMMUNOHISTOCHEMISTRY

Similar to tubular carcinomas, invasive cribriform carcinomas are classically uniformly ER positive, variably PR positive, and ERBB2 (HER2) negative.[69,70]

MOLECULAR TESTING

Not of current clinical relevance in the diagnosis of these tumors.

DIFFERENTIAL DIAGNOSIS

Cribriform DCIS: DCIS with cribriform morphology shows generally rounded contours and retains an intact rim of myoepithelium, which is absent in invasive cribriform carcinoma.

Adenoid cystic carcinoma: Invasive cribriform carcinoma lacks the characteristic cylindromatous-like architecture of adenoid cystic carcinoma. Invasive cribriform carcinoma is ER/PR positive, while adenoid cystic carcinoma is usually triple negative.

PROGNOSIS

Patients with invasive cribriform carcinoma, similar to those with tubular carcinoma, have a generally favorable long-term outcome and it is also considered a "favorable histologic subtype."[68,69,71,72] An isolated case of a patient with an invasive cribriform carcinoma that was left untreated for more than a decade presenting with osseous metastasis is on record.[73]

CLINICS CARE POINTS

- Cribriform "islands" of tumor cells
- Grade 1
- ER positive, HER2 negative
- Favorable prognosis; genomic testing (OncotypeDX) and chemotherapy not recommended

MUCINOUS CARCINOMA

CLINICAL FINDINGS AND EPIDEMIOLOGY

Mucinous carcinoma of the breast, which accounts for approximately 1% to 3% of all breast cancers,[74] commonly arises in older patients, with a median age of 71.[74–76] Mammography may reveal a relatively well-circumscribed mass.

MACROSCOPIC FEATURES

Gross findings depend on the proportion of mucin versus fibrous stroma. Mucin-rich tumors show a glistening, gelatinous cut appearance, with "pushing" margins.

HISTOLOGY

Two classic types of mucinous carcinoma were described by Capella and colleagues[77]: type A, comprising scant clusters of tumor cells suspended within abundant extracellular mucin; and type B, composed of hypercellular epithelial groups and sheets [**Fig. 4**], often with neuroendocrine differentiation[77] demonstrable by appropriate immunohistochemical evaluation. Fine fibrous septa and delicate blood vessels may be perceived amidst pools of mucin.

Mucinous carcinoma may also assume a micropapillary pattern[78–83]: morules and ring-like formations of neoplastic epithelial cells are set within mucin pools; in this pattern, pronounced nuclear atypia may be appreciated, as well as hobnail cells and psammomatous calcifications. The micropapillary pattern of mucinous carcinoma may present in younger patients, with a higher occurrence of lymphovascular invasion and nodal metastases.[79–81]

It is important to note that high-grade carcinomas can produce mucin and this does not equate with a diagnosis of a pure mucinous carcinoma. In fact, the WHO criteria for a diagnosis of a pure mucinous carcinoma has > 90% pattern purity requirement; lesser extents of the mucinous pattern should also be reported in mixed carcinomas and if a high-grade or HER2 positive component is present, the mucinous carcinoma label should not be used since they are best classified as "no special type with mucin production." Associated DCIS is often present.

IMMUNOHISTOCHEMISTRY

Mucinous carcinomas are most commonly ER and PR positive.[74–76] ERBB2 (HER2) overexpression is rare,[84] except in mucinous carcinomas with micropapillary pattern.[79,81] Of note, the micropapillary pattern may exhibit a distinct basolateral ("U-shaped") pattern of HER2 staining, which should be considered as 2+ (equivocal) and reflexed to in situ hybridization.

MOLECULAR TESTING

Not of current clinical relevance in the diagnosis of these tumors.

DIFFERENTIAL DIAGNOSIS

Mucocele-like lesion: *Mucocele-like lesion* (MLLs) consist of mucin-containing cysts that may rupture, with spillage of mucin into stroma; it is a descriptive term, with the exact classification of the lesion determined by the nature of the associated epithelium (benign, atypical, or malignant).[85] The distinction of benign MLL with abundant extravasated mucin from paucicellular mucinous carcinoma may be challenging. The lack of atypia and presence of immunohistochemically demonstrated myoepithelium within detached epithelial clusters, as well as lining the associated duct space, can help favor a benign process.

Secretory carcinoma (SC): *Secretory carcinoma* (SC) contains intracellular and "bubbly" extracellular secretions, which are pale, eosinophilic, or amphophilic in appearance, displays a variety of architectural patterns (microcystic, tubular, papillary), and a pathognomonic *ETV6-NTRK3* gene fusion.

Foreign material: Injected material for breast augmentation, such as polyacrylamide, may mimic the appearance of mucin. The presence of a foreign body-type giant cell reaction, and a thorough knowledge of the clinical picture, will aid in the correct diagnosis.

PROGNOSIS

When the classic diagnostic criteria are met, pure mucinous carcinomas are considered a favorable histologic subtype associated with a generally favorable long-term outcome,[74,76,86,87] although late metastases may develop.[88] Similar to pure tubular and cribriform carcinomas, the NCCN has a different treatment pathway for these favorable histologic types, without consideration of chemotherapy or testing to determine chemotherapy benefit. Treatment most often involves lumpectomy with radiation and endocrine therapy. No significant prognostic difference is observed between Type A and Type B tumors.[89] Mixed carcinomas with a mucinous pattern do not retain the same excellent prognoses as pure mucinous

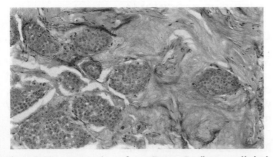

Fig. 4. An example of a Type B (hypercellular) mucinous carcinoma, with cellular tumor nests suspended within abundant extracellular mucin.

carcinomas.[89,90] A micropapillary pattern, if it accounts for more than 50% of the tumor, was shown to confer a worse prognosis.[79] Again, if a mucin-producing carcinoma is high-grade or HER2 positive, it is not likely to have the same favorable prognosis as a classic mucinous carcinoma, and therefore should not be diagnosed or treated as such.

CLINICS CARE POINTS

- Low-intermediate grade tumor epithelial cells suspended within abundant extracellular mucin
- Mucinous carcinoma with micropapillary pattern tends to occur in younger patients, with a higher incidence of lymphovascular invasion and lymph node metastases
- Classic mucinous carcinoma has a favorable prognosis; genomic testing (OncotypeDX) is not required, and chemotherapy is not recommended
- A high-grade or HER2 positive carcinoma with mucinous features should be diagnosed as "invasive carcinoma NST with mucin production" (rather than "mucinous carcinoma") due to prognostic implications

MUCINOUS CYSTADENOCARCINOMA

CLINICAL FINDINGS AND EPIDEMIOLOGY

This is a very rare and newly recognized form of breast cancer, with most cases reported in women of postmenopausal age,[91–93] with many from Asian countries.[94–98]

MACROSCOPIC FEATURES

A relatively circumscribed solid-cystic mass, with gelatinous areas.

HISTOLOGY

Tall, stratified columnar cells with papillary, micropapillary, and cribriform architecture are seen lining and projecting in excrescent fashion into mucin-distended cystic spaces, which generally show rounded contours but lack myoepithelial rimming. The neoplastic cells demonstrate basally located nuclei and intracytoplasmic mucin, with variable atypia [**Fig. 5**]. Associated DCIS may be present.

IMMUNOHISTOCHEMISTRY

Unlike conventional mucinous carcinoma and encapsulated papillary carcinoma, mucinous

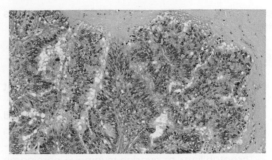

Fig. 5. Tall columnar cells with intracytoplasmic mucin and basally-oriented nuclei line papillary cores in mucinous cystadenocarcinoma. (*From* Hannah Wen, MD, PhD and *WHO Classification of Tumors Editorial Board. Breast Tumors.* 5th ed. International Agency for Research on Cancer; 2019; 2019. https://publications.iarc.fr/581, with permission)

cystadenocarcinomas are usually negative for ER, PR, and ERBB2 (HER2).[91–93] Rare HER2-amplified cases have been reported.[96,99] Of note, the neoplastic cells are CK7-positive, while being negative for CK20 and CDX-2, which may help in the diagnostic distinction from metastatic pancreatobiliary carcinoma. GATA3 was negative in one case of mucinous cystadenocarcinoma studied.[92]

MOLECULAR TESTING

Not of current clinical relevance in the diagnosis of these tumors.

DIFFERENTIAL DIAGNOSIS

Mucinous carcinoma (MC): In addition to the morphologic differences, mucinous cystadenocarcinoma tends to be ER and PR negative, in contrast to MC. Mammary MCs express MUC4 and MUC6 mucins, while mucinous cystadenocarcinoma is positive for MUC5.[100]

Metastatic mucinous carcinoma: Close clinical and radiological correlation is required to exclude metastasis from a pancreatobiliary or ovarian primary. The presence of associated DCIS favors origin from the breast.

PROGNOSIS

Most of the reported cases seem to show relatively good prognoses, although one case of local recurrence after lumpectomy was reported.[92] Lymph node spread is uncommon.[92] It may be important to emphasize to clinicians that although this is a triple-negative form of breast cancer, it is not a typical form and may not warrant the same aggressive treatment that clinical treatment pathways currently recommend based on its triple-negative status alone.

INVASIVE MICROPAPILLARY CARCINOMA

CLINICAL FINDINGS AND EPIDEMIOLOGY

An uncommon tumor in its pure form,[101,102] it is more often seen as a component pattern mixed with invasive carcinoma of NST.[103–105] It may affect patients of any biological sex, with an age range of patients that overlaps with that of invasive carcinoma (NST).[103,106–108] Invasive micropapillary carcinoma has a pronounced propensity for axillary lymph node involvement and angiolymphatic spread.[104,109–111]

MACROSCOPIC FEATURES

It consists of a solid, soft-to-firm, whitish-gray mass with irregular margins and may be multifocal.

HISTOLOGY

Morules and "hollow" nests of cuboidal-to-columnar neoplastic epithelial cells, devoid of true fibrovascular cores, are surrounded by clear, empty clefts [**Fig. 6**] within a delicate fibroblastic and connective tissue stromal framework.[112] The

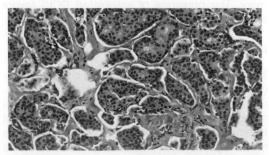

Fig. 6. Morules of tumor cells are surrounded by clear clefts in this invasive micropapillary carcinoma.

apical poles of tumor cells, occasionally forming blebs or associated with secretions, are oriented toward the outward aspect of the morular clusters (facing the surrounding empty spaces rather than the center).

The neoplastic cells are usually of intermediate to high nuclear grade.[103,108,113–115] Rarely, a micropapillary pattern may be associated with the presence of mucin (see "Mucinous carcinoma" section above). Multinucleated giant cells may be seen.[116] Associated micropapillary or cribriform intermediate-to-high-grade DCIS is often present.

IMMUNOHISTOCHEMISTRY

Most invasive micropapillary carcinomas are ER and PR positive,[115,117–119] with some cases showing ERBB2 (HER2) overexpression and amplification.[115,117,118,120] Micropapillary carcinoma may exhibit HER2 staining in a unique "U-shaped" basolateral pattern with sparing of the luminal cell membrane; this staining pattern should be considered as HER2 2+ (equivocal) and submitted for in situ hybridization testing.[65,121]

The use of EMA (MUC1) immunohistochemistry displays a distinctive pattern of "reversed polarity" (stroma-facing) staining,[111,122] resulting in linear staining by EMA of the outer aspect of micropapillary tumor clusters, as well as a mutually exclusive, that is, "basolateral," expression of adhesion proteins (p120, E-cadherin).[123]

MOLECULAR TESTING

Not of current clinical relevance in the diagnosis of these tumors.

DIFFERENTIAL DIAGNOSIS

The distinct morphology of invasive micropapillary carcinoma usually makes for straightforward diagnosis. In the presence of a significant past medical history, metastatic micropapillary carcinoma from other anatomic sites (such as bladder, female genital tract, and lung) should be excluded; the presence of DCIS favors a breast origin.

PROGNOSIS

Lymphovascular invasion and axillary lymph node spread are common. However, meta-analysis has shown no statistically significant differences in overall, disease-specific, or distant metastasis-free survival of micropapillary carcinoma than invasive carcinoma (NST), despite a higher rate of locoregional recurrence.[124] In one study, when matched for patient age, tumor size, tumor grade, lymphovascular invasion, immunohistochemically defined molecular subtype, and number of positive lymph nodes, the presence of micropapillary histology did not contribute independent information toward the risk of local relapse, distant relapse, and overall survival, as compared with invasive carcinoma (NST).[118] Therefore, current clinical treatment guidelines do not differ from standard invasive carcinoma NST and are based on ER and HER2 status, lymph node status, size, etc.

CLINICS CARE POINTS

- Micropapillary tumor clusters with a "reversed polarity" pattern surrounded by clear, "empty" clefts
- EMA highlights stroma-facing border of tumor clusters
- Lymphovascular invasion and lymph node metastases are frequent
- Treatment is similar to invasive carcinoma NST, and based on ER and HER2 status, lymph node status, size, etc.

CARCINOMA WITH APOCRINE DIFFERENTIATION

CLINICAL FINDINGS AND EPIDEMIOLOGY

A rare tumor[125] with an older patient profile than that of invasive carcinoma (NST).[126–128]

MACROSCOPIC FEATURES

No specific characteristic gross morphologic features.

HISTOLOGY

Abundant, eosinophilic, granular cytoplasm distinguishes the tumor cells of this entity.[129,130] Nuclei are round-to-oval, variably enlarged, and contain prominent nucleoli [Fig. 7]. The tumor most often

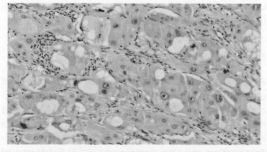

Fig. 7. The tumor cells of carcinoma with apocrine differentiation possess abundant, eosinophilic cytoplasm with a granular quality, and enlarged nuclei with prominent nucleoli.

proliferates in a solid fashion, although any architectural pattern may be encountered. An uncommon, histiocytoid variant has been described.[131] Associated intermediate-to- high-grade DCIS of apocrine morphology is often present.[132]

IMMUNOHISTOCHEMISTRY

Androgen receptor (AR)[125,126,133,134] and GCDFP-15[135] expression are observed in the neoplastic cells, which are usually ER and PR negative. ERBB2 (HER2) overexpression and/or amplification may be seen.[133,136–138]

MOLECULAR TESTING

Not of current clinical relevance in the diagnosis of these tumors.

DIFFERENTIAL DIAGNOSIS

Metastatic cutaneous apocrine carcinoma: Apocrine carcinomas originating from the skin and breast are histologically similar. Diffuse CK5/6 staining may favor an apocrine carcinoma of cutaneous origin,[139] while calretinin staining may favor a mammary tumor.[140] Clinical correlation is essential in the distinction.

Metastatic renal cell carcinoma: Renal cell carcinoma may be highlighted by PAX2, PAX8, and RCC antigens, while mammary apocrine carcinoma is positive for CK7, AR, and GCDFP-15.

Granular cell tumor: These tumors are keratin-negative and CD68-positive, in contrast to apocrine carcinomas which are keratin-positive and CD68-negative. S100 highlights granular cell tumors in a strong, diffuse fashion, while it may stain apocrine carcinoma focally.[141]

PROGNOSIS

Due to variable diagnostic criteria, the reported outcomes of carcinomas with apocrine differentiation have been controversial, with some studies demonstrating a worse prognosis of these tumors than invasive carcinoma (NST),[126,142] although the difference was diminished once demographic and clinicopathologic factors were matched.[142] Some studies have found invasive apocrine carcinoma to show better overall survival outcomes than other triple-negative carcinomas,[128,143–145] while others showed no significant differences.[146,147] Currently, prognosis and treatment are determined by conventional criteria, that is, ER and HER2 status, tumor size, grade, and nodal status. However, lower grade triple-negative cancers with apocrine differentiation are often a topic of tumor board discussions as more aggressive triple-negative treatments are designed for the more classic high-grade triple-negative cancer. Whether low-grade triple-negative apocrine carcinomas should be handled differently is still a matter of debate with limited data available.

CLINICS CARE POINTS

- Tumor cells with apocrine morphology: large cells with ample, eosinophilic, granular cytoplasm, and enlarged nuclei with prominent nucleoli
- AR-positive, ER- and PR-negative
- Most current clinical treatment pathways do not differentiate apocrine triple-negative cancers from other triple-negative cancers; there is debate/limited data on how low-grade apocrine cancers should be treated

METAPLASTIC CARCINOMA

CLINICAL FINDINGS AND EPIDEMIOLOGY

Metaplastic carcinomas, a heterogeneous group of rare tumors with different prognoses, most often present as a palpable lump or radiologically-detected mass. They are uncommon, accounting for up to 1% of all invasive breast cancers,[148–150] and may occur in any anatomic region of the breast.

MACROSCOPIC FEATURES

Most metaplastic carcinomas are firm-to-hard nodules, with variably infiltrative borders. Tumors with chondroid metaplasia may show whitish-gray, glistening cut appearances. Areas of osseous differentiation may be gritty or so unyielding to routine sectioning that decalcification is required.

HISTOLOGY

The diagnosis of metaplastic carcinoma requires the presence of an associated invasive carcinoma of conventional mammary-type histology and/or ductal carcinoma-in-situ (DCIS), or unequivocal evidence of epithelial differentiation on immunohistochemical analysis.

A descriptive classification system used by the WHO Classification of Tumors categorizes these tumors based on the type of the metaplastic elements, namely: epithelial-only carcinomas (low-grade adenosquamous carcinoma [LGASC], high-grade adenosquamous carcinoma, pure squamous cell carcinoma), pure sarcomatoid carcinomas (spindle cell carcinoma, matrix-producing

carcinoma), or biphasic epithelial and sarcomatoid carcinomas.[2]

There may be 1 (monophasic) or 2 and more (biphasic) metaplastic components. The proportion of each metaplastic component (if more than one is identified) should be noted in the pathologic report.

LOW-GRADE ADENOSQUAMOUS CARCINOMA

Neoplastic glands, tubules, and cords of epithelial cells are intermingled with solid squamous nests in a desmoplastic background containing peripheral lymphocytic aggregates [Fig. 8A,B]. The tumor often infiltrates among non-neoplastic breast structures. The glandular structures in LGASC may show variable expression of p63 and basal keratins along the basal layer. It should be distinguished from a squamous cell (metaplastic) carcinoma admixed with invasive carcinoma (NST), that is, a high-grade adenosquamous carcinoma pattern, due to its generally favorable prognosis.[151] Limited adenosquamous foci seen in sclerosing lesions should not be over-interpreted as LGASC.

FIBROMATOSIS-LIKE METAPLASTIC CARCINOMA

Most (>95%) of the tumor should comprise bland, spindled cells within a collagenized stroma. Lesional cells have slender, tapered nuclei, and a fine chromatin pattern, with pale eosinophilic cytoplasm disposed as interlacing, wavy, or long fascicles infiltrating into adjacent normal breast tissue. Close scrutiny reveals nests or cords of plump, epithelioid cells, sometimes with focal squamous differentiation.[152–155]

Fibromatosis-like metaplastic carcinoma must enter into the differential diagnostic evaluation of any bland spindled breast proliferation. The diagnosis may be made by the evidence of epithelial differentiation in the tumor, which includes the use of a panel of immunohistochemical markers (detailed later in discussion).

SPINDLE CELL CARCINOMA

Atypical spindled cells proliferate in a variety of architectural patterns, including short-to-long fascicles or storiform formations [Fig. 8C]. There is moderate to marked nuclear pleomorphism. Foci of epithelioid morphology or frank squamous differentiation may be discerned.[156–158] Evidence of epithelial differentiation, with immunohistochemical aid (see later in discussion), confirms the diagnosis [Fig. 8D].

Fig. 8. (*A*) Angular nests and tubules within a desmoplastic stroma characterize low-grade adenosquamous carcinoma (LGASC). There is an irregular tumor border, associated with peripheral lymphoid aggregates. (*B*) Squamoid nests, composed of polygonal cells with densely eosinophilic cytoplasm, are seen in LGASC. (*C*) In this example of a spindle cell carcinoma, atypical cells form haphazard fascicles. Immunohistochemical analysis is necessary for the definitive evaluation of this tumor. (*D*) The tumor cells are highlighted by pancytokeratin MNF116 immunohistochemical stain, confirming the diagnosis of a spindle cell carcinoma. (*E*) Neoplastic glands are present in proximity to abnormal squamous nests

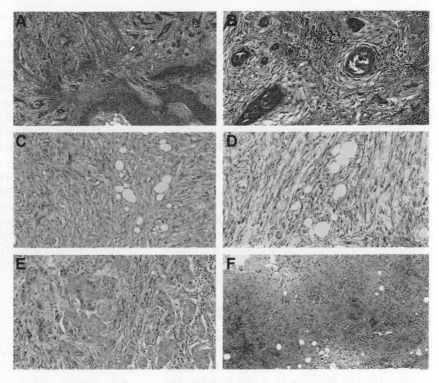

in this case of a metaplastic carcinoma with squamous differentiation. (*F*) Chondroid stroma can be a component of metaplastic carcinoma with heterologous mesenchymal differentiation.

SQUAMOUS CELL CARCINOMA

Pure squamous cell carcinoma of the breast often forms a cystic structure lined by variably atypical squamous cells, with infiltrative nests and sheets at the periphery.[159,160] Pseudoangiomatous and acantholytic features may be present. There may be admixture with other types of metaplastic carcinoma, such as spindle cell carcinoma, or with invasive carcinoma (NST). The finding of a pure squamous cell carcinoma in the breast warrants exclusion of origin from the skin, or metastasis from another site such as the cervix or lung.

METAPLASTIC CARCINOMA WITH HETEROLOGOUS MESENCHYMAL DIFFERENTIATION

Carcinomatous areas (such as glands, tubules, solid nests, or squamous foci [**Fig. 8**E]) are admixed with mesenchymal components (which may include chondroid [**Fig. 8**F], rhabdomyoid, osseous, or glial elements).[161–164] The latter component may be relatively well-differentiated or markedly atypical.

The term "matrix-producing carcinoma" was used to refer to tumors containing chondroid or osteoid matrix material, whereby an abrupt transition, devoid of an intervening spindle cell component, was observed between epithelial and mesenchymal components. However, it is now felt that the presence of some spindle cells should not detract from this diagnosis.

MIXED METAPLASTIC CARCINOMAS

Many metaplastic carcinomas contain varying admixtures of the above-described tumor patterns, as well as conventional (glandular) carcinoma. They may be diagnosed as mixed metaplastic carcinomas, with explanatory notes detailing the different tumor components.

IMMUNOHISTOCHEMISTRY

Most metaplastic carcinomas are negative for ER, PR, and ERRB (HER2).[148,150,165,166]

A panel of immunohistochemical markers may be employed to elucidate evidence of epithelial differentiation, including: p63, CK5/6, AE1/3, MNF116, and 34betaE12. This is of critical diagnostic importance in tumors that otherwise lack conventional histologic evidence of epithelial differentiation or associated DCIS.

Low-molecular-weight keratins, such as CK8/18, CK7, and CK19, are less commonly positive. Myoepithelial markers, such as CD10 and SMA, may be expressed.

MOLECULAR TESTING

Not of current clinical relevance in the diagnosis of these tumors.

DIFFERENTIAL DIAGNOSIS

Low-grade spindle cell proliferation: Differentials include fibromatosis, nodular fasciitis, pseudoangiomatous stromal hyperplasia (PASH), and myofibroblastoma. Fibromatosis forms broad, sweeping fascicles; aberrant nuclear localization of beta-catenin expression is present, while no expression of p63 or keratins should be seen. Of note, some metaplastic carcinomas may also display nuclear staining for beta-catenin,[167,168] warranting caution in the evaluation of low-grade mammary spindle cell lesions with this stain. Nodular fasciitis presents as a rapidly enlarging, sometimes painful mass; lesional cells show a "tissue culture"-like appearance and stain with SMA while showing no keratin expression. It is now regarded as a transient neoplastic phenomenon, with a characteristic *MYH9-USP6* gene fusion.[169] The cells of PASH and myofibroblastoma are CD34 positive and may express PR/ER, while metaplastic carcinoma is usually negative for the aforementioned markers.

High-grade spindle cell proliferation: Differentials include phyllodes tumor with stromal overgrowth, primary mammary sarcoma, and metastatic sarcoma from another anatomic site. Evaluation of a wholly high-grade spindle cell breast lesion on core biopsy demands prudence on the part of the pathologist, and often requires assessment of an excisional specimen for additional diagnostic clues, such as the characteristic "fronds" of phyllodes tumor, as well as close clinical and radiological correlation.

PROGNOSIS

The specific subtype of metaplastic carcinoma influences prognosis, with LGASC and fibromatosis-like carcinomas associated with less aggressive behavior.[151,170] Matrix-producing carcinomas may have a better prognosis, while (high-grade) spindle cell carcinoma and squamous cell carcinoma are associated with worse outcomes.[171,172] The presence of more than 3 distinct morphologic elements seems to be correlated with a poorer prognosis.[173]

In the NCCN breast cancer guidelines (BINV-10, version 5.2021), metaplastic carcinomas are listed in the triple-negative treatment pathways but with a footnote recognizing that there are rare subtypes of metaplastic carcinoma (eg, low-grade adenosquamous and low-grade fibromatosis like carcinoma) that are considered to have a favorable prognosis without adjuvant systemic therapies. In a way, these are actually considered to be triple-negative cancers with favorable histology similar to adenoid cystic carcinomas/salivary forms and secretory carcinomas (described later in discussion). The NCCN lists these triple-negative forms in their favorable histologies treatment pathways (BINV-11, version 5.2021), with consideration for treatment beyond surgical excision only in lymph node-positive disease.

CLINICS CARE POINTS

- A heterogeneous group of tumors characterized by differentiation toward mesenchymal or squamous elements
- In tumors lacking conventional mammary-type carcinoma or DCIS components, demonstration of epithelial differentiation by immunohistochemistry (cytokeratins, p63) is crucial
- Triple-negative form of breast cancer but with different treatments depending on subtype (low-grade forms not treated aggressively)

ACINIC CELL CARCINOMA

CLINICAL FINDINGS AND EPIDEMIOLOGY

A rare type of breast cancer, with fewer than 50 reported cases in the literature,[174] which predominantly affects adult women.

MACROSCOPIC FEATURES

A firm-to-hard mass with irregular borders.

HISTOLOGY

Cytologic features are key to the recognition of this tumor, which may display a wide variety of architectural patterns, including solid foci with necrosis, and microglandular areas [**Fig. 9**A]. Abundant, eosinophilic, basophilic, or clear cytoplasm with a granular quality, that is, serous acinar features [**Fig. 9**B], characterizes the tumor cells.[175] On PAS/D staining, large, eosinophilic, intracellular granules may be seen. The tumor cells show variable atypia with prominent nucleolation. Associated in-situ carcinoma may be present.

Fig. 9. (*A*)Acinic cell carcinoma comprises nests and tubules of tumor cells, sometimes containing colloid-like luminal material. (*B*) The neoplas-tic cells of acinic cell carcinoma possess ample cytoplasm with a granular quality, akin to those of salivary serous acini. (*C*) Positive cytoplasmic reactivity with lysozyme immunohistochemistry is present in acinic cell carcinoma.

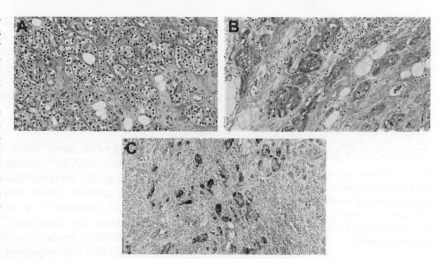

IMMUNOHISTOCHEMISTRY

Serous acinar differentiation may be demonstrated by strong immunopositivity for lysozyme [**Fig. 9**C] and alpha-1-antichymotrypsin.[176] Tumor cells also express S100, EMA, and low-molecular-weight keratins; ER, PR, and ERBB2 (HER2) are negative.

MOLECULAR TESTING

Not of current clinical relevance in the diagnosis of these tumors. There is evidence that acinic cell carcinoma and MGA may exist along a spectrum of so-called "low-grade triple negative" breast lesions that frequently harbor *TP53* mutations.[177,178]

DIFFERENTIAL DIAGNOSIS

Secretory carcinoma: Acinic cell carcinoma does not contain prominent intracellular and extracellular secretions, is highlighted by markers for serous acinar differentiation, and lacks the *ETV6-NTRK3* gene fusion characteristic of secretory carcinoma.

Granular cell tumor: Granular cell tumor lacks keratin staining, in contrast to acinic cell carcinoma. Both tumors may express S100 and CD68.[179]

PROGNOSIS

Due to the rarity of this tumor, prognostic information is limited.[174] Axillary nodal metastases and distant organ metastases with resultant mortality have been reported in a small number of cases,[174] with most patients remaining recurrence-free at 6 to 184 months post-diagnosis. Similar to other forms of salivary-like cancer in the breast, they may warrant less aggressive treatment than typical high-grade triple-negative cancers.

CLINICS CARE POINTS

- Tumor cells with clear, eosinophilic, or basophilic cytoplasm with a granular quality and PAS/D-positive intracytoplasmic granules
- Evidence of serous acinar differentiation on immunohistochemistry: lysozyme, alpha-1-antichymotrypsin
- Triple negative but not necessarily treated similar to classic high-grade triple-negative breast cancers of NST

ADENOID CYSTIC CARCINOMA

CLINICAL FINDINGS AND EPIDEMIOLOGY

A rare tumor in the breast, accounting for 0.1% to 3.5%[180,181] of all breast tumors, that predominantly affects elderly women. Rarely occurs in men[182–184] and adolescents.[185]

MACROSCOPIC FEATURES

A solid, nodular tumor that may contain cystic areas. Despite microscopic infiltration, gross examination often gives an impression of circumscribed borders.[186,187]

HISTOLOGY

The histologic appearances of mammary adenoid cystic carcinoma parallel those observed in the salivary gland tumors. Three main subtypes are recognized:

Classic adenoid cystic carcinoma

This tumor is composed of a heterogeneous distribution of gland-forming luminal epithelial and myoepithelial/abluminal cells intimately associated with basement membrane material and

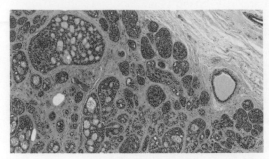

Fig. 10. Classic adenoid cystic carcinoma can display a variety of architectural patterns and contains admixed populations of epithelial and myoepithelial (abluminal) cells. Basement membrane and stromal material are incorporated into the tumor, which may contain luminal mucin.

stroma [**Fig. 10**]. Cribriform, tubular, reticular/trabecular, solid, and cylindromatous architecture can be observed. Luminal spaces may contain mucin that can be demonstrated by Alcian blue (pH 2.5) staining. Myoepithelial cells form so-called "pseudolumina" filled with stromal cells, basement membrane, and occasional capillary-sized blood vessels. Classic AdCC lacks significant nuclear atypia or necrosis, with infrequent mitotic activity. Most AdCCs show an infiltrative growth pattern. Squamous[188] and sebaceous metaplasia[189] may be present in rare tumors.

Solid-basaloid adenoid cystic carcinoma

SB-AdCC contains solid nests of basaloid cells with pronounced nuclear atypia, necrosis, and brisk mitoses, in addition to areas of classic AdCC which may be present.[190] Perineural invasion is commonly seen.

Adenoid cystic carcinoma with high-grade transformation

A well-recognized entity in the salivary gland,[191] rare cases of AdCC with high-grade transformation have been described in the breast. Differentiation into invasive ductal carcinoma (NST),[192] small cell carcinoma,[193] and malignant adenomyoepithelioma[194] have been reported.

IMMUNOHISTOCHEMISTRY

Most breast AdCCs are negative for ER, PR, and ERRB (HER2). Rarely, focal ER and PR expression may be observed in classic AdCC,[195,196] within the epithelial component.

Epithelial cells can be highlighted by low-molecular-weight keratins CK7, CK8, as well as EMA and occasionally CK5/6.[197] CD117 (c-kit) also stains the luminal epithelial cells. Myoepithelial cells are decorated by CK14, CK5/6, p63,[198] S100, and heavy-chain myosin. SOX10 staining has been demonstrated in both luminal epithelial and myoepithelial/abluminal cells of AdCC.[199] MYB immunohistochemistry can be a valuable aid in the diagnosis of these tumors.[200,201]

MOLECULAR TESTING

MYB-NFIB gene fusion characterizes most reported AdCCs,[202] similar to that seen in the salivary gland, demonstrable by FISH. This fusion is also present, albeit less frequently, in the SB-AdCC subtype[203]; a negative result does not exclude the diagnosis.[204,205] AdCCs that lack *MYB-NFIB* fusion may show *MYB* amplification or *MYBL1* rearrangement.[202,205]

DIFFERENTIAL DIAGNOSIS

Collagenous spherulosis: Collagenous spherulosis is usually an incidental finding, compared with AdCC which is a mass-forming lesion. CD117 stains AdCC, while being largely negative in collagenous spherulosis.

Invasive carcinoma with prominent cribriform pattern: Conventional invasive carcinoma lacks myoepithelial participation and intimate involvement of stroma/basement membrane material. Invasive cribriform carcinoma is usually strongly positive for ER, while AdCC is triple negative.

PROGNOSIS

The histologic subtype of AdCC has an important bearing on prognosis. Classic AdCC has a generally excellent outcome,[206] with complete surgical excision being the treatment of choice. Nodal and distant metastases are rare.[206] Similar to other forms of salivary-like cancer in the breast, they may warrant less aggressive treatment than typical high-grade triple-negative cancers and the NCCN recognizes them as a favorable histology (BINV-11, version 5.2021), with consideration for treatment beyond surgical excision only in lymph node-positive disease. SB-AdCCs, on the other hand, can more frequently present with axillary disease and distant metastases and may warrant more aggressive treatment although data are very limited. The rare cases of breast AdCC with high-grade transformation have mostly resulted in mortality.[190,207]

CLINICS CARE POINTS

- A biphasic tumor composed of epithelial and myoepithelial cells, with cribriform, tubular, and occasional solid architectural patterns

- Gland lumina contain epithelial mucins
- Pseudolumina associated with myoepithelial cells contain stromal matrix material, basal lamina, and fibroblasts
- 3 subtypes: classic AdCC, solid-basaloid AdCC, and AdCC with high-grade transformation; only the classic type is associated with a favorable prognosis
- Characteristic *MYB-NFIB* gene fusion may be present but other *MYB*related amplification or rearrangements can also occur. Demonstration of these alterations is not required for the diagnosis.
- Triple negative but not necessarily treated similar to classic high-grade triple-negative breast cancers of NST

SECRETORY CARCINOMA

CLINICAL FINDINGS AND EPIDEMIOLOGY

This rare tumor, accounting for less than 0.05% of all invasive breast cancers,[208,209] occurs predominantly in adult women, with juvenile[210] and male[211] cases described. It most often presents as a slow-growing, relatively circumscribed mass.[212,213]

MACROSCOPIC FEATURES

A tan, grayish-white mass with a solid, glistening cut surface, as well as tiny-to-larger cysts containing colorless to brown, viscous secretions.

HISTOLOGY

The constituent tumor cells of this unusual tumor possess ample, eosinophilic cytoplasm with a granular or vacuolated quality, with at most mild-to-moderate nuclear atypia. Rare high-grade tumors, with marked nuclear atypia, necrosis, and numerous mitoses, have been described.[214] Mixed architectural patterns are usually present, including solid, papillary, tubular, and microcystic areas, the last of which may simulate thyroid follicles. Secretions are a prominent feature, displaying eosinophilic to amphophilic hues, accumulated intracytoplasmically as well as located extracellularly [**Fig. 11**]; these characteristic secretions may be highlighted by PAS, mucicarmine, and Alcian blue stains.

IMMUNOHISTOCHEMISTRY

The tumor cells are mostly negative for ER, PR, and ERBB2 (HER2), although weak ER/PR expression may be observed. The tumor cells may express S100, polyclonal CEA, mammaglobin, SOX10, MUC4, CK5/6, EGFR, GATA3, and CD117 (c-kit).[212,214-216] The use of myoepithelial stains may highlight an in situ component,[216,217] which is usually of low-to-intermediate nuclear grade and of solid or cribriform patterns.

MOLECULAR TESTING

ETV6-NTRK3 gene fusion is the sine qua non of secretory carcinoma[215,216,218]; currently, RT-PCR, FISH, and next-generation sequencing may be used for its detection, although the use of a pan-*TRK* antibody for immunohistochemical analysis shows promise.[219-221] Detection of the gene fusion is of particular importance in light of the development of therapeutic pan-*TRK* inhibitors.[222-225]

DIFFERENTIAL DIAGNOSIS

Apocrine carcinoma: Apocrine carcinoma does not contain the characteristic secretions of secretory carcinoma. Lacks *ETV6-NTRK3* gene fusion.

Mucinous carcinoma: Consists of neoplastic epithelium associated with abundant extracellular mucin. Lacks *ETV6-NTRK3* gene fusion.

PROGNOSIS

The prognosis is generally favorable, particularly in young patients[213,215]; some tumors in older adults may behave more aggressively,[226] with late recurrences[227] and rare deaths.[213,214,227] It is recognized as a favorable histologic type by the NCCN, with more conservative treatment than a typical high-grade triple-negative breast cancer recommended, similar to breast salivary gland like-tumors (NCCN BINV-11, version 5.2021), unless there is metastatic spread. In the metastatic setting, the presence of an NTRK fusion would make the patient a potential candidate for available targeted therapy with tropomyosin kinase receptor inhibitors (NCCN BINV-R, version 5.2021).

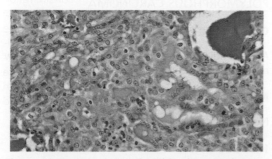

Fig. 11. Secretions, located within the cytoplasm as well as extracellularly, are prominent in secretory carcinoma, which is composed of cells with ample, eosinophilic cytoplasm with a vacuolated quality.

- Tumor cells with ample, eosinophilic, granular cytoplasm containing intracytoplasmic secretions
- Extracellular "bubbly" secretions
- Variety of architectural patterns, including microcystic, solid, tubular, and papillary
- Characteristic *ETV6-NTRK3* gene fusion present (targeted therapy with tropomyosin kinase receptor inhibitors available in the metastatic setting)
- Favorable outcomes, despite triple-negative status and not necessarily treated similar to classic high-grade triple-negative breast cancers of NST

MUCOEPIDERMOID CARCINOMA

CLINICAL FINDINGS AND EPIDEMIOLOGY

Mucoepidermoid carcinoma (MEC) of the breast arises in adult women. A common tumor of the salivary glands, it is rare in the breast, with fewer than 50 cases reported in the literature.[228]

MACROSCOPIC FEATURES

A solid mass. Cystic areas may be present.

HISTOLOGY

The hallmark of this tumor is the presence of 3 different cellular populations, namely mucous, squamoid, and intermediate cells. Squamoid cells have ample, eosinophilic cytoplasm with an epidermoid or polygonal morphology; crucially, true keratinization is not seen. Mucous cells, which may require diligence to detect in some tumors, contain mucin-filled vacuoles. Intermediate cells may range in appearance from small, basaloid cells with scanty cytoplasm to oval cells with abundant, palely eosinophilic cytoplasm that merge imperceptibly with squamoid or mucous cells. The different cell types, in varying proportions, may yield a wide spectrum of histologic patterns. Solid and cystic architecture may be present, with low-grade tumors being more commonly cystic. High-grade tumors, which tend to be solid, display appreciable cytologic atypia, frequent mitoses, and necrosis.[229]

IMMUNOHISTOCHEMISTRY

Immunohistochemistry is of aid in delineating the different cellular components. Low-molecular-weight keratins (such as CK7) highlight mucous cells, while p63 and high-molecular-weight keratins (eg, CK14) stain squamoid and intermediate cells.[229–231]

Most MECs show a triple-negative phenotype. However, ER, PR, and AR positivity have been described in some cases of low-grade breast MEC.[232]

MOLECULAR TESTING

Low-grade MEC of the salivary gland characteristically shows *CRTC1-MAML2* fusion resulting from t(11;19) (q21;p13) translocation. Breast MECs have been reported to show *MAML2* rearrangement and partial deletion of 11q21(*MAML2*).[232–234]

DIFFERENTIAL DIAGNOSIS

Recognition of the constituent cellular populations of this distinctive neoplasm usually establishes the diagnosis.

PROGNOSIS

The clinical behavior of breast MEC correlates with tumor grade, which may be determined based on cellular atypia, mitotic count, and architecture (using the established criteria for breast cancer, as well as those used to grade salivary gland MECs).[228,229,232] Low- and intermediate-grade breast MECs generally have favorable prognoses, while high-grade MECs can present with nodal or distant metastases resulting in mortality.[228]

- Presence of mucous, intermediate (transitional/basaloid), and squamoid (epidermoid) cells
- Absence of true keratinization

Favorable outcome, despite triple-negative status and not necessarily treated similar to classic high-grade triple-negative breast cancers of NST.

POLYMORPHOUS CARCINOMA

CLINICAL FINDINGS AND EPIDEMIOLOGY

An exceedingly rare tumor of the breast,[235] the few reported cases range in age from 37 to 74.[236]

MACROSCOPIC FEATURES

Nodule(s) within breast parenchyma.

HISTOLOGY

Monomorphic, small, rounded tumor cells with a modest amount of eosinophilic cytoplasm form a central solid mass, surrounded by peripheral cribriform nests and slender strands. In contradistinction to adenoid cystic carcinoma, only 1 neoplastic cell type constitutes this tumor.

IMMUNOHISTOCHEMISTRY

Polymorphous adenocarcinoma has a triple-negative phenotype. Positivity for BCL2 has been reported, as well as focal CK7 positivity. Weak, partial membranous E-cadherin staining is present.

MOLECULAR TESTING

Not of current clinical relevance in the diagnosis of these tumors.

DIFFERENTIAL DIAGNOSIS

Invasive lobular carcinoma: Polymorphous adenocarcinoma is BCL2 positive and ER/PR negative, in contrast to invasive lobular carcinoma which is ER and PR positive.

Adenoid cystic carcinoma: Polymorphous adenocarcinoma consists of a single population of neoplastic cells. Adenoid cystic carcinoma is a biphasic tumor with a prominent stromal component.

PROGNOSIS

Out of the 3 reported cases, one patient had metastatic disease, resulting in death. Due to its rarity, there are insufficient data regarding the clinical behavior of this tumor; the designation "low grade" should therefore not be used.[236]

CLINICS CARE POINTS

- A monotonous population of neoplastic cells, forming a central, solid area surrounded by cribriform nests and thin strands, morphologically similar to polymorphous adenocarcinoma of the salivary gland
- BCL-2 positive; E-cadherin shows weak, partial staining
- Triple negative with limited data on outcomes

TALL CELL CARCINOMA WITH REVERSED POLARITY

CLINICAL FINDINGS AND EPIDEMIOLOGY

A rare subtype of invasive breast carcinoma,[237,238] tall cell carcinoma with reversed polarity (TCCRP) presents as a clinically palpable or radiologic mass. The mean age of patients is 64 years (range: 39–89 years),[239–241] with axillary nodal metastases reported in a few cases.[242–245]

MACROSCOPIC FEATURES

A relatively circumscribed, firm, grayish-white mass.

HISTOLOGY

TCCRPs comprise tall, columnar epithelial cells with eosinophilic cytoplasm, with distinctive placement of nuclei at the apical (as opposed to the basal) pole, often arranged as a "back to back" bilayer, forming solid nests that contain delicate fibrovascular cores, attesting to an underlying papillary architecture.[239,241–243] Occasional foamy histiocytes may be observed within the cores. Nuclear grade is low-to-intermediate; nuclear grooves and intranuclear cytoplasmic inclusions may be present.[246] The tumor nests are disposed haphazardly or in a "jigsaw" fashion within a densely collagenous stroma.

IMMUNOHISTOCHEMISTRY

Most TCCRPs are triple-negative in phenotype, with a low (<20%) Ki67 proliferative index; occasional weak, focal hormone receptor expression may be seen.[237,239,242,245] The tumor cells show focal-to-diffuse calretinin staining,[239] as well as variable immunoreactivity for GATA3, mammaglobin, and GCDFP-15. Expression of both low-molecular-weight keratins (CK7) and high-molecular keratins (CK5/6) can be observed. There is no TTF-1, thyroglobulin, synaptophysin, or chromogranin A staining in typical cases. An anti-*IDH2* R172 antibody shows promise for diagnostic immunohistochemical use.[239,247]

MOLECULAR TESTING

TCCRPs, unique among breast carcinomas, frequently harbor *IDH2* p.Arg172 hotspot mutations,[237,239,241,248,249] which have been described in cholangiocarcinoma, acute myeloid leukemia, chrondosarcoma, and glioma. In addition, more than half of TCCRPs have been desc-ribed to contain *PIK3CA* missense muta-tions.[239,241,248]

DIFFERENTIAL DIAGNOSIS

Solid-papillary carcinoma: Solid-papillary carcinoma comprises circumscribed, solid nodules of ovoid-to-spindled neoplastic cells harboring delicate, barely perceptible intratumoral fibrovascular cores. Neuroendocrine differentiation may be present. They are commonly ER and PR positive.

Metastatic thyroid carcinoma: A carcinoma of thyroid origin would be expected to express TTF-1 and thyroglobulin, which are absent in tall cell carcinoma with reversed polarity.

PROGNOSIS

Prognosis is generally favorable, with most documented cases being disease-free during follow-up.[239,245,248] Only a single case of bone metastasis has been reported thus far.[244]

CLINICS CARE POINTS

- Tall columnar neoplastic cells, with abundant eosinophilic cytoplasm and nuclei oriented toward the apical (rather than basal) poles, arranged in solid-papillary architectural pattern
- Characteristic *IDH2* p.Arg172 hotspot mutations
- Triple negative but favorable prognosis with limited treatment

DISCLOSURE

The authors have nothing to disclose.

REFERENCES

1. Bray F, Ferlay J, Soerjomataram I, et al. Global cancer statistics 2018: GLOBOCAN estimates of incidence and mortality worldwide for 36 cancers in 185 countries. CA Cancer J Clin 2018;68(6): 394–424.
2. WHO Classification of Tumours Editorial Board. WHO classification of tumours of the breast, Breast tumours, 2019, 5th edition, 2019, Lyon: International Agency for Research on Cancer; Available at: https://publications.iarc.fr/581.
3. Li CI, Uribe DJ, Daling JR. Clinical characteristics of different histologic types of breast cancer. Br J Cancer 2005;93(9):1046–52.
4. Sastre-Garau X, Jouve M, Asselain B, et al. Infiltrating lobular carcinoma of the breast: clinicopathologic analysis of 975 cases with reference to data on conservative therapy and metastatic patterns. Cancer 1996;77(1):113–20.
5. Winchester DJ, Chang HR, Graves TA, et al. A comparative analysis of lobular and ductal carcinoma of the breast: presentation, treatment, and outcomes. J Am Coll Surg 1998;186(4):416–22.
6. Wilson N, Ironside A, Diana A, et al. Lobular breast cancer: a review. Front Oncol 2021;10. https://doi.org/10.3389/fonc.2020.591399.
7. Rakha EA, Ellis IO. Lobular breast carcinoma and its variants. Semin Diagn Pathol 2010;27(1):49–61.
8. Arpino G, Bardou VJ, Clark GM, et al. Infiltrating lobular carcinoma of the breast: tumor characteristics and clinical outcome. Breast Cancer Res 2004; 6(3). https://doi.org/10.1186/bcr767.
9. Broët P, De La Rochefordière A, Scholl SM, et al. Contralateral breast cancer: annual incidence and risk parameters. J Clin Oncol 1995;13(7):1578–83.
10. Lesser ML, Rosen PP, Kinne DW. Multicentricity and bilaterality in invasive breast carcinoma. Surgery 1982;91(2):234–40.
11. DiCostanzo D, Rosen PP, Gareen I, et al. Prognosis in infiltrating lobular carcinoma. An analysis of "classical" and variant tumors. Am J Surg Pathol 1990;14(1):12–23.
12. Ilić IR, Petrović A, Živković VV, et al. Immunohistochemical features of multifocal and multicentric lobular breast carcinoma. Adv Med Sci 2017; 62(1):78–82.
13. Kanumuri P, Hayse B, Killelea BK, et al. Characteristics of Multifocal and Multicentric Breast Cancers. Ann Surg Oncol 2015;22(8):2475–82.
14. Butler RS, Venta LA, Wiley EL, et al. Sonographic evaluation of infiltrating lobular carcinoma. Am J Roentgenol 1999;172(2):325–30.
15. Selinko VL, Middleton LP, Dempsey PJ. Role of sonography in diagnosing and staging invasive lobular carcinoma. J Clin Ultrasound 2004;32(7): 323–32.
16. Albayrak ZK, Onay HK, Karatağ GY, et al. Invasive lobular carcinoma of the breast: mammographic and sonographic evaluation. Diagn Interv Radiol 2011;17(3):232–8.
17. Dietzel M, Baltzer PA, Vag T, et al. Magnetic resonance mammography of invasive lobular versus ductal carcinoma: Systematic comparison of 811 patients reveals high diagnostic accuracy irrespective of typing. J Comput Assist Tomogr 2010;34(4): 587–95.
18. Corso G, Intra M, Trentin C, et al. CDH1 germline mutations and hereditary lobular breast cancer. Fam Cancer 2016;15(2):215–9.
19. Foote FW, Stewart FW. A histologic classification of carcinoma of the breast. Surgery 1946;19(1): 74–99.
20. Esposito NN, Chivukula M, Dabbs DJ. The ductal phenotypic expression of the E-cadherin/catenin complex in tubulolobular carcinoma of the breast: an immunohistochemical and clinicopathologic study. Mod Pathol 2007;20(1):130–8.
21. Kuroda H, Tamaru JI, Takeuchi I, et al. Expression of E-cadherin, α-catenin, and β-catenin in tubulolobular carcinoma of the breast. Virchows Arch 2006;448(4):500–5.
22. Acs G, Lawton TJ, Rebbeck TR, et al. Differential expression of E-Cadherin in lobular and ductal neoplasms of the breast and its biologic and diagnostic implications. Am J Clin Pathol 2001;115(1): 85–98.
23. Silva L Da, Parry S, Reid L, et al. Aberrant expression of e-cadherin in lobular carcinomas of the breast. Am J Surg Pathol 2008;32(5):773–83.
24. El Sharouni MA, Postma EL, van Diest PJ. Correlation between E-cadherin and p120 expression in invasive ductal breast cancer with a lobular

component and MRI findings. Virchows Arch 2017;
471(6):707–12.

25. Dabbs DJ, Bhargava R, Chivukula M. Lobular
versus ductal breast neoplasms: The diagnostic
utility of P120 catenin. Am J Surg Pathol 2007;
31(3):427–37.

26. Sarrió D, Pérez-Mies B, Hardisson D, et al. Cytoplasmic localization of p120ctn and E-cadherin
loss characterize lobular breast carcinoma from
preinvasive to metastatic lesions. Oncogene
2004;23(19):3272–83.

27. Simpson PT, Reis-Filho JS, Lambros MBK, et al.
Molecular profiling pleomorphic lobular carcinomas of the breast: Evidence for a common molecular genetic pathway with classic lobular
carcinomas. J Pathol 2008;215(3):231–44.

28. Middleton LP, Palacios DM, Bryant BR, et al. Pleomorphic lobular carcinoma: Morphology, immunohistochemistry, and molecular analysis. Am J
Surg Pathol 2000;24(12):1650–6.

29. Christgen M, Steinemann D, Kühnle E, et al.
Lobular breast cancer: Clinical, molecular and
morphological characteristics. Pathol Res Pract
2016;212(7):583–97.

30. Moran MS, Yang Q, Haffty BG. The Yale University
Experience of Early-Stage Invasive Lobular Carci-
noma (ILC) and Invasive Ductal Carcinoma (IDC)
Treated with Breast Conservation Treatment
(BCT): analysis of clinical-pathologic features,
long-term outcomes, and molecular expression of
COX-2, Bcl-2, and p53 as a Function of Histology.
Breast J 2009;15(6):571–8.

31. Ferlicot S, Vincent-Salomon A, Médioni J, et al. Wide
metastatic spreading in infiltrating lobular carcinoma
of the breast. Eur J Cancer 2004;40(3):336–41.

32. Bane AL, Tjan S, Parkes RK, et al. Invasive lobular
carcinoma: to grade or not to grade. Mod Pathol
2005;18(5):621–8.

33. Mokbel K. Grading of infiltrating lobular carcinoma
[1]. Eur J Surg Oncol 2001;27(6):609.

34. Rakha EA, El-Sayed ME, Powe DG, et al. Invasive
lobular carcinoma of the breast: Response to hormonal therapy and outcomes. Eur J Cancer 2008;
44(1):73–83.

35. Pestalozzi BC, Zahrieh D, Mallon E, et al. Distinct
clinical and prognostic features of infiltrating
lobular carcinoma of the breast: combined results
of 15 International Breast Cancer Study Group clinical trials. J Clin Oncol 2008;26(18):3006–14.

36. Conforti F, Pala L, Pagan E, et al. Endocrine-
responsive lobular carcinoma of the breast: features associated with risk of late distant recurrence.
Breast Cancer Res 2019;21(1). https://doi.org/10.
1186/S13058-019-1234-9.

37. Weidner N, Semple JP. Pleomorphic variant of invasive lobular carcinoma of the breast. Hum Pathol
1992;23(10):1167–71.

38. Buchanan CL, Flynn LW, Murray MP, et al. Is pleomorphic lobular carcinoma really a distinct clinical
entity? J Surg Oncol 2008;98(5):314–7.

39. Bentz JS, Yassa N, Clayton F. Pleomorphic lobular
carcinoma of the breast: Clinicopathologic features
of 12 cases. Mod Pathol 1998;11(9):814–22.

40. Dixon JM, Renshaw L, Dixon J, et al. Invasive
lobular carcinoma: response to neoadjuvant letrozole therapy. Breast Cancer Res Treat 2011;
130(3):871–7.

41. Luveta J, Parks RM, Heery DM, et al. Invasive
Lobular Breast Cancer as a Distinct Disease: Implications for Therapeutic Strategy. Oncol Ther 2020;
8(1):1.

42. Sullivan PS, Apple SK. Should histologic type be
taken into account when considering neoadjuvant
chemotherapy in breast carcinoma? Breast J
2009;15(2):146–54.

43. Truin W, Vugts G, Roumen RMH, et al. Differences
in response and surgical management with neoadjuvant chemotherapy in invasive lobular versus
ductal breast cancer. Ann Surg Oncol 2015;23(1):
51–7.

44. Dillon MF, Hill ADK, Fleming FJ, et al. Identifying
patients at risk of compromised margins following
breast conservation for lobular carcinoma. Am J
Surg 2006;191(2):201–5.

45. Smitt MC, Horst K. Association of clinical and pathologic variables with lumpectomy surgical margin
status after preoperative diagnosis or excisional biopsy of invasive breast cancer. Ann Surg Oncol
2007;14(3):1040–4.

46. Mann RM, Loo CE, Wobbes T, et al. The impact of
preoperative breast MRI on the re-excision rate in
invasive lobular carcinoma of the breast. Breast
Cancer Res Treat 2010;119(2):415–22.

47. Lau B, Romero LM. Does preoperative magnetic resonance imaging beneficially alter surgical management of invasive lobular carcinoma? 2011;77(10):
1368–71.

48. Cormier WJ, Gaffey TA, Welch JM, et al. Linitis
plastica caused by metastatic lobular carcinoma
of the breast. Mayo Clin Proc 1980;55(12):
747–53. Available at: http://europepmc.org/article/
med/6261047. Accessed July 17, 2021.

49. Whitty LA, Crawford DL, Woodland JH, et al. Metastatic breast cancer presenting as linitis plastica of
the stomach. Gastric Cancer 2005;8(3):193–7.

50. Bitter MA, Fiorito D, Corkill ME, et al. Bone marrow
involvement by lobular carcinoma of the breast
cannot be identified reliably by routine histological
examination alone. Hum Pathol 1994;25(8):781–8.

51. Lyda MH, Tetef M, Carter NH, et al. Keratin immunohistochemistry detects clinically significant metastases in bone marrow biopsy specimens in
women with lobular breast carcinoma. Am J Surg
Pathol 2000;24(12):1593–9.

52. Groisman GM. Lobular carcinoma of the breast metastatic to the spleen and accessory spleen: report of a case. Case Rep Pathol 2016;2016:1–5.

53. Patel A, D'Alfonso T, Cheng E, et al. Sentinel lymph nodes in classic invasive lobular carcinoma of the breast: cytokeratin immunostain ensures detection, and precise determination of extent, of involvement. Am J Surg Pathol 2017;41(11):1499–505.

54. Anderson WF, Pfeiffer RM, Dores GM, et al. Comparison of age distribution patterns for different histopathologic types of breast carcinoma. Cancer Epidemiol Biomarkers Prev 2006;15(10):1899–905.

55. Rakha EA, Lee AHS, Evans AJ, et al. Tubular carcinoma of the breast: Further evidence to support its excellent prognosis. J Clin Oncol 2010;28(1): 99–104.

56. Carstens PHB, Gfeenberg RA, Francis D, et al. Tubular carcinoma of the breast. A long term follow-up. Histopathology 1985;9(3):271–80.

57. Poirier É, Desbiens C, Poirier B, et al. Characteristics and long-term survival of patients diagnosed with pure tubular carcinoma of the breast. J Surg Oncol 2018;117(6):1137–43.

58. Romano AM, Wages NA, Smolkin M, et al. Tubular carcinoma of the breast: Institutional and SEER database analysis supporting a unique classification. Breast Dis 2015;35(2):103–11.

59. Abdel-Fatah TMA, Powe DG, Hodi Z, et al. High frequency of coexistence of columnar cell lesions, lobular neoplasia, and low grade ductal carcinoma in situ with invasive tubular carcinoma and invasive lobular carcinoma. Am J Surg Pathol 2007;31(3): 417–26.

60. Aulmann S, Elsawaf Z, Penzel R, et al. Invasive tubular carcinoma of the breast frequently is clonally related to flat epithelial atypia and low-grade ductal carcinoma in situ. Am J Surg Pathol 2009; 33(11):1646–53.

61. Kunju LP, Ding Y, Kleer CG. Tubular carcinoma and grade 1 (well-differentiated) invasive ductal carcinoma: Comparison of flat epithelial atypia and other intra-epithelial lesions. Pathol Int 2008;58(10): 620–5.

62. Alvarado-Cabrero I, Valencia-Cedillo R, Estevez-Castro R. Preneoplasia of the Breast and Molecular Landscape. Arch Med Res 2020;51(8):845–50.

63. Fernández-Aguilar S, Simon P, Buxant F, et al. Tubular carcinoma of the breast and associated intra-epithelial lesions: A comparative study with invasive low-grade ductal carcinomas. Virchows Arch 2005;447(4):683–7.

64. Collins LC. precursor lesions of the low-grade breast neoplasia pathway. Surg Pathol Clin 2018; 11(1):177–97.

65. Wolff AC, Elizabeth Hale Hammond M, Allison KH, et al. Human epidermal growth factor receptor 2 testing in breast cancer: American society of clinical oncology/college of American pathologists clinical practice guideline focused update. J Clin Oncol 2018;36(20):2105–22.

66. Rosen PP, Saigo PE, Braun DW, et al. Predictors of recurrence in stage I (T1N0M0) breast carcinoma. Ann Surg 1981;193(1):15–25.

67. Li B, Chen M, Nori D, et al. Adjuvant radiation therapy and survival for pure tubular breast carcinoma - experience from the SEER database. Int J Radiat Oncol Biol Phys 2012;84(1):23–9.

68. Page DL, Dixon JM, Anderson TJ, et al. Invasive cribriform carcinoma of the breast. Histopathology 1983;7(4):525–36.

69. Venable JG, Schwartz AM, Silverberg SG. Infiltrating cribriform carcinoma of the breast: A distinctive clinicopathologic entity. Hum Pathol 1990;21(3):333–8.

70. Liu XY, Jiang YZ, Liu YR, et al. Clinicopathological characteristics and survival outcomes of invasive cribriform carcinoma of breast: A SEER population-based study. Medicine (Baltimore) 2015;94(31): e1309.

71. Zhang W, Zhang T, Lin Z, et al. Invasive cribriform carcinoma in a Chinese population: comparison with low-grade invasive ductal carcinoma-not otherwise specified. Int J Clin Exp Pathol 2013; 6(3):445. Available at: /pmc/articles/PMC3563205/. Accessed July 21, 2021.

72. Mo C-H, Ackbarkhan Z, Gu Y-Y, et al. Invasive cribriform carcinoma of the breast: a clinicopathological analysis of 12 cases with review of literature. Int J Clin Exp Pathol 2017;10(9):9917. Available at: /pmc/articles/PMC6965980/. Accessed July 21, 2021.

73. Zhang W, Lin Z, Zhang T, et al. A pure invasive cribriform carcinoma of the breast with bone metastasis if untreated for thirteen years: A case report and literature review. World J Surg Oncol 2012; 10. https://doi.org/10.1186/1477-7819-10-251.

74. Di Saverio S, Gutierrez J, Avisar E. A retrospective review with long term follow up of 11,400 cases of pure mucinous breast carcinoma. Breast Cancer Res Treat 2008;111(3):541–7.

75. Barkley CR, Ligibel JA, Wong JS, et al. Mucinous breast carcinoma: a large contemporary series. Am J Surg 2008;196(4):549–51.

76. Diab SG, Clark GM, Osborne CK, et al. Tumor characteristics and clinical outcome of tubular nad mucinous breast carcinomas. J Clin Oncol 1999; 17(5):1442–8.

77. Capella C, Eusebi V, Mann B, et al. Endocrine differentiation in mucoid carcinoma of the breast. Histopathology 1980;4(6):613–30. Available at: http://www.ncbi.nlm.nih.gov/pubmed/6254868. Accessed December 16, 2015.

78. Bal A, Joshi K, Sharma SC, et al. Prognostic significance of micropapillary pattern in pure mucinous

carcinoma of the breast. Int J Surg Pathol 2008; 16(3):251–6.

79. Liu F, Yang M, Li Z, et al. Invasive micropapillary mucinous carcinoma of the breast is associated with poor prognosis. Breast Cancer Res Treat 2015;151(2):443–51.

80. Ranade AC, Batra R, Sandhu G, et al. Clinicopathological evaluation of 100 cases of mucinous carcinoma of breast with emphasis on axillary staging and special reference to a micropapillary pattern. J Clin Pathol 2010;63(12):1043–7.

81. Barbashina V, Corben AD, Akram M, et al. Mucinous micropapillary carcinoma of the breast: an aggressive counterpart to conventional pure mucinous tumors. Hum Pathol 2013;44(8):1577–85.

82. Asano Y, Kashiwagi S, Nagamori M, et al. Pure mucinous breast carcinoma with micropapillary pattern (MUMPC): a case report. Case Rep Oncol 2019;12(2):554–9.

83. Collins K, Ricci A. Micropapillary variant of mucinous breast carcinoma: a distinct subtype. Breast J 2018;24(3):339–42.

84. Zhao X, Yang X, Gao R, et al. HER2-positive pure mucinous breast carcinoma: A case report and literature review. Medicine (Baltimore) 2020; 99(33):e20996.

85. Ginter PS, Tang X, Shin SJ. A review of mucinous lesions of the breast. Breast J 2020;26(6):1168–78.

86. Louwman MWJ, Vriezen M, Van Beek MWPM, et al. Uncommon breast tumors in perspective: Incidence, treatment and survival in the Netherlands. Int J Cancer 2007;121(1):127–35.

87. Marrazzo E, Frusone F, Milana F, et al. Mucinous breast cancer: a narrative review of the literature and a retrospective tertiary single-centre analysis. Breast 2020;49:87–92.

88. Toikkanen S, Kujari H. Pure and mixed mucinous carcinomas of the breast: a clinicopathologic analysis of 61 cases with long-term follow-up. Hum Pathol 1989;20(8):758–64.

89. Rasmussen BB, Rose C, Christensen I. Prognostic factors in primary mucinous breast carcinoma. Am J Clin Pathol 1987;87(2):155–60.

90. Komaki K, Sakamoto G, Sugano H, et al. Mucinous carcinoma of the breast in Japan. A prognostic analysis based on morphologic features. Cancer 1988;61(5):989–96.

91. Koenig C, Tavassoli FA. Mucinous cystadenocarcinoma of the breast. Am J Surg Pathol 1998;22(6): 698–703.

92. Nayak A, Bleiweiss IJ, Dumoff K, et al. Mucinous cystadenocarcinoma of the breast: report of 2 cases including one with long-term local recurrence. Int J Surg Pathol 2018;26(8):749–57.

93. Koufopoulos N, Goudeli C, Syrios J, et al. Mucinous cystadenocarcinoma of the breast: The challenge of diagnosing a rare entity. Rare Tumors 2017; 9(3):98–100.

94. Lee SH, Chaung CR. Mucinous metaplasia of breast carcinoma with macrocystic transformation resembling ovarian mucinous cystadenocarcinoma in a case of synchronous bilateral infiltrating ductal carcinoma. Pathol Int 2008;58(9):601–5.

95. Honma N, Sakamoto G, Ikenaga M, et al. Mucinous cystadenocarcinoma of the breast: a case report and review of the literature. Arch Pathol Lab Med 2003;127(8):1031–3.

96. Petersson F, Pang B, Thamboo TP, et al. Mucinous cystadenocarcinoma of the breast with amplification of the HER2-gene confirmed by FISH: the first case reported. Hum Pathol 2010;41(6):910–3.

97. Chen WY, Chen CS, Chen HC, et al. Mucinous cystadenocarcinoma of the breast coexisting with infiltrating ductal carcinoma. Pathol Int 2004;54(10): 781–6.

98. Gulwani H, Bhalla S. Mucinous cystadenocarcinoma: a rare primary malignant tumor of the breast. Indian J Pathol Microbiol 2010;53(1):200–2.

99. Kucukzeybek BB, Yigit S, Sari AA, et al. Primary mucinous cystadenocarcinoma of the breast with amplification of the HER2 gene confirmed by FISH - case report and review of the literature. Pol J Pathol 2014;65(1):70–3.

100. Kim SE, Park JH, Hong S, et al. Primary mucinous cystadenocarcinoma of the breast: cytologic finding and expression of MUC5 are different from mucinous carcinoma. Korean J Pathol 2012; 46(6):611–6.

101. Chen H, Wu K, Wang M, et al. Invasive micropapillary carcinoma of the breast has a better long-term survival than invasive ductal carcinoma of the breast in spite of its aggressive clinical presentations: a comparison based on large population database and case–control analysis. Cancer Med 2017;6(12):2775–86.

102. Paterakos M, Watkin WG, Edgerton SM, et al. Invasive micropapillary carcinoma of the breast: a prognostic study. Hum Pathol 1999;30(12): 1459–63.

103. Guo X, Chen L, Lang R, et al. Invasive micropapillary carcinoma of the breast : association of pathologic features with lymph node metastasis. Am J Clin Pathol 2006;126(5):740–6.

104. Zekioglu O, Erhan Y, Çiris M, et al. Invasive micropapillary carcinoma of the breast: high incidence of lymph node metastasis with extranodal extension and its immunohistochemical profile compared with invasive ductal carcinoma. Histopathology 2004;44(1):18–23.

105. Walsh MM, Bleiweiss IJ. Invasive micropapillary carcinoma of the breast: Eighty cases of an under-recognized entity. Hum Pathol 2001;32(6):583–9.

106. Adrada B, Arribas E, Gilcrease M, et al. Invasive micropapillary carcinoma of the breast: mammographic, sonographic, and MRI features. Am J Roentgenol 2009;193(1). https://doi.org/10.2214/AJR.08.1537.

107. Erhan Y, Erhan Y, Zekioğlu O. Pure invasive micropapillary carcinoma of the male breast: report of a rare case. Can J Surg 2005;48(2):156–7.

108. Luna-Moré S, Casquero S, Pérez-Mellado A, et al. Importance of estrogen receptors for the behavior of invasive micropapillary carcinoma of the breast. Review of 68 cases with follow-up of 45. Pathol Res Pract 2000;196(1):35–9.

109. Yun SU, Choi BB, Shu KS, et al. Imaging findings of invasive micropapillary carcinoma of the breast. J Breast Cancer 2012;15(1):57–64.

110. Alsharif S, Daghistani R, Kamberoğlu EA, et al. Mammographic, sonographic and MR imaging features of invasive micropapillary breast cancer. Eur J Radiol 2014;83(8):1375–80.

111. Pettinato G, Manivel CJ, Panico L, et al. Invasive micropapillary carcinoma of the breast : clinicopathologic study of 62 cases of a poorly recognized variant with highly aggressive behavior. Am J Clin Pathol 2004;121(6):857–66.

112. Yang YL, Liu BB, Zhang X, et al. Invasive micropapillary carcinoma of the breast: an update. In: Borczuk AC editor, editor. Archives of pathology and laboratory medicineVol 140, 8th. College of American Pathologists; 2016. p. 799–805.

113. Yu J II, Choi DH, Park W, et al. Differences in prognostic factors and patterns of failure between invasive micropapillary carcinoma and invasive ductal carcinoma of the breast: Matched case-control study. Breast 2010;19(3):231–7.

114. Yu JI, Choi DH, Huh SJ, et al. Differences in prognostic factors and failure patterns between invasive micropapillary carcinoma and carcinoma with micropapillary component versus invasive ductal carcinoma of the Breast: Retrospective Multicenter Case-Control Study (KROG 13-06). Clin Breast Cancer 2015;15(5):353–61.e2.

115. Marchiò C, Iravani M, Natrajan R, et al. Genomic and immunophenotypical characterization of pure micropapillary carcinomas of the breast. J Pathol 2008;215(4):398–410.

116. Marchiò C, Pietribiasi F, Castiglione R, et al. "Giants in a microcosm": multinucleated giant cells populating an invasive micropapillary carcinoma of the breast. Int J Surg Pathol 2015;23(8):654–5.

117. Marchiò C, Iravani M, Natrajan R, et al. Mixed micropapillary-ductal carcinomas of the breast: a genomic and immunohistochemical analysis of morphologically distinct components. J Pathol 2009;218(3):301–15.

118. Vingiani A, Maisonneuve P, Dell'Orto P, et al. The clinical relevance of micropapillary carcinoma of the breast: a case-control study. Histopathology 2013;63(2):217–24.

119. Tang SL, Yang JQ, Du ZG, et al. Clinicopathologic study of invasive micropapillary carcinoma of the breast. Oncotarget 2017;8(26):42455–65.

120. Yamaguchi R, Tanaka M, Kondo K, et al. Characteristic morphology of invasive micropapillary carcinoma of the breast: an immunohistochemical analysis. Jpn J Clin Oncol 2010;40(8):781–7.

121. Stewart RL, Caron JE, Gulbahce EH, et al. HER2 immunohistochemical and fluorescence in situ hybridization discordances in invasive breast carcinoma with micropapillary features. Mod Pathol 2017;30(11):1561–6.

122. Troxell ML. Reversed MUC1/EMA polarity in both mucinous and micropapillary breast carcinoma. Hum Pathol 2014;45(2):432–4.

123. Lepe M, Kalife ET, Ou J, et al. 'Inside-out' p120 immunostaining pattern in invasive micropapillary carcinoma of the breast; additional unequivocal evidence of reversed polarity. Histopathology 2017;70(5):832–4.

124. Wu Y, Zhang N, Yang Q. The prognosis of invasive micropapillary carcinoma compared with invasive ductal carcinoma in the breast: a meta-analysis. BMC Cancer 2017;17(1). https://doi.org/10.1186/s12885-017-3855-7.

125. Mills AM, Gottlieb CE, Wendroth SM, et al. Pure apocrine carcinomas represent a clinicopathologically distinct androgen receptor-positive subset of triple-negative breast cancers. In: Mills SE editor, editor. American journal of surgical pathologyVol 40. Lippincott Williams and Wilkins; 2016. p. 1109–16.

126. Dellapasqua S, Maisonneuve P, Viale G, et al. Immunohistochemically defined subtypes and outcome of apocrine breast cancer. Clin Breast Cancer 2013;13(2):95–102.

127. Imamovic D, Bilalovic N, Skenderi F, et al. A clinicopathologic study of invasive apocrine carcinoma of the breast: A single-center experience. Breast J 2018;24(6):1105–8.

128. Mills MN, Yang GQ, Oliver DE, et al. Histologic heterogeneity of triple negative breast cancer: A National Cancer Centre Database analysis. Eur J Cancer 2018;98:48–58.

129. Page DL. Apocrine carcinomas of the breast. Breast 2005;14(1):1–2.

130. D'Arcy C, Quinn CM. Apocrine lesions of the breast: part 2 of a two-part review. Invasive apocrine carcinoma, the molecular apocrine signature and utility of immunohistochemistry in the diagnosis of apocrine lesions of the breast. J Clin Pathol 2019;72(1):7–11.

131. Eusebi V, Foschini MP, Bussolati G, et al. Myoblastomatoid (histiocytoid) carcinoma of the breast: a type of apocrine carcinoma. Am J Surg Pathol 1995;19(5):553–62.

132. Vranic S, Schmitt F, Sapino A, et al. Apocrine carcinoma of the breast: A comprehensive review. Histol Histopathol 2013;28(11):1393–409.

133. Vranic S, Tawfik O, Palazzo J, et al. EGFR and HER-2/neu expression in invasive apocrine carcinoma of the breast. Mod Pathol 2010;23(5):644–53.

134. Gatalica Z. Immunohistochemical analysis of apocrine breast lesions. Pathol Res Pract 1997; 193(11–12):753–8.

135. Pagani A, Sapino A, Bergnolo P, et al. PIP/GCDFP-15 gene expression and apocrine differentiation in carcinomas of the breast. Virchows Arch 1994; 425(5):459–65.

136. Daemen A, Manning G. HER2 is not a cancer subtype but rather a pan-cancer event and is highly enriched in AR-driven breast tumors. Breast Cancer Res 2018;20(1):8.

137. De Mattos Lima Lin F, Pincerato KM, Bacchi CE, et al. Coordinated expression of oestrogen and androgen receptors in HER2-positive breast carcinomas: Impact on proliferative activity. J Clin Pathol 2012;65(1):64–8.

138. Alvarenga CA, Paravidino PI, Alvarenga M, et al. Reappraisal of immunohistochemical profiling of special histological types of breast carcinomas: a study of 121 cases of eight different subtypes. J Clin Pathol 2012;65(12):1066–71.

139. Fernandez-Flores A. Immunohistochemical and morphologic evaluation of primary cutaneous apocrine carcinomas and cutaneous metastases from ductal breast carcinoma. Rom J Morphol Embryol 2012;53(4):879–92.

140. Fernandez-Flores A. Cutaneous metastases from breast carcinoma: Calretinin expression and estrogen, progesterone and Her2/neu status of the metastases, compared to primary cutaneous apocrine tumors. Rom J Morphol Embryol 2013;54(3 Suppl):695–9.

141. Celis JE, Gromova I, Gromov P, et al. Molecular pathology of breast apocrine carcinomas: A protein expression signature specific for benign apocrine metaplasia. FEBS Lett 2006;580(12):2935–44.

142. Zhang N, Zhang H, Chen T, et al. Dose invasive apocrine adenocarcinoma has worse prognosis than invasive ductal carcinoma of breast: Evidence from SEER database. Oncotarget 2017;8(15): 24579–92.

143. Zhao S, Ma D, Xiao Y, et al. Clinicopathologic features and prognoses of different histologic types of triple-negative breast cancer: A large population-based analysis. Eur J Surg Oncol 2018;44(4):420–8.

144. Liao HY, Zhang WW, Sun JY, et al. The clinicopathological features and survival outcomes of different histological subtypes in triple-negative breast cancer. J Cancer 2018;9(2):296–303.

145. Meattini I, Pezzulla D, Saieva C, et al. Triple negative apocrine carcinomas as a distinct subtype of triple negative breast cancer: a case-control study. Clin Breast Cancer 2018;18(5):e773–80.

146. Montagna E, Maisonneuve P, Rotmensz N, et al. Heterogeneity of triple-negative breast cancer: Histologic subtyping to inform the outcome. Clin Breast Cancer 2013;13(1):31–9.

147. Dreyer G, Vandorpe T, Smeets A, et al. Triple negative breast cancer: Clinical characteristics in the different histological subtypes. Breast 2013;22(5): 761–6.

148. Schroeder MC, Rastogi P, Geyer CE, et al. Early and locally advanced metaplastic breast cancer: presentation and survival by receptor status in surveillance, epidemiology, and end results (SEER) 2010–2014. Oncologist 2018;23(4):481–8.

149. Nelson RA, Guye ML, Luu T, et al. Survival Outcomes of Metaplastic Breast Cancer Patients: Results from a US Population-based Analysis. Ann Surg Oncol 2015;22(1):24–31.

150. Paul Wright G, Davis AT, Koehler TJ, et al. Hormone receptor status does not affect prognosis in metaplastic breast cancer: a population-based analysis with comparison to infiltrating ductal and lobular carcinomas. Ann Surg Oncol 2014;21(11):3497–503.

151. Van Hoeven KH, Drudis T, Cranor ML, et al. Low-grade adenosquamous carcinoma of the breast: a clinicopathologic study of 32 cases with ultrastructural analysis. Am J Surg Pathol 1993;17(3):248–58.

152. Gobbi H, Simpson JF, Borowsky A, et al. Metaplastic breast tumors with a dominant fibromatosis-like phenotype have a high risk of local recurrence. Cancer 1999;85(10):2170–82.

153. Gobbi H, Simpson JF, Jensen RA, et al. Metaplastic spindle cell breast tumors arising within papillomas, complex sclerosing lesions, and nipple adenomas. Mod Pathol 2003;16(9):893–901.

154. Sneige N, Yaziji H, Mandavilli SR, et al. Low-grade (fibromatosis-like) spindle cell carcinoma of the breast. Am J Surg Pathol 2001;25(8):1009–16.

155. Davis WG, Hennessy B, Babiera G, et al. Metaplastic sarcomatoid carcinoma of the breast with absent or minimal overt invasive carcinomatous component: a misnomer. Am J Surg Pathol 2005; 29(11):1456–63.

156. Carter MR, Hornick JL, Lester S, et al. Spindle cell (sarcomatoid) carcinoma of the breast: a clinicopathologic and immunohistochemical analysis of 29 cases. Am J Surg Pathol 2006;30(3):300–9.

157. Gersell DJ, Katzenstein ALA. Spindle cell carcinoma of the breast. A clinocopathologic and ultrastructural study. Hum Pathol 1981;12(6):550–61.

158. Wargotz ES, Does PH, Norris HJ. Metaplastic carcinomas of the breast. II. Spindle cell carcinoma. Hum Pathol 1989;20(8):732–40.

159. Jones EL. Primary squamous-cell carcinoma of breast with pseudosarcomatous stroma. J Pathol 1969;97(2):383–5.

160. Wargotz ES, Norris HJ. Metaplastic carcinomas of the breast. IV. Squamous cell carcinoma of ductal origin. Cancer 1990;65(2):272–6.

161. Wargotz ES, Norris HJ. Metaplastic carcinomas of the breast. I. Matrix-producing carcinoma. Hum Pathol 1989;20(7):628–35.

162. Wargotz ES, Norris HJ. Metaplastic carcinomas of the breast. III. Carcinosarcoma. Cancer 1989; 64(7):1490–9.

163. Oberman HA. Metaplastic carcinoma of the breast. A clinicopathologic study of 29 patients. Am J Surg Pathol 1987;11(12):918–29.

164. Downs-Kelly E, Nayeemuddin KM, Albarracin C, et al. Matrix-producing carcinoma of the breast: an aggressive subtype of metaplastic carcinoma. Am J Surg Pathol 2009;33(4):534–41.

165. Rakha EA, Coimbra NDM, Hodi Z, et al. Immuno-profile of metaplastic carcinomas of the breast. Histopathology 2017;70(6):975–85.

166. Reis-Filho JS, Milanezi F, Steele D, et al. Meta-plastic breast carcinomas are basal-like tumours. Histopathology 2006;49(1):10–21.

167. Lacroix-Triki M, Geyer FC, Lambros MB, et al. β-Catenin/Wnt signalling pathway in fibromatosis, metaplastic carcinomas and phyllodes tumours of the breast. Mod Pathol 2010;23(11):1438–48.

168. Lee AHS. Recent developments in the histological diagnosis of spindle cell carcinoma, fibromatosis and phyllodes tumour of the breast. Histopathology 2008;52(1):45–57.

169. Erickson-Johnson MR, Chou MM, Evers BR, et al. Nodular fasciitis: a novel model of transient neoplasia induced by MYH9-USP6 gene fusion. Lab Invest 2011;91(10):1427–33.

170. Rakha EA, Badve S, Eusebi V, et al. Breast lesions of uncertain malignant nature and limited metastatic potential: Proposals to improve their recognition and clinical management. Histopathology 2016; 68(1):45–56.

171. Rakha EA, Tan PH, Varga Z, et al. Prognostic factors in metaplastic carcinoma of the breast: A multi-institutional study. Br J Cancer 2015;112(2): 283–9.

172. Yamaguchi R, Horii R, Maeda I, et al. Clinicopathologic study of 53 metaplastic breast carcinomas: their elements and prognostic implications. Hum Pathol 2010;41(5):679–85.

173. McCart Reed AE, Kalaw E, Nones K, et al. Phenotypic and molecular dissection of metaplastic breast cancer and the prognostic implications. J Pathol 2019;247(2):214–27.

174. Foschini MP, Morandi L, Asioli S, et al. The morphological spectrum of salivary gland type tumours of the breast. Pathology 2017;49(2):215–27.

175. Conlon N, Adri N, Orben AD, et al. Acinic cell carcinoma of breast: Morphologic and

176. Coyne JD, Dervan PA. Primary acinic cell carcinoma of the breast. J Clin Pathol 2002;55(7):545–7.

177. Geyer FC, Berman SH, Marchiò C, et al. Genetic analysis of microglandular adenosis and acinic cell carcinomas of the breast provides evidence for the existence of a low-grade triple-negative breast neoplasia family. Mod Pathol 2017;30(1): 69–84.

178. Guerini-Rocco E, Piscuoglio S, Ng CKY, et al. Microglandular adenosis associated with triple-negative breast cancer is a neoplastic lesion of triple-negative phenotype harbouring TP53 somatic mutations. J Pathol 2016;238(5):677–88.

179. Zhao Y, Li W, Lang R, et al. Primary acinic cell carcinoma of the breast: a case report and review of the literature. Int J Surg Pathol 2014;22(2):177–81.

180. Bhutani N, Kajal P, Singla S. Adenoid cystic carcinoma of the breast: experience at a tertiary care centre of Northern India. Int J Surg Case Rep 2018;51:204–9.

181. Boujelbene N, Khabir A, Boujelbene N, et al. Clinical review - breast adenoid cystic carcinoma. Breast 2012;21(2):124–7.

182. Pang W, Wang Z, Jin X, et al. Adenoid cystic carcinoma of the breast in a male: a case report. Med (United States). 2019;98(32). https://doi.org/10.1097/MD.0000000000016760.

183. Tang P, Yang S, Zhong X, et al. Breast adenoid cystic carcinoma in a 19-year-old man: A case report and review of the literature. World J Surg Oncol 2015;13(1). https://doi.org/10.1186/s12957-015-0442-8.

184. Yoo SJ, Lee DS, Oh HS, et al. Male breast adenoid cystic carcinoma. Case Rep Oncol 2013;6(3): 514–9.

185. Liu J, Jia W, Zeng Y, et al. Adolescent male adenoid cystic breast carcinoma. Am Surg 2012;78(5). https://doi.org/10.1177/000313481207800519.

186. Rosen PP. Adenoid cystic carcinoma of the breast. A morphologically heterogeneous neoplasm. Pathol Annu 1989;24(Pt 2):237–54.

187. Cavaxzo FJ, Taylor HB. Adenoid cystic carcinoma of the breast. An analysis of 21 cases. Cancer 1969;24(4):740–5.

188. Lamovec J, Us-Krašovec M, Zidar A, et al. Adenoid cystic carcinoma of the breast: a histologic, cytologic, and immunohistochemical study. Semin Diagn Pathol 1989;6(2):153–64.

189. Tavassoli FA, Norris HJ. Mammary adenoid cystic carcinoma with sebaceous differentiation. A morphologic study of the cell types. Arch Pathol Lab Med 1986;110(11):1045–53.

190. Shin SJ, Rosen PP. Solid variant of mammary adenoid cystic carcinoma with basaloid features:

a study of nine cases. Am J Surg Pathol 2002; 26(4):413–20.

191. Seethala RR, Hunt JL, Baloch ZW, et al. Adenoid cystic carcinoma with high-grade transformation: a report of 11 cases and a review of the literature. Am J Surg Pathol 2007;31(11):1683–94.

192. Righi A, Lenzi M, Morandi L, et al. Adenoid cystic carcinoma of the breast associated with invasive duct carcinoma: A case report. Int J Surg Pathol 2011;19(2):230–4.

193. Cabibi D, Cipolla C, Florena AM, et al. Solid variant of mammary "adenoid cystic carcinoma with basaloid features" merging with "small cell carcinoma. Pathol Res Pract 2005;201(10):705–11.

194. Yang Y, Wang Y, He J, et al. Malignant adenomyoepithelioma combined with adenoid cystic carcinoma of the breast: a case report and literature review. Diagn Pathol 2014;9(1). https://doi.org/10.1186/1746-1596-9-148.

195. Ghabach B, Anderson WF, Curtis RE, et al. Adenoid cystic carcinoma of the breast in the United States (1977 to 2006): a population-based cohort study. Breast Cancer Res 2010;12(4). https://doi.org/10.1186/bcr2613.

196. Arpino G, Clark GM, Mohsin S, et al. Adenoid cystic carcinoma of the breast: Molecular markers, treatment, and clinical outcome. Cancer 2002; 94(8):2119–27.

197. Nakai T, Ichihara S, Kada A, et al. The unique luminal staining pattern of cytokeratin 5/6 in adenoid cystic carcinoma of the breast may aid in differentiating it from its mimickers. Virchows Arch 2016;469(2):213–22.

198. Mastropasqua MG, Maiorano E, Pruneri G, et al. Immunoreactivity for c-kit and p63 as an adjunct in the diagnosis of adenoid cystic carcinoma of the breast. Mod Pathol 2005;18(10):1277–82.

199. Yang C, Zhang L, Sanati S. SOX10 is a sensitive marker for breast and salivary gland adenoid cystic carcinoma: immunohistochemical characterization of adenoid cystic carcinomas. Breast Cancer (Auckl) 2019;13. https://doi.org/10.1177/1178223419842185.

200. Cimino-Mathews A. Novel uses of immunohistochemistry in breast pathology: interpretation and pitfalls. Mod Pathol 2021;34(Suppl 1):62–77.

201. Poling JS, Yonescu R, Subhawong AP, et al. MYB Labeling by immunohistochemistry is more sensitive and specific for breast adenoid cystic carcinoma than MYB labeling by FISH. Am J Surg Pathol 2017;41(7):973–9.

202. Kim J, Geyer FC, Martelotto LG, et al. MYBL1 rearrangements and MYB amplification in breast adenoid cystic carcinomas lacking the MYB–NFIB fusion gene. J Pathol 2018;244(2):143–50.

203. D'Alfonso TM, Mosquera JM, Macdonald TY, et al. MYB-NFIB gene fusion in adenoid cystic carcinoma of the breast with special focus paid to the solid variant with basaloid features. Hum Pathol 2014;45(11):2270–80.

204. Wetterskog D, Lopez-Garcia MA, Lambros MB, et al. Adenoid cystic carcinomas constitute a genomically distinct subgroup of triple-negative and basal-like breast cancers. J Pathol 2012;226(1): 84–96.

205. Webb DV, Mentrikoski MJ, Verduin L, et al. Analysis of MYB expression and MYB-NFIB gene fusions in adenoid cystic carcinoma and other salivary neoplasms. Mod Pathol 2011;24(9): 1169–76.

206. Treitl D, Radkani P, Rizer M, et al. Adenoid cystic carcinoma of the breast, 20 years of experience in a single center with review of literature. Breast Cancer 2018;25(1):28–33.

207. Foschini MP, Rizzo A, De Leo A, et al. Solid Variant of Adenoid Cystic Carcinoma of the Breast: A Case Series with Proposal of a New Grading System. Int J Surg Pathol 2016;24(2):97–102.

208. Horowitz DP, Sharma CS, Connolly E, et al. Secretory carcinoma of the breast: Results from the survival, epidemiology and end results database. Breast 2012;21(3):350–3.

209. Jacob JD, Hodge C, Franko J, et al. Rare breast cancer: 246 invasive secretory carcinomas from the National Cancer Data Base. J Surg Oncol 2016;113(7):721–5.

210. Botta G, Fessia L, Ghiringhello B. Juvenile milk protein secreting carcinoma. Virchows Arch A Pathol Anat Histol 1982;395(2):145–52.

211. Arce C, Cortes-Padilla D, Huntsman DG, et al. Secretory carcinoma of the breast containing the ETV6-NTRK3 fusion gene in a male: case report and review of the literature. World J Surg Oncol 2005;3:35.

212. Li D, Xiao X, Yang W, et al. Secretory breast carcinoma: a clinicopathological and immunophenotypic study of 15 cases with a review of the literature. Mod Pathol 2012;25(4):567–75.

213. Tavassoli FA, Norris HJ. Secretory carcinoma of the breast. Cancer 1980;45(9):2404–13.

214. Del Castillo M, Chibon F, Arnould L, et al. Secretory breast carcinoma : A histopathologic and genomic spectrum characterized by a joint specific ETV6-NTRK3 gene fusion. Am J Surg Pathol 2015; 39(11):1458–67.

215. Laé M, Fréneaux P, Sastre-Garau X, et al. Secretory breast carcinomas with ETV6-NTRK3 fusion gene belong to the basal-like carcinoma spectrum. Mod Pathol 2009;22(2):291–8.

216. Krings G, Joseph NM, Bean GR, et al. Genomic profiling of breast secretory carcinomas reveals distinct genetics from other breast cancers and similarity to mammary analog secretory carcinomas. Mod Pathol 2017;30(8):1086–99.

217. Diallo R, Schaefer KL, Bankfalvi A, et al. Secretory carcinoma of the breast: a distinct variant of invasive ductal carcinoma assessed by comparative genomic hybridization and immunohistochemistry. Hum Pathol 2003;34(12):1299–305.

218. Tognon C, Knezevich SR, Huntsman D, et al. Expression of the ETV6-NTRK3 gene fusion as a primary event in human secretory breast carcinoma. Cancer Cell 2002;2(5):367–76.

219. Solomon JP, Hechtman JF. Detection of NTRK fusions: merits and limitations of current diagnostic platforms. Cancer Res 2019;79(13):3163–8.

220. Hechtman JF, Benayed R, Hyman DM, et al. Pan-Trk immunohistochemistry is an efficient and reliable screen for the detection of NTRK fusions. Am J Surg Pathol 2017;41(11):1547–51.

221. Gatalica Z, Xiu J, Swensen J, et al. Molecular characterization of cancers with NTRK gene fusions. Mod Pathol 2019;32(1):147–53.

222. Cocco E, Scaltriti M, Drilon A. NTRK fusion-positive cancers and TRK inhibitor therapy. Nat Rev Clin Oncol 2018;15(12):731–47.

223. Drilon A, Laetsch TW, Kummar S, et al. Efficacy of larotrectinib in TRK fusion–positive cancers in adults and children. N Engl J Med 2018;378(8):731–9.

224. Kheder ES, Hong DS. Emerging targeted therapy for tumors with NTRK fusion proteins. Clin Cancer Res 2018;24(23):5807–14.

225. Shukla N, Roberts SS, Baki MO, et al. Successful targeted therapy of refractory pediatric ETV6-NTRK3 fusion-positive secretory breast carcinoma. JCO Precis Oncol 2017;1:1–8.

226. Hoda RS, Brogi E, Pareja F, et al. Secretory carcinoma of the breast: clinicopathologic profile of 14 cases emphasising distant metastatic potential. Histopathology 2019;75(2):213–24.

227. Krausz T, Jenkins D, Grontoft O, et al. Secretory carcinoma of the breast in adults: emphasis on late recurrence and metastasis. Histopathology 1989;14(1):25–36.

228. Basbug M, Akbulut S, Arikanoglu Z, et al. Mucoepidermoid carcinoma in a breast affected by burn scars: comprehensive literature review and case report. Breast Care 2011;6(4):293–7.

229. Di Tommaso L, Foschini MP, Ragazzini T, et al. Mucoepidermoid carcinoma of the breast. Virchows Arch 2004;444(1):13–9.

230. Lüchtrath H, Moll R. Mucoepidermoid mammary carcinoma - Immunohistochemical and biochemical analyses of intermediate filaments. Virchows Arch A Pathol Anat Histopathol 1989;416(2):105–13.

231. Rached Palermo MH, Pinto MB, Zanetti JS, et al. Primary mucoepidermoid carcinoma of the breast: a case report with immunohistochemical analysis and comparison with salivary gland mucoepidermoid carcinomas. Polish J Pathol 2013;64(3):210–5.

232. Bean GR, Krings G, Otis CN, et al. CRTC1–MAML2 fusion in mucoepidermoid carcinoma of the breast. Histopathology 2019;74(3):463–73.

233. Camelo-Piragua SI, Habib C, Kanumuri P, et al. Mucoepidermoid carcinoma of the breast shares cytogenetic abnormality with mucoepidermoid carcinoma of the salivary gland: a case report with molecular analysis and review of the literature. Hum Pathol 2009;40(6):887–92.

234. Yan M, Gilmore H, Harbhajanka A. Mucoepidermoid carcinoma of the breast with MAML2 rearrangement: a case report and literature review. Int J Surg Pathol 2020;28(7):787–92.

235. Trihia HJ, Valavanis C, Novkovic N, et al. Polymorphous adenocarcinoma of the breast—an exceptionally rare entity: clinicopathological description of a case and brief review. Breast J 2020;26(2):261–4.

236. Asioli S, Marucci G, Ficarra G, et al. Polymorphous adenocarcinoma of the breast. Report of three cases. Virchows Arch 2006;448(1):29–34.

237. Chiang S, Weigelt B, Wen HC, et al. IDH2 mutations define a unique subtype of breast cancer with altered nuclear polarity. Cancer Res 2016;76(24):7118–29.

238. Shea EKH, Koh VCY, Tan PH. Invasive breast cancer: Current perspectives and emerging views. Pathol Int 2020;70(5):242–52.

239. Alsadoun N, MacGrogan G, Truntzer C, et al. Solid papillary carcinoma with reverse polarity of the breast harbors specific morphologic, immunohistochemical and molecular profile in comparison with other benign or malignant papillary lesions of the breast: a comparative study of 9 additional cases. Mod Pathol 2018;31(9):1367–80.

240. Lozada JR, Basili T, Pareja F, et al. Solid papillary breast carcinomas resembling the tall cell variant of papillary thyroid neoplasms (solid papillary carcinomas with reverse polarity) harbour recurrent mutations affecting IDH2 and PIK3CA: a validation cohort. Histopathology 2018;73(2):339–44.

241. Zhong E, Scognamiglio T, D'Alfonso T, et al. Breast tumor resembling the tall cell variant of papillary thyroid carcinoma: molecular characterization by next-generation sequencing and histopathological comparison with tall cell papillary carcinoma of thyroid. Int J Surg Pathol 2019;27(2):134–41.

242. Toss MS, Billingham K, Egbuniwe IU, et al. Breast tumours resembling the tall cell variant of thyroid papillary carcinoma: are they part of the papillary carcinoma spectrum or a distinct entity? Pathobiology 2019;86(2–3):83–91.

243. Foschini MP, Asioli S, Foreid S, et al. Solid papillary breast carcinomas resembling the tall cell variant

of papillary thyroid neoplasms. Am J Surg Pathol 2017;41(7):887–95.

244. Cameselle-Teijeiro J, Abdulkader I, Barreiro-Morandeira F, et al. Breast tumor resembling the tall cell variant of papillary thyroid carcinoma: a case report. Int J Surg Pathol 2006;14(1):79–84.

245. Tosi AL, Ragazzi M, Asioli S, et al. Breast tumor resembling the tall cell variant of papillary thyroid carcinoma: report of 4 cases with evidence of malignant potential. Int J Surg Pathol 2007;15(1):14–9.

246. Eusebi V, Damiani S, Ellis IO, et al. Breast tumor resembling the tall cell variant of papillary thyroid carcinoma: report of 5 cases. Am J Surg Pathol 2003;27(8):1114–8.

247. Pareja F, da Silva EM, Frosina D, et al. Immunohistochemical analysis of IDH2 R172 hotspot mutations in breast papillary neoplasms: applications in the diagnosis of tall cell carcinoma with reverse polarity. Mod Pathol 2020;33(6):1056–64.

248. Bhargava R, Florea AV, Pelmus M, et al. Breast tumor resembling tall cell variant of papillary thyroid carcinoma: a solid papillary neoplasm with characteristic immunohistochemical profile and few recurrent mutations. Am J Clin Pathol 2017;147(4):399–410.

249. Haefliger S, Muenst S, Went P, et al. Tall cell carcinoma of the breast with reversed polarity (TCCRP) with mutations in the IDH2 and PIK3CA genes: a case report. Mol Biol Rep 2020;47(6):4917–21.

Neoadjuvant Therapy in Breast Cancer
Histologic Changes and Clinical Implications

Megan L. Troxell, MD, PhD[1],*, Tanya Gupta, MD[2]

KEYWORDS

• Breast carcinoma • Neoadjuvant • Chemotherapy • Endocrine therapy • Residual cancer

Key points

- Chemotherapy before surgery (neoadjuvant) is increasingly prescribed for breast cancer (T2, N1+); response to neoadjuvant therapy is prognostic and may guide further therapy.
- Correlation with radiology, detailed gross, and histologic evaluation with cassette mapping of the tumor bed and residual carcinoma is essential in the analysis of postneoadjuvant specimens.
- Histologic features of tumor bed are variable but often include loose collagenized to myxoid stroma with overabundant vessels and paucity of normal epithelial structures.
- Histologic features of posttherapy residual carcinoma are variable (hyperchromatic pleomorphic nuclei; clear, vacuolated, to eosinophilic cytoplasm; small dyscohesive lobular-like cells), and can blend into the tumor bed or lymph node.
- Semi-quantitative estimate of residual carcinoma using residual cancer burden (RCB) or other algorithms provides clinically useful data.

ABSTRACT

Cytotoxic or endocrine therapy before surgery (neoadjuvant) for breast cancer has become standard of care, affording the opportunity to assess and quantify response in the subsequent resection specimen. Correlation with radiology, cassette mapping, and histologic review with a semi-quantitative reporting system such as residual cancer burden (RCB) provides important prognostic data that may guide further therapy. The tumor bed should be identified histologically, often as a collagenized zone devoid of normal breast epithelium, with increased vasculature. Identification of residual treated carcinoma may require careful high power examination, as residual tumor cells may be small and dyscohesive; features are widely variable and include hyperchromatic small, large, or multiple nuclei with clear, foamy, or eosinophilic cytoplasm. Calculation of RCB requires residual carcinoma span in 2 dimensions, estimated carcinoma cellularity (% area), number of involved lymph nodes, and span of largest nodal carcinoma. These RCB parameters may differ from AJCC staging measurements, which depend on only contiguous carcinoma in breast and lymph nodes.

INTRODUCTION

Invasive breast cancer is generally treated with some form of systemic "adjuvant" therapy, including combinations of cytotoxic chemotherapy, HER2 targeted therapy, immunotherapy, other emerging targeted therapies, and/or antihormonal therapy (endocrine therapy), based on the biomarker profiles of the carcinoma. Neoadjuvant therapy entails systemic treatment before definitive surgical therapy. Neoadjuvant therapy has become standard of care for high-risk local-regional breast

[1] Department of Pathology, Stanford University School of Medicine, Stanford Pathology, 300 Pasteur Drive, H2110, Stanford, CA 94305, USA; [2] Department of Medicine, Division of Oncology, Stanford University School of Medicine, 900 Blake Wilbur Drive, Palo Alto, CA 94304 USA
* Corresponding author.
E-mail address: megant@stanford.edu

Surgical Pathology 15 (2022) 57–75
https://doi.org/10.1016/j.path.2021.11.004

Table 1
Postneoadjuvant chemotherapy pathologic reporting schemes, published since 2000[6,11,15,16,17]

Scheme or Author, year	Score in Breast	Requires Correlate w/Core?	Lymph Nodes Included?	# Categories of Partial Response
Fisher, B-18, 2002	Sparse cellularity and fibrosis	No	Yes, size	1
Miller-Payne, 2003	Presence of invasive, cellularity	Yes	No	4
Chollett, MNPI, 2003	Size of invasive, grade	No	Yes, #	3
Pinder, 2007	% tumor remaining in breast	Yes	Yes, TE	3
Symanns RCB, 2007	**Span in 2-dimensions, cellularity**	**No**	**Yes, # & size**	**3 (& numerical score)**
Ellis, PEPI, 2008	For ER+ & neoendocrine therapy: ypT stage, ER, Ki-67	No	ypN stage	2 groups (0–12 points)
Chollet, RDBN, 2008	Residual tumor size, grade	No	Yes	3
Sherri, RPCB, 2015	RCB and Ki-67	No	Yes	3
AJCC (y)	**Size of invasive, 1 dimension, contiguous only**	**No**	**Yes (#, level)**	**Standard pT, N**

Abbreviations: MNPI, modified Nottingham prognostic index; PEPI, preoperative endocrine prognostic index; RCB, residual cancer burden; RDBN, residual disease in breast and nodes; RPCB, residual proliferative cancer burden; TE, Treatment Effect.

cancer, and patients with 2 cm or larger tumors (T2), or positive nodes (N1) are considered candidates.[1] Outcome is generally equivalent in the adjuvant and neoadjuvant paradigms, while neoadjuvant chemotherapy has advantages in potentially converting to breast-conserving surgery (instead of mastectomy), allowing for the monitoring of clinical and radiologic response during treatment, and assessing histopathologic response at the time of surgery.[2,3] Response to chemotherapy is prognostic in terms of disease-free survival and overall survival,[4–7] and facilitates tailoring of additional systemic therapy, for example, escalation/deescalation.[1,7] Patients achieving a "pathologic complete response" (pCR), with no residual carcinoma in lymph nodes and no stromal invasive or intralymphatic carcinoma in breast have the most favorable outcome (ypT0/ypTis), especially in the setting of HER2 positive or triple-negative breast cancer.[4,5,7–9] Additional chemotherapy may provide a survival benefit for patients with residual carcinoma at surgery.[1,7,10] Further, the rate of pCR has been used as an endpoint in modern therapy trials, greatly accelerating drug regimen evaluation.[1,3,6,7] In the absence of pCR, several scoring systems have emerged to measure

and convey the degree of response and amount of residual carcinoma after chemotherapy (**Table 1**). The "Residual Cancer Burden" (RCB) scoring has been shown to be prognostic in several studies, is relatively reproducible, and has been widely adopted within and outside of clinical trials.[5,7,8,11–14] Careful pathologic assessment and understanding of the gross and histologic changes after systemic therapy are important in guiding therapy and prognosis, and are the subject of this section. **Box 1** outlines the basic pathologic approach to postneoadjuvant therapy breast resection specimens.

PRELUDE TO NEOADJUVANT THERAPY

Any patient considered for neoadjuvant therapy should have a diagnosis of invasive breast cancer and its biomarker panel (estrogen receptor (ER), progesterone receptor (PR), HER2, +/-Ki-67) well-established by core needle biopsy, with adequate tissue available for additional assays as needed (eg mutational or gene expression profiling).[6,8,13,15,18,19] Patients with a high fraction of ductal carcinoma in situ (DCIS), microinvasive carcinoma, or uncertainties on biopsy might benefit from additional sampling or up-front

---

Box 1
Steps to evaluate postneoadjuvant breast specimens

1. Recognize the posttherapy setting

2. Correlate with pre- and posttherapy imaging

3. Identify residual tumor/tumor bed/clips grossly

4. Judiciously sample with measurements and mapping (see **Fig. 1**)

5. Assess residual carcinoma and/or tumor bed histologically

    a. Identify residual carcinoma, clip or biopsy site, histologic tumor bed

    b. Measure largest contiguous carcinoma focus, number of foci (for AJCC pT stage)

    c. Measure residual carcinoma span in 2 dimensions (for RCB)

    d. Estimate residual tumor cellularity (% cells per area, for RCB, see **Fig. 7**)

    e. Report margins and other standard parameters

6. Evaluate lymph nodes

    a. Number with residual carcinoma as each of itc, micrometastasis, metastasis, and size of largest (measure contiguous carcinoma only, not include fibrosis, for AJCC pN stage)

    b. Measure span of residual carcinoma in largest (including intervening fibrosis, for RCB)

    c. Evaluate extranodal extension

7. Report according to local requirements, custom (AJCC stage, CAP template, +/-RCB elements, or other systems)

Abbreviations: AJCC, American joint committee on cancer; CAP, College of American pathologists; RCB, Residual Cancer Burden.

---

surgery for further characterization, before embarking on systemic therapy.[8,15] A radiopaque marker ("clip") at the site of the primary carcinoma should be considered mandatory before therapy, such that the tumor site can be identified and resected even in the case of complete clinical/radiologic response.[6,8,13,15,18,19] Many of these patients with high-risk breast cancer have abnormal lymph nodes identified on axillary ultrasound, and at least one of these is typically sampled by either fine needle aspiration (FNA) or core biopsy.[7,8] Clip or other marker in the sampled (positive) lymph node is also recommended.[7,8,18] Surgical sentinel lymph node biopsy before therapy precludes the assessment of some of the neoadjuvant response scores such as RCB, and is disfavored.[18]

APPROACH TO NEOADJUVANT THERAPY GROSS SPECIMENS

In the current era of the electronic medical record, the surgical specimen requisition almost never contains information about breast tumor number, location, size, associated clips, calcifications, nodes, or prior treatment.[7,11,15] This data is essential in approaching any breast resection, but even

moreso in the posttherapy setting. A helpful clue to neoadjuvant therapy is a long time interval between core biopsy and resection (4–6 months).[7] The correlative radiologic data listed above should be obtained from the medical record, requisition, or surgeon, and in the case of neoadjuvant therapy, should also include the *pretherapy* size.[6] Posttherapy clinical and imaging size and characteristics provide additional context, but they may not be well correlated with histopathologic findings (**Box 2**).[6,11,19]

After orientation and inking, the specimen should be thinly sliced (0.3–0.5 cm intervals). Slices should be laid out sequentially and uniformly oriented (**Fig. 1**). Ideally, the specimen should be x-rayed to facilitate the identification of marker clips and calcifications.[6,13,18,19] If specimen radiography is not available, a gross photo may instead serve to document and map sampling,[13,18] but the identification of clips or tumor bed can be very difficult. The sectioned specimen is then examined to identify marker clip(s), tumor bed(s), and residual tumor (if any). Palpation of the sections may also be helpful in discriminating tumor (hard, gritty), tumor bed (fibrous to soft), and fibrocystic disease (rubbery). The grossly estimated size and margin distances of the tumor bed and

---

Box 2
Correlative radiologic and clinical data essential in the gross examination of postneoadjuvant therapy specimens

Pretherapy number of tumors

Pretherapy location of each tumor (esp. o'clock, distance from nipple, depth)

Pretherapy size of each tumor

Posttherapy size of each tumor

Clip placement and localization

   Including shape/type location of each clip if multiple

   Location/diagnosis of any "benign" biopsies/clips

   Displacement of clip from targets, if any

   Axillary lymph node clips, if any

   Localization approach (wires, scouts, Magseed, radioactive marker strategy if multiple eg, goalpost vs marking each lesion)

Calcifications, if any

Orientation guides for surgical specimen (suture or inking key)

Any special clinical trial parameters

---

residual tumor should be documented. All clips and radiologic lesions should be grossly accounted for,[8] with the practical caveat that rarely clips can be displaced during surgical or pathologic manipulation.

The gross tumor bed (gTB) is defined as the grossly apparent area of fibrosis or scarring at the tumor site, and includes areas of gross residual tumor. The microscopic tumor bed (mTB) is defined as the area of discernible (stromal) histologic changes in the tumor site. The histologic span of residual invasive carcinoma (RIC) may be larger or smaller than the gTB or mTB (described in more detail later in discussion and in **Fig. 2**), and is generally the size entered into the RCB system.

After therapy, breast carcinoma may disappear completely (pCR), partially resolve concentrically or eccentrically, or leave a patchwork of tumor clusters; some tumors show little response, or very rarely, continue to growly during therapy (see **Figs. 1** and **2**;).[7,15,18,20] In the latter situations, gross sampling is similar to that of any grossly or radiologically apparent breast cancer. In the former, judicious representative sampling and mapping, guided by gross and radiologic findings, is necessary for complete diagnosis and prognostication (see **Figs. 1–3**). Paradoxically, the less the residual tumor, the more sampling/sections may be needed. Some institutions sample the entire tumor bed in the case of apparent complete

pathologic response, although exhaustive sampling of the entire gTB is not mandated by all experts.[8,13,15]

If the resection specimen is small, it can be completely submitted; mapping or a detailed cassette key is still needed. For larger specimens (mastectomy, large lumpectomy), sampling recommendations vary; at least one (largest) cross-section of the gTB should be fully blocked in for histologic review (up to 5 cassettes in some centers).[8,11,13] Then, one to several cassettes of each tumor bed slice should be submitted, with consideration for sampling a full cross-section every 1 to 2 cm of tumor bed, (up to about 25 blocks in some centers).[8,11,13] Sampling should extend beyond the gross residual tumor/tumor bed, as guided by the *pretherapy tumor size*, given the propensity for occult microscopic extension of carcinoma.[8,11,18] Large cassettes could be advantageous for these cases, but are seldom available.[13] gTB at the margin should certainly be submitted for accurate histologic margin review. If multiple tumors were recognized pretreatment, each area should be handled similarly, with attention to the submission of intervening sections to substantiate separate versus contiguous lesions. As depicted in **Fig. 1**, the location of each section should be documented on a radiograph or photograph of the specimen, preserving the relationship of the sections to one another, and to landmarks such as biopsy clips, skin, margin, etc.[5,7,11,13,18]

Fig. 1. Specimen mapping. The specimen radiograph depicts 3 slices from the center of a skin and nipple-sparing mastectomy, laid out in order (white #s-slice #; each slice oriented as superior-top, inferior-bottom; anterior right and posterior left; staple at nipple bed). Obvious residual tumor is present in slices 11 and 12, with the clip in slice 12. Submitting only sections A7 and A12 would represent undersampling, as the pretherapy radiologic abnormality was 5 cm in the superior-inferior dimension, beginning just superior to the nipple. Blocking in 2 full cross-sections of the expected tumor bed is illustrated. Sampling would continue on slices medial to 10 and lateral to 12 as guided by the medial-lateral dimensions on radiology, and by the gross findings. Histologic sections demonstrated chemotherapy-resistant

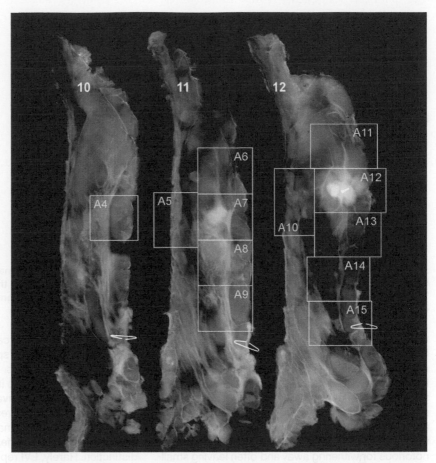

carcinoma in the visible nodule (1.4 cm), with microscopic tumor extending across adjacent histologic sections 3 cm in the superior-inferior and 2.3 cm in the medial-lateral dimensions, a stage ypT2.

Handling of lymph node specimens is discussed later in discussion; attention to clips or other markers remains imperative.

APPROACH TO NEOADJUVANT THERAPY HISTOLOGIC SECTIONS

In the posttherapy setting, it is important to identify at least one of: (1) residual viable carcinoma, (2) definite histologic evidence of tumor bed (mTB), or (3) histologic/gross evidence of biopsy site/clip, to confirm appropriate histologic sampling and surgical resection. In very rare instances, treated carcinoma may vanish with little stromal reaction (see **Fig. 3**)[11]; in these cases, one is left with the biopsy site/clip (radiology reports should document any displacement relative to the pretreatment tumor). Although tumor bed changes are variable in posttherapy specimens, they become familiar with experience (see **Fig. 1, Table 2**). Often, the tumor bed demonstrates a lack or paucity of normal breast structures, especially

lobules, as compared with the background breast parenchyma (**Fig. 3**).[15] Normal structures are replaced by a swath of loose to collagenized fibrosis with a relative abundance of small vessels.[6,11,19,15,16] Calcifications, histiocytes, fat necrosis, multi-nucleated giant cells, hemosiderin, or mucin make the tumor bed more obvious (see **Fig. 3**).[6,11,19,16] Biopsy sites may be identified by a cluster of giant cells and foreign material, or depending on the type of marker, a lucent area surrounded by synovial-like histiocytes (see **Fig. 3**). Given the time interval between biopsy and surgery, biopsy sites will also be "older" for example, more resolved and less obvious as compared with those we are familiar with in untreated surgical specimens. Small collections of histiocytes do not qualify as the biopsy site.

Chemotherapy-related cytoarchitectural changes in breast carcinoma are many and varied (**Fig. 4, Table 2, Box 3**). Commonly described alterations include greater nuclear pleomorphism, hyperchromasia, or multinucleation.[4,11,13,19,16] A decrease in

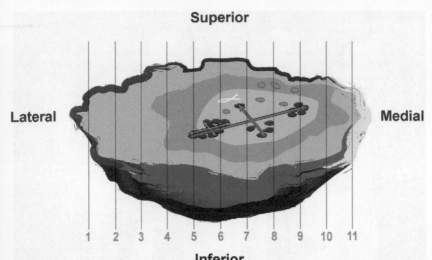

Superior

Lateral

Medial

1 2 3 4 5 6 7 8 9 10 11

Inferior

Fig. 2. Residual carcinoma in tumor bed. The darker gray shading indicates the extent of pretherapy carcinoma by imaging, with biopsy clip (white ribbon). The yellow shading indicates the grossly apparent fibrous scar (gTB), which does not necessarily match the distribution of residual carcinoma. Residual invasive carcinoma is depicted by red circles, with residual ductal carcinoma in situ (DCIS) as blue circles. The span of residual invasive carcinoma (RIC) is indicated by green arrows, and represents the 2-dimensional size for residual cancer burden (RCB) calculation. The percent cellularity for RCB would be averaged over this area (also see **Fig. 10**). The largest contiguous extent of invasive carcinoma (RIC) is indicated by gray arrows and is used for AJCC staging, with the designation of multifocality (m) in this example.

the mitotic rate is expected.[13,15] The cytoplasm may be more or less abundant, with eosinophilia, clearing, or vacuolization.[4,6,11,16] The cells may become less cohesive, even plasmacytoid, histiocytoid, or lobular carcinoma-like.[11,16] A ductal carcinoma with dyshesive features after therapy should not be reclassified as lobular.[16] ER-positive tumors treated with neoadjuvant endocrine therapy are notorious for withering away and often leaving small cells scattered across the tumor bed that can be extremely hard to recognize (**Fig. 5**). In contrast, postchemotherapy carcinoma may demonstrate anaplasia, metaplasia, heterogeneity, or other features that were not apparent on core biopsy (see **Fig. 4**). This could reflect an artifact of biopsy sampling, chemotherapy-induced changes, or selection of chemotherapy-resistant clone(s).[13]

Sections of tumor bed and surround should be examined diligently at medium to high power, as low cellularity residual carcinoma can blend into the background and be extremely tricky to identify (see **Figs. 4** and **5**, **Table 2**, **Box 3**).[6,13,15] Residual single or small clusters of carcinoma tend to trickle through the stroma and any remnant normal structures; they may also be obscured by the collections of lymphocytes or histiocytes.[16] Clues to carcinoma include epithelial clusters "out of place" relative to benign breast architecture, as well as subtle cytologic differences from the benign background epithelium. Once occult residual cancers cells are discovered, it may be helpful to re-review the tumor bed searching for more of the same, to best capture their extent and confirm margin status. Judicious immunostains may be helpful, as described later.

Islands of cohesive carcinoma cells may be rimmed by retraction space, mimicking lymphvascular tumor clusters. Conversely, large proliferative tumor collections in lymphatics (see **Fig. 4**) may mimic DCIS or invasive carcinoma.[16] The staging and outcome of residual DCIS and residual intralymphatic carcinoma (lymphvascular invasion, LVI), are vastly different, so this is a crucial distinction. Rarely, LVI represents the only residual in-breast tumor; additional sampling may be warranted for confirmation. Patients with no to minimal RIC and considerable residual LVI have guarded prognosis.[21–24] Complexities in reporting of these unusual cases are discussed later.

Occasionally keratin immunostaining (+/-histiocyte markers) is needed to confirm carcinoma and distinguish tumor cells from inflammatory cells (histocytes, plasma cells, mast cells), or endothelial or other stromal nuclei (see **Figs. 4** and **5**).[6,11,15,16] Myoepithelial immunostains can aid in confirming invasion for small cell clusters in an around lobules or sclerosing adenosis. Immunostains may be useful in discriminating DCIS from invasive carcinoma from LVI, including the myoepithelial stains p63 or p40 (nuclear), calponin or smooth muscle myosin heavy chain (cytoplasmic), and the lymphatic/endothelial stains D2-40 and/or CD31, with the caveat that D2-40 may label the subset of myoepithelial cells in treated and untreated specimens.[25]

DCIS is traditionally thought to be somewhat less chemotherapy sensitive than invasive carcinoma.[6] Residual DCIS should be distinguished from reactive, inflammatory, or treatment-related atypia within "benign" ductal or lobular spaces. Features

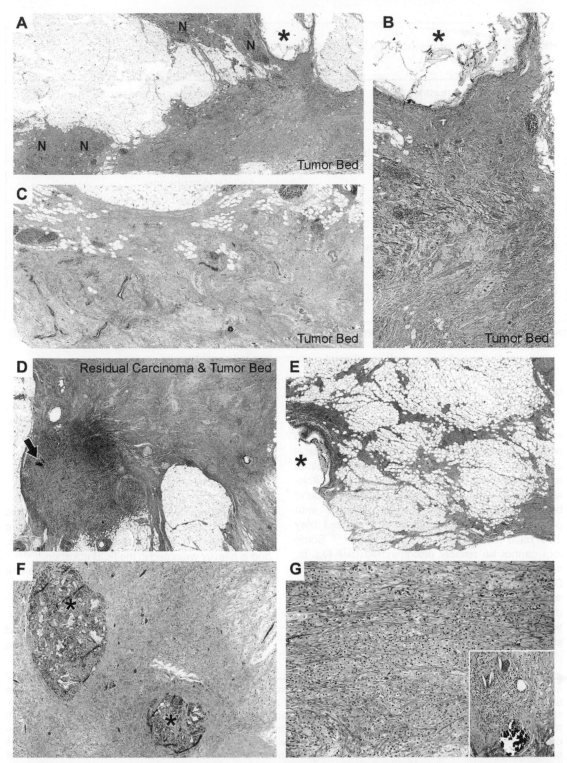

Fig. 3. Histologic features of tumor bed. (*A*) At low power, normal postchemotherapy breast parenchyma (N) in a young woman shows regularly spaced ducts and lobules in a dense fibrous stroma. This contrasts with the tumor bed occupying most of the bottom portion of the panel, where normal breast structures are markedly diminished and replaced by loose fibrosis, vessels, scattered inflammation. The biopsy site is denoted by an asterisk. (*B*) Higher power of the biopsy site (*) and underlying tumor bed. Vessels, collagen, and fibromyxoid change are prominent, and normal breast architecture is effaced. (*C*) Edge of tumor bed from another patient. Several

Table 2
Histologic features of tumor bed and treated breast carcinoma

Tumor Bed	Residual Carcinoma
Paucity of normal breast structures	Cytoplasmic clearing or vacuolization (even histiocyte-like)
Increase of vessels	Cytoplasmic hypereosinophilia

Stromal fibrosis
    Nonuniform, different from the rubbery
        homogeneous stroma of fibrocystic change
	Nuclear enlargement, hyperchromasia, pleomorphism, multinucleation, or alternatively pyknosis[a]

Stromal edema, myxoid change	Cellular dyscohesion
Stromal histocytes or other inflammatory cells	Decrease in cell size (even plasmacytoid or lobular like features)[a]
Cholesterol clefts	Retraction spaces
Fat necrosis (tumor necrosis may resolve by surgery)	Increased heterogeneity
Multinucleated giant cells	Reduced mitotic rate
Hemosiderin	Reduced cellularity[a]
Biopsy site remnant	

This list captures the wide spectrum of possible findings. Treatment response is highly variable; tumors may show varying combinations of the listed features.

[a] Indicates features often seen with neoadjuvant endocrine (neoendocrine) therapy.

favoring residual DCIS include high-grade nuclei and cytologic features similar to residual invasive or pretherapy carcinoma (**Fig. 6**). Residual DCIS may even have a clinging (single layer) pattern within ducts or manifest as rare markedly atypical cells within lobules (see **Fig. 6**). It may be helpful to consider the spectrum of therapy-related epithelial change within other areas of the background breast, which typically seems atrophic with pyknotic nuclei and increased fibrosis, but may also have low grades of atypia.[4,6,11,13,19] Some foci cannot be reliably discriminated (see **Fig. 6**), and there are no defining immunostains of residual DCIS, although HER2 positive DCIS may maintain its phenotype.[6,11,15] In this situation, a descriptive diagnosis such as "atypical intraductal proliferation" may be prudent, with a discussion of the considerations of treated DCIS versus reactive atypia.[15] There would not be clinical treatment implications unless the involved ducts are close to final margins. Residual in situ carcinoma is considered pCR in most but not all countries (see **Table 3**).

LOCALIZATION AND PATHOLOGIC EVALUATION OF SENTINEL LYMPH NODES

In the postneoadjuvant therapy setting, pathologic evaluation of axillary lymph nodes is very important in AJCC staging as well as prognostic schemes, and is heavily weighted in the RCB equation.[4,5,13,18] In the initial clinical workup, patients with high-risk tumors often have axillary lymph nodes evaluated by ultrasound, with tissue sampling of radiologically suspicious nodes by FNA or core biopsy. The sampled (positive) lymph node should be marked (tattooed or clipped), such that it can be identified

normal lobules are seen in the upper portion of the panel within fatty parenchyma, whereas tumor bed in the bottom of the panel is collagenized and elastotic with a rare large purple calcification (bottom, near center). There was no residual carcinoma, but the tumor bed must be carefully examined for rare glands and cells. (*D*) Treated carcinoma can be very heterogeneous. At bottom left, a densely cellular carcinoma nodule with calcification (*arrow*). At far right, residual carcinoma with low cellularity, and at the center, tumor bed with only rare carcinoma cells. The cellularity should be averaged across the span of treated carcinoma for residual cancer burden (RCB) calculations. (*E*) From a different case, the tumor bed does not stand out by gross or histologic examination. The biopsy marker (*) was essential in identifying tumor bed. There may still be occult carcinoma within the mostly fatty stroma. (*F*) A different type of biopsy site marker (*) is seen within collagenized stroma at slightly higher power. Other examples of biopsy markers are shown in the lymph node **Fig. 8**. (*G*) An obvious tumor bed consisting of fibrosis and foamy histiocytes. The cytologic features should be examined to rule out histiocytoid or admixed carcinoma (see **Fig. 4E**). The inset shows prominent calcifications and cholesterol clefts associated with multinucleated giant cells.

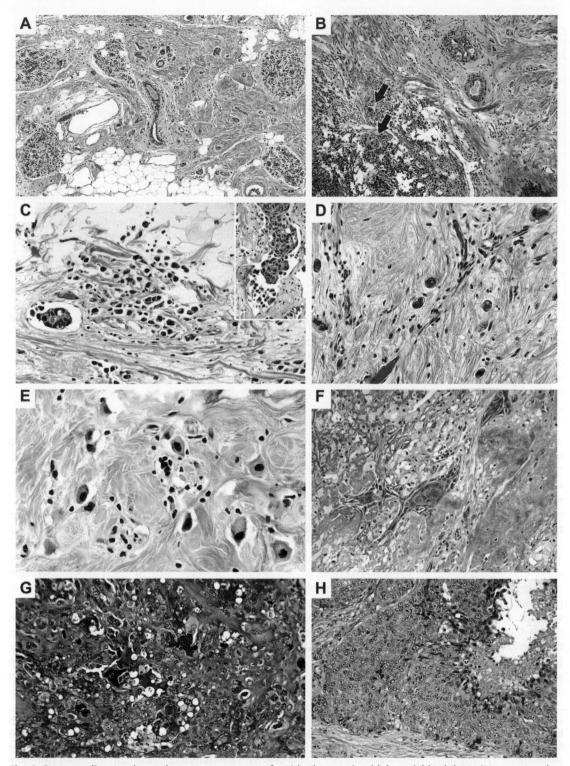

Fig. 4. Postneoadjuvant chemotherapy appearance of residual tumor is widely variable. (*A*) Medium power view of residual carcinoma clusters trickling through breast lobules at the edge of the tumor bed. Residual carcinoma can be considerably more occult. These normal breast structures show epithelial atrophy and increased intralobular fibrosis due to chemotherapy. (*B*) Medium power view of another tumor bed demonstrates residual DCIS. However, there is also invasive carcinoma obscured by the inflammation (*arrows*), requiring careful high power examination. (*C*) From a different case, one of numerous residual satellite invasive foci is shown, consisting of

Table 3
Definitions of pathologic complete response (pCR)[7,8,18]

Residual Pathology	pCR	NOT pCR	Comment
Breast: invasive carcinoma		X	
Breast: Ductal carcinoma in situ (DCIS)	X		AJCC 8th allows DCIS in pCR; some European systems do not
Breast: Lobular carcinoma in situ (LCIS)	X		
Breast: acellular mucin pools	X		Generous sections or levels to exclude residual carcinoma cells
Breast: necrosis without viable tumor	X		Generous sections or levels to exclude viable carcinoma
Breast: Intralymphatic carcinoma (LVI)		X	If LVI without residual invasive (rare), suggest ypTX or ypTX-lvi[16,24] Consider additional sampling
Lymph nodes: macro- & micro- met		X	Residual carcinoma in lymph node worse prognosis irrespective of breast status
Lymph nodes: isolated tumor cells		X	ypN0(i+) different significance than in untreated nodes

Data from Bossuyt V, Spring L. Pathologic evaluation of response to neoadjuvant therapy drives treatment changes and improves long-term outcomes for breast cancer patients. Breast J. 2020;26(6):1189-1198., Bossuyt V. Processing and Reporting of Breast Specimens in the Neoadjuvant Setting. Surg Pathol Clin. 2018;11(1):213-230., Bossuyt V, Provenzano E, Symmans WF, et al. Recommendations for standardized pathological characterization of residual disease for neoadjuvant clinical trials of breast cancer by the BIG-NABCG collaboration. Ann Oncol. 2015;26(7):1280-1291. cite references as from reference section, not as table footnote

after therapy.[8,10,11,26–29] At the time of surgery, patients with good clinical response undergo sentinel lymph node biopsy, with dual tracer method and collection of multiple nodes recommended to reduce false-negative rates (**Fig. 7**).[10,26–29] Whether or not it localizes as a sentinel node, a previously positive clipped node should be also be collected (clipped = sentinel in 75%–90% of cases).[10,11,26–29] This node may be localized preoperatively with wires, scouts, Magseed, or radioactive markers according to local custom.[10,26–29] Thus, the pathologist may be confronted by a specimen with a wire/scout, biopsy clip and biopsy site change **Fig. 8**. It is important to keep track of which node the biopsy clip/site is associated with, both for surgical correlation and prognostic purposes, and to avoid pitfalls in intraoperative or final diagnosis.

Other than the identification of markers, gross evaluation and sectioning of lymph nodes is similar to untreated axillary node biopsies or dissections. As in other organ systems, both positive and negative nodes may be grossly smaller posttherapy.[6,11,19,15] It is important to dissect all candidate nodes, section them at 2 mm thickness, and completely submit, maintaining the identity of each node, such that the total number of nodes, number positive, size of each metastasis, and the presence of extranodal extension can be synthesized after histologic examination.[8,11]

Lymph nodes may show a similar histologic spectrum of tumor-related changes as seen in breast tissue. Carcinoma in previously positive lymph nodes may completely resolve with therapy, leaving a histologically normal node without a hint

small dyscohesive cells with hyperchromatic nuclei. There was prominent intralymphatic tumor, seen at left, with large tumor emboli distending lymphatic channels elsewhere, in the higher power inset. (*D*) From another case at higher power, many carcinoma cells have hyperchromatic multi-lobed or multiple nuclei and varying amounts of amphophilic cytoplasm. (*E*) These individual carcino-ma cells have a histiocytoid flavor, with abundant pale cytoplasm. However, they have large hyperchromatic nuclei, and keratin immunostaining was positive (not shown), confirming the diagnosis. (*F*) This carcinoma had areas of conventional high-grade invasive ductal carcinoma (not shown), as well as extensive squamous differentiation, not seen on the prechemotherapy core biopsy. (*G*) A tumor that grew during treatment demonstrates very large pleomorphic nuclei and chondroid matrix after chemotherapy (*H*) This field shows a chemoresistant dermal nodule that was growing through chemotherapy. The necrosis is likely related to rapid tumor growth rather than chemotherapy effect. Other foci of tumor had an excellent response (see **Fig. 3**G).

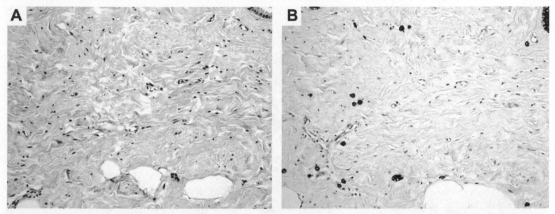

Fig. 5. Lobular breast cancer after neoadjuvant endocrine therapy "Neoendocrine therapy." (*A*) Medium power view shows relatively pauci-cellular tumor bed with a fewdarker nuclei that could be easily missed on scanning power. (*B*) Keratin immunohistochemical stain of a serial section highlights residual single or small clusters of tumor cells.

of prior involvement.[6,11,13,16] Alternatively, an area of prior involvement may be replaced by fibrous tissue and/or histiocytes (treatment effect, **Fig. 8**). As with the fibrous tumor bed in the breast specimen, is very important to carefully evaluate this area, as occult individual cells or tumor clusters may remain (see **Fig. 8**).[6,11,16] The prior nodal biopsy site may mimic or obscure residual

Box 3
Histologic clues to minimal residual invasive carcinoma

Architectural clues to occult carcinoma: Small clusters of epithelioid cells

　Within tumor bed stroma

　In stroma between residual lobules/adenosis; especially out of place versus normal structures

　In between acini of splayed lobule

　Obscured by lymphoid aggregates, histiocytes

Cytology of occult carcinoma

　Nuclei larger and more hyperchromatic than normal breast epithelium with treatment effect

　Cytoplasm often scant

　Endocrine treated (lobular) carcinoma may closely resemble plasma cells or lymphocytes and require immunohistochemical confirmation

Ancillary studies for occult carcinoma, if needed

　Ensure cells of concern are on immunohistochemical levels; if absent, stains are uninformative and uninterpretable

　Keratin immunostain to confirm epithelial differentiation; *the most crucial*

　Lack of myoepithelial cell staining to support invasive carcinoma

　　Recommend 1 nuclear (p63 or p40) along with 1 cytoplasmic (smooth muscle myosin heavy chain, calponin)

　In HER2+ carcinoma, HER2 immunostaining can be diagnostic to reveal and confirm residual HER2+ carcinoma

　Lymphatic endothelial (D2-40) or endothelial (CD31/CD34) immunostains if concern for lymphvascular carcinoma

　With any immunostain order, cutting additional unstained is recommend; refacing the tissue block has a risk of cutting through target cells

If low cellularity carcinoma is discovered, *re-review tumor bed* with specific attention to features of residual cells

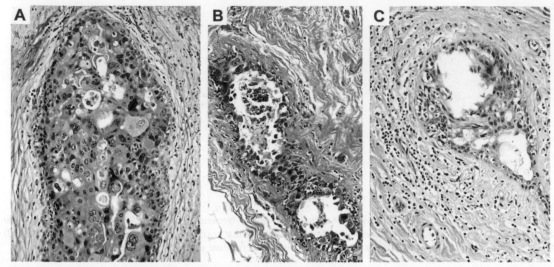

Fig. 6. Intraductal carcinoma postneoadjuvant chemotherapy. (*A*) Residual DCIS with marked nuclear pleomorphism, abundant eosinophilic cytoplasm, focal necrosis, and several atypical mitotic figures. There is surrounding inflammation. (*B*) Residual clinging DCIS with high-grade cytology; elsewhere in the specimen, invasive and in situ carcinoma had similar cytology. (*C*) This duct is partially filled by cells with enlarged nuclei, fine chromatin, nucleoli, and wispy cytoplasm, along with admixed macrophages and lymphocytes. It may not be possible to definitively distinguish residual intraductal carcinoma from chemotherapy-related changes in proliferative breast in such foci; comparison with other foci of residual carcinoma (invasive, in situ, if any), as well as changes in background benign breast may be informative.

carcinoma (see **Fig. 8**).[18] In such sections, keratin immunostains may be helpful, but are not recommended for all treated nodes.[4,6,14] In some cases, residual tumor in lymph nodes seems virtually untouched by treatment. In rare cases, treated tumor may resemble granulomas, germinal centers, or otherwise blend in with the lymph node (**Fig. 9**). Other complexities include nodal extramedullary hematopoiesis,[14] benign breast glandular or Mullerian inclusions, or nodal nevi.[30]

Patients whose sentinel lymph nodes are negative following neoadjuvant therapy may forego completion axillary dissection.[10,11,26–29] In contrast, patients with clinical/radiologic indications of residual disease will generally be recommended for nodal dissection, along with patients having pathologic

Fig. 7. Post chemotherapy management of the axilla

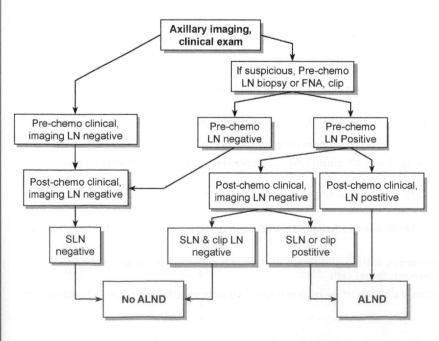

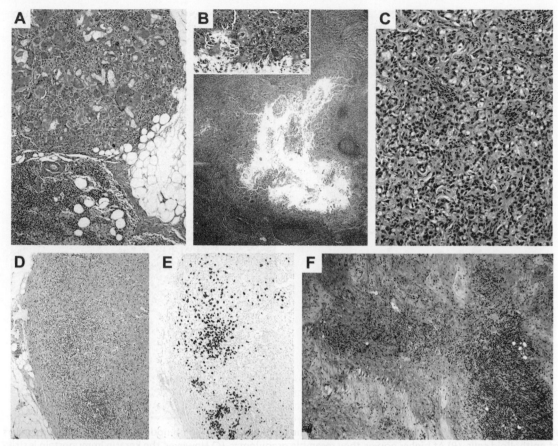

Fig. 8. Lymph nodes postneoadjuvant chemotherapy. (*A*) At medium power, a large biopsy clip site occupies the top of the field. A negative lymph node with prominent histiocytes is below. (*B*) At lower power, a different type of biopsy marker change is seen in this lymph node. The edge of the biopsy site shows epithelioid histiocytes and multinucleated giant cells (inset) which can appear quite atypical without the context of prior biopsy. (*C*) Elsewhere in the same lymph node specimen shown in B, residual carcinoma is associated with fibrosis. (*D*) A typical area of posttreatment scarring should be carefully evaluated for residual carcinoma. While these lobular cells are somewhat apparent on H&E, the keratin stain (shown in *E*) may reveal more than meets the eye. Keratin stains can be helpful in select cases, but are not considered routine or mandatory. (*F*) This area of treatment effect demonstrates fibrosis, elastosis, and hemosiderin. A careful search was negative for residual carcinoma.

chemotherapy-resistant nodal disease (see **Fig. 7**).[11,26] Randomized studies of axillary surgery and radiotherapy in the neoadjuvant therapy setting are underway and will inform future management, which may differ by intrinsic type of breast cancer.[10,27–29,31]

APPROACH TO NEOADJUVANT THERAPY REPORTING

All of the standard breast cancer reporting elements apply to postchemotherapy surgical specimens, including size, margins, lymph node status, AJCC stage, etc.[6] However, supplemental data are added to stratify response and calculate RCB or other prognostic parameters. In addition to numerical parameters, a concise description is

recommended and may prove invaluable to the treatment team.[8,11] Residual carcinoma should be graded using the standard Nottingham system (tubules, nuclei, mitosis), although pretherapy grade may be more relevant,[16] and may not change overall (for instance, if the mitotic score decreases and the nuclear pleomorphism score increases).[11,15] Some groups recommend reporting tumor bed at the margin when present, especially if spare carcinoma cells are widely dispersed.[6] As in untreated settings, LVI carcinoma at the margin should not be reported as a positive surgical margin, yet some groups prefer to describe this finding.

Several post-(cytotoxic) chemotherapy reporting schemes have been published (see **Table 1**), some with demonstrated long-term prognostic value.

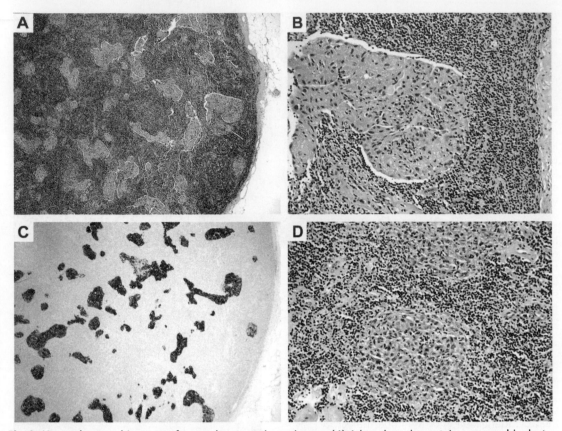

Fig. 9. Unusual cytoarchitecture of treated metastatic carcinoma. (*A*) A lymph node contains geographic clusters of epithelioid cells. (*B*) At higher power, they resemble granulomas. (*C*) However, the keratin immunostain is strikingly positive, confirming that the epithelioid clusters represent treated tumor. (*D*) In another node from the same patient, residual tumor closely resembled the size, distribution, and cytology of germinal centers; again, the foci were all keratin positive (not shown). These images also demonstrate artifact from prior frozen section evaluation; not surprisingly, the unusual carcinoma was not recognized at the time of intraoperative consultation.

Further discussion and examples pertain to the RCB system[5]. The RCB score was published in 2007 by Symmans and colleagues based on outcome data, and is accompanied by links to detailed instructions for reporting pathologists, and an online calculator, which is available at http://www3.mdanderson.org/app/medcalc/index.cfm?pagename=jsconvert35. Derivation of RCB requires the span of residual carcinoma in 2 dimensions, the percentage of residual carcinoma, as well as the number of residual involved lymph nodes and largest span nodal involvement. These parameters are entered into a mathematical equation (which is quite heavily weighted to nodal involvement), available as an online calculator which generates both and RCB numerical score, and assigns a grouping from RCB-0 (pCR) to RCB-III (more residual tumor, less favorable prognosis).

The tumor span (size) used for RCB may be different than the tumor size in the postchemotherapy AJCC stage (ypT) in some cases (see **Fig. 2**).

The RCB uses the span of residual (invasive) carcinoma in each of the 2 largest dimensions, including intervening fibrosis (RIC as described above).[5,7,8,11,13,18,16] This is not the size of the gTB, but the span of histologically confirmed (invasive) carcinoma (RIC). In contrast, the AJCC ypT stage is based on the largest contiguous focus of invasive carcinoma, excluding fibrosis.[7,8,11,13,18,16] For instance, if a single pretherapy tumor mass evolves to nodules of carcinoma separated by fibrosis, only the largest nodule is measured for AJCC ypT stage (with the m modifier), whereas the span of all of them would be considered for RCB (see **Fig. 2**).[7,8,11,13,18,16] Reporting as separate tumors requires documentation of intervening "abundant" negative breast, fibrous, or adipose tissue.[18] For hypercellular residual nodules separated by areas of less cellular but continuous tumor, the full span is measured as the ypT size/stage. Pathologist judgment is certainly required in this determination. The section mapping is particularly useful in

Fig. 10. Estimation of cellularity for RCB versus Molecular studies. For residual cancer burden (RCB), cellularity assessment involves cancer cells and area, regardless of the presence of other cell types such as lymphocytes (tumor-infiltrating lymphocytes, TILS) or normal breast. For molecular studies, the emphasis is on the number/percentage of nuclei that are cancer cells. In the examples shown here, red tumor cells occupy about 10% of the area in both panels

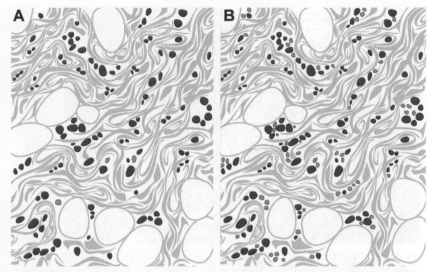

(*A* and *B*) (RCB cellularity = 10%). In panel (*A*), the vast majority of cells are tumor (red), with only a few blue stromal cells or lymphocytes, and the % tumor cellularity for molecular studies is greater than 90%. In panel (*B*), the number of smaller blue lymphocytes is equal to the number of tumor cells, such that the percent tumor cellularity for molecular is about 45%, while the RCB cellularity is unchanged at 10%.

reconstructing 3-dimensional sizes and lining up adjacent sections for the measurement of continuous span of carcinoma. In the rare cases having LVI carcinoma without any residual invasive tumor, an AJCC stage of ypTX or ypTX-lvi + has been proposed[16,23,24]; other authors suggest using the span and cellularity of LVI to derive an RCB value.[8,24]

The tumor cellularity is estimated as the percentage of the RIC area occupied by tumor cells. Symmans and colleagues provide some handy visual calibrations and they recommend estimation in deciles down to 10% (10%, 20%, 30%, etc.), with tighter intervals for very low cellularity tumors (5%, 1%)[5,7]; values less than 1% may be entered into the calculator for particularly pauci-cellular cases.[7,8] Again, the relevant area is the span of microscopic carcinoma (RIC), *not* the span of gross or microscopic fibrotic tumor bed. The authors suggest dotting the outline of residual carcinoma, estimating cellularity for each slide, and averaging across involved slides. The original publication and the online calculator suggest estimating the percentage of carcinoma, including invasive and in situ carcinoma, then subtracting the fraction of tumor that is DCIS in a separate line of the online calculator. However, the same result can be derived by including only the invasive cellularity and entering 0 (zero) for DCIS.[7,8] Another distinction involves cellularity estimates as per RCB versus cellularity estimates for molecular studies, illustrated in **Fig. 10.**

For AJCC ypN staging, positive nodes are each categorized by the size of largest contiguous metastatic tumor cluster, without associated or intervening fibrosis into isolated tumor cells (itc =<0.2 mm or 200 cells), micrometastasis (>0.2–2 mm), and metastasis (>2 mm). Although itc are considered pN0(i+) in AJCC staging, they indicate lack of pCR (see **Table 3**). For the RCB score, the number of positive nodes and span of carcinoma in the largest involved node is entered, which may include fibrosis, different from the AJCC schema.[7,8,13]

INTRINSIC TYPES, THERAPY RESPONSE, AND BIOMARKERS AFTER THERAPY

Experience with neoadjuvant chemotherapy has clarified the chemosensitivity of different biologic types of breast carcinoma. The ER positive, HER2 negative carcinomas (so called "luminal" intrinsic types) have the most favorable overall prognosis, yet they tend to be the least sensitive to cytotoxic chemotherapy, with pCR rates of about 20%.[6,11,15,16,26] The role of endocrine therapy is increasingly recognized in this group, either in lieu of or after cytotoxic chemotherapy. Indeed, a subset of patients may be treated with neoadjuvant endocrine therapy ("neoendocrine").[32–35] Antihormonal treatment is given for a prolonged period and typically results in decreased cell size and cell density, although decreases in overall tumor size may not be as dramatic.[32,33] As mentioned, in the neoendocrine setting, residual cancer cells may remain scattered across the tumor bed and may be particularly difficult to discern

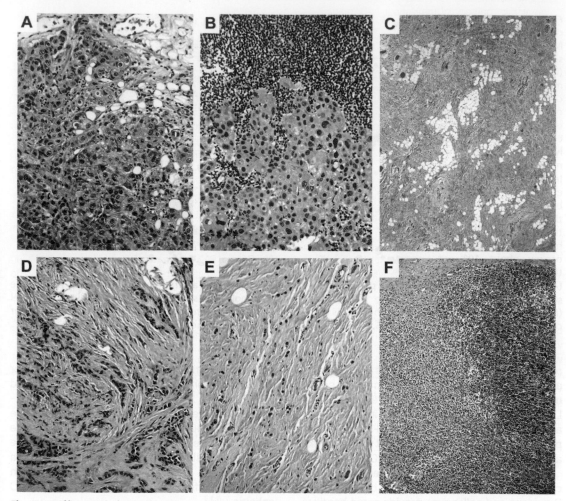

Fig. 11. Differential chemotherapy response according to tumor biology. This patient had 2 concurrent carcinomas, and both were exposed to cytotoxic chemotherapy. The high-grade triple-negative invasive ductal carcinoma had a pathologic complete response (pCR). (*A*) Invasive ductal carcinoma on initial core biopsy. (*B*) Lymph node metastasis of the invasive ductal carcinoma on core biopsy before therapy. (*C*) Tumor bed at the site of ductal carcinoma in the breast, low power. There was no evidence of residual ductal carcinoma in the breast or lymph nodes. From the same patient, a concurrent lobular carcinoma did not achieve pathologic complete response (pCR) with chemotherapy. (*D*) Invasive lobular carcinoma on core biopsy. This tumor was E-cadherin negative, positive for both ER and PR, and HER2 negative (not shown). (*E*) The postchemotherapy resection had residual invasive lobular carcinoma with a decrease in cellularity. (*F*) At lower power, abundant metastatic lobular carcinoma remained in a lymph node (left portion of image). Luminal A tumors, such as invasive lobular carcinoma, often show less response to cytotoxic chemotherapy.

histologically. A dedicated prognostic algorithm was proposed by Ellis and colleagues for neoendocrine treatment, which integrates residual T stage, N stage, ER status, and proliferation as assayed by Ki-67 immunostaining, the Preoperative Endocrine Prognostic Index, or PEPI score **Table 1**.[36]

In contrast, HER2 positive tumors treated with modern targeted therapy and chemotherapy, along with high grade, highly proliferative, "triple negative" (ER, PR, HER2 negative) carcinomas have considerably higher pCR rates of up to or exceeding 60% in very recent studies.[11,15,26,37]

The difference in chemotherapy response is strikingly illustrated in patients with concurrent tumors of different intrinsic types (**Fig. 11**).

Neoadjuvant therapy may result in a shift in the biomarker or even mutational profile of the residual carcinoma, possibly due to the selection and outgrowth of resistant subclones.[1,6] It is our current practice to repeat the immunohistochemical biomarker panel after chemotherapy (ER, PR, HER2, Ki-67). Published estimates cite widely variable postchemotherapy discordance rates, with an average of 5% to 10% of cases for HER2, 10% to 15% for ER, and higher for

PR.[14,15,16,38,39] PR expression is expected to diminish setting of neoendocrine aromatase inhibitor therapy (letrozole, anastrozole, exemestane), and both ER and PR should decrease with fulvestrant.[34,40,41] "Gain" of ER or HER2 has potential implications for postoperative therapy. Posttherapy assessment of tumor-infiltrating lymphocytes (TILS) has shown some interest with small, early studies suggesting more favorable outcomes with more abundant TILS.[42,43]

PATHOLOGIC RESPONSE AND TAILORED POSTSURGICAL THERAPY

Pathologic response to neoadjuvant therapy allows for tailored selection of postneoadjuvant treatment, particularly in triple-negative and Her2+ breast cancer.[1] After neoadjuvant chemotherapy for early-stage triple-negative breast cancer, the addition of adjuvant capecitabine in patients with residual disease leads to prolonged disease-free survival and improved overall survival. The CREATE-X trial evaluated 910 patients with Her2-negative residual disease after neoadjuvant chemotherapy who were randomized to adjuvant capecitabine or placebo for up to 6 months.[1,44] In the subset of patients with triple-negative breast cancer, the disease-free survival at 5 years was 69.8% with capecitabine as compared with 56.1% with placebo, with a hazard ratio for recurrence, second cancer, or death of 0.58 (95% confidence interval (CI): 0.39–0.87). The overall survival with capecitabine was 78.8% as compared with 70.3% with placebo, with hazard ratio for death of 0.52 (95% CI: 0.30–0.90).[1,44]

After neoadjuvant treatment of early-stage Her2+ breast cancer, the addition of trastuzumab emtansine (TDM1) in patients with residual disease leads to prolonged invasive disease-free survival. TDM1 is an antibody–drug conjugate comprised of trastuzumab linked to the microtubule inhibitor DM1. In the KATHERINE trial, 1486 patients with a residual disease were randomized to adjuvant TDM1 or trastuzumab to complete 1 year of Her2-targeted therapy.[45] The 3-year invasive disease-free survival with TDM1 was 88.3% as compared with 77.0% with trastuzumab.[45] Trials are ongoing for other agents including immunotherapies, and this is a rapidly evolving field.

SUMMARY

Neoadjuvant systemic therapy represents a well-established advance in breast cancer treatment, importantly allowing for the assessment of response. This paradigm has not only facilitated studies of novel chemotherapy protocols but also

allows tailoring of therapy for individual patients (escalation or de-escalation of surgery, radiotherapy, further chemotherapy). Careful pathologic analysis of the postneoadjuvant therapy specimen is central to these advances, including radiologic correlation, judicious sampling and mapping, identification, and measurement of residual tumor in breast and lymph node specimens, standardized reporting, and consideration for repeat biomarker testing.

CLINICS CARE POINTS

- Gross examination and cassette mapping tailored to the chemotherapy setting with knowledge of prechemotherapy size is essential.

- Postchemotherapy carcinoma can be relatively occult and diligent examination of the tumor bed is mandatory.

- The degree of treatment response to chemotherapy is prognostic, particularly in ER-negative carcinomas.

- Treatment response can be meaningfully stratified using the Residucal Cancer Burden (RCB) or other systems.

- Studies have shown benefit of additional chemotherapy in certain groups of patients who do not achieve a pathologic complete response (pCR), see Tailored Postsurgical Therapy Section.

DISCLOSURE

The authors have nothing to disclose.

REFERENCES

1. Pelizzari G, Gerratana L, Basile D, et al. Post-neoadjuvant strategies in breast cancer: from risk assessment to treatment escalation. Cancer Treat Rev 2019;72:7–14.

2. Manguso N, Gangi A, Giuliano AE. Neoadjuvant chemotherapy and surgical management of the axilla in breast cancer: a review of current data. Oncology (Williston Park) 2015;29(10):733–8.

3. Kummel S, Holtschmidt J, Loibl S. Surgical treatment of primary breast cancer in the neoadjuvant setting. Br J Surg 2014;101(8):912–24.

4. Fisher ER, Wang J, Bryant J, et al. Pathobiology of preoperative chemotherapy: findings from the National Surgical Adjuvant Breast and Bowel (NSABP) protocol B-18. Cancer 2002;95(4):681–95.

5. Symmans WF, Peintinger F, Hatzis C, et al. Measurement of residual breast cancer burden to predict survival after neoadjuvant chemotherapy. J Clin Oncol 2007;25(28):4414–22.

6. Sahoo S, Lester SC. Pathology considerations in patients treated with neoadjuvant chemotherapy. Surg Pathol Clin 2012;5(3):749–74.

7. Bossuyt V, Spring L. Pathologic evaluation of response to neoadjuvant therapy drives treatment changes and improves long-term outcomes for breast cancer patients. Breast J 2020;26(6):1189–98.

8. Bossuyt V. Processing and reporting of breast specimens in the neoadjuvant setting. Surg Pathol Clin 2018;11(1):213–30.

9. Cortazar P, Zhang L, Untch M, et al. Pathological complete response and long-term clinical benefit in breast cancer: the CTNeoBC pooled analysis. Lancet 2014;384(9938):164–72.

10. Pilewskie M, Morrow M. Axillary nodal management following neoadjuvant chemotherapy: a review. JAMA Oncol 2017;3(4):549–55.

11. Mrkonjic M, Berman HK, Done SJ, et al. Breast specimen handling and reporting in the post-neoadjuvant setting: challenges and advances. J Clin Pathol 2019;72(2):120–32.

12. Peintinger F, Sinn B, Hatzis C, et al. Reproducibility of residual cancer burden for prognostic assessment of breast cancer after neoadjuvant chemotherapy. Mod Pathol 2015;28(7):913–20.

13. Provenzano E, Bossuyt V, Viale G, et al. Standardization of pathologic evaluation and reporting of post-neoadjuvant specimens in clinical trials of breast cancer: recommendations from an international working group. Mod Pathol 2015;28(9):1185–201.

14. Provenzano E, Pinder SE. Modern therapies and iatrogenic changes in breast pathology. Histopathology 2017;70(1):40–55.

15. Pinder SE, Rakha EA, Purdie CA, et al. Macroscopic handling and reporting of breast cancer specimens pre- and post-neoadjuvant chemotherapy treatment: review of pathological issues and suggested approaches. Histopathology 2015;67(3):279–93.

16. Baker GM, King TA, Schnitt SJ. Evaluation of breast and axillary lymph node specimens in breast cancer patients treated with neoadjuvant systemic therapy. Adv Anat Pathol 2019;26(4):221–34.

17. Sejben A, Koszo R, Kahan Z, et al. Examination of tumor regression grading systems in breast cancer patients who received neoadjuvant therapy. Pathol Oncol Res 2020;26(4):2747–54.

18. Bossuyt V, Provenzano E, Symmans WF, et al. Recommendations for standardized pathological characterization of residual disease for neoadjuvant clinical trials of breast cancer by the BIG-NABCG collaboration. Ann Oncol 2015;26(7):1280–91.

19. Sahoo S, Lester SC. Pathology of breast carcinomas after neoadjuvant chemotherapy: an overview with recommendations on specimen processing and reporting. Arch Pathol Lab Med 2009; 133(4):633–42.

20. Zombori T, Cserni G. Patterns of regression in breast cancer after primary systemic treatment. Pathol Oncol Res 2019;25(3):1153–61.

21. Rabban JT, Glidden D, Kwan ML, et al. Pure and predominantly pure intralymphatic breast carcinoma after neoadjuvant chemotherapy: an unusual and adverse pattern of residual disease. Am J Surg Pathol 2009;33(2):256–63.

22. Cheng E, Ko D, Nguyen M, et al. Residual pure intralymphatic breast carcinoma following neoadjuvant chemotherapy is indicative of poor clinical outcome, even in node-negative patients. Am J Surg Pathol 2017;41(9):1275–82.

23. MacColl CE, Pare G, Salehi A, et al. Postneoadjuvant pure and predominantly pure intralymphatic breast carcinoma: case series and literature review. Am J Surg Pathol 2021;45(4):537–42.

24. Guilbert MC, Overmoyer B, Lester SC. Pure intralymphatic invasion in the absence of stromal invasion after neoadjuvant therapy: a rare pattern of residual breast carcinoma. Am J Surg Pathol 2018;42(5):679–86.

25. Rabban JT, Chen YY. D2-40 expression by breast myoepithelium: potential pitfalls in distinguishing intralymphatic carcinoma from in situ carcinoma. Hum Pathol 2008;39(2):175–83.

26. Balasubramanian R, Morgan C, Shaari E, et al. Wire guided localisation for targeted axillary node dissection is accurate in axillary staging in node positive breast cancer following neoadjuvant chemotherapy. Eur J Surg Oncol 2020;46(6):1028–33.

27. Dixon JM, Cartlidge CWJ. Twenty-five years of change in the management of the axilla in breast cancer. Breast J 2020;26(1):22–6.

28. Bear HD, McGuire KP. Sentinel node biopsy after neoadjuvant systemic therapy for breast cancer: the method matters. Ann Surg Oncol 2019;26(8): 2316–8.

29. Rubio IT. Sentinel lymph node biopsy after neoadjuvant treatment in breast cancer: work in progress. Eur J Surg Oncol 2016;42(3):326–32.

30. Cimino-Mathews A. Axillary lymph node inclusions. Surg Pathol Clin 2018;11(1):43–59.

31. Morrow M, Van Zee KJ, Patil S, et al. Axillary dissection and nodal irradiation can be avoided for most node-positive Z0011-eligible breast cancers: a prospective validation study of 793 patients. Ann Surg 2017;266(3):457–62.

32. Weiss A, King TA, Mittendorf EA. The landmark series: neoadjuvant endocrine therapy for breast cancer. Ann Surg Oncol 2020;27(9):3393–401.

33. Pariser AC, Sedghi T, Soulos PR, et al. Utilization, duration, and outcomes of neoadjuvant endocrine therapy in the United States. Breast Cancer Res Treat 2019;178(2):110 20.

34. Ellis MJ, Ma C. Letrozole in the neoadjuvant setting: the P024 trial. Breast Cancer Res Treat 2007; 105(Suppl 1):33–43.

35. Spring LM, Gupta A, Reynolds KL, et al. Neoadjuvant endocrine therapy for estrogen receptor-positive breast cancer: a systematic review and meta-analysis. JAMA Oncol 2016;2(11):1477–86.

36. Ellis MJ, Tao Y, Luo J, et al. Outcome prediction for estrogen receptor-positive breast cancer based on postneoadjuvant endocrine therapy tumor characteristics. J Natl Cancer Inst 2008;100(19):1380–8.

37. Tasoulis MK, Lee HB, Yang W, et al. Accuracy of post-neoadjuvant chemotherapy image-guided breast biopsy to predict residual cancer. JAMA Surg 2020;55(12):e204103.

38. Rey-Vargas L, Mejia-Henao JC, Sanabria-Salas MC, et al. Effect of neoadjuvant therapy on breast cancer biomarker profile. BMC Cancer 2020;20(1):675.

39. Gahlaut R, Bennett A, Fatayer H, et al. Effect of neoadjuvant chemotherapy on breast cancer phenotype, ER/PR and HER2 expression - Implications for the practising oncologist. Eur J Cancer 2016;60:40–8.

40. Kurosumi M, Takatsuka Y, Watanabe T, et al. Histopathological assessment of anastrozole and tamoxifen as preoperative (neoadjuvant) treatment in postmenopausal Japanese women with hormone receptor-positive breast cancer in the PROACT trial. J Cancer Res Clin Oncol 2008;134(6):715–22.

41. Agrawal A, Robertson JF, Cheung KL, et al. Biological effects of fulvestrant on estrogen receptor positive human breast cancer: short, medium and long-term effects based on sequential biopsies. Int J Cancer 2016;138(1):146–59.

42. Luen SJ, Salgado R, Dieci MV, et al. Prognostic implications of residual disease tumor-infiltrating lymphocytes and residual cancer burden in triple-negative breast cancer patients after neoadjuvant chemotherapy. Ann Oncol 2019;30(2):236–42.

43. Pinard C, Debled M, Ben Rejeb H, et al. Residual cancer burden index and tumor-infiltrating lymphocyte subtypes in triple-negative breast cancer after neoadjuvant chemotherapy. Breast Cancer Res Treat 2020;179(1):11–23.

44. Masuda N, Lee SJ, Ohtani S, et al. Adjuvant capecitabine for breast cancer after preoperative chemotherapy. N Engl J Med 2017;376(22):2147–59.

45. von Minckwitz G, Huang CS, Mano MS, et al. Trastuzumab emtansine for residual invasive HER2-positive breast cancer. N Engl J Med 2019;380(7):617–28.

High-Grade Spindle Cell Lesions of the Breast
Key Pathologic and Clinical Updates

Esther Yoon, MD[a],*, Qingqing Ding, MD, PhD[a],
Kelly Hunt, MD[b], Aysegul Sahin, MD[a]

KEYWORDS

- Breast • High-grade spindle cells • Malignant phyllodes tumor • Metaplastic breast carcinoma
- Primary breast sarcomas • *MED12*

Key points

- Malignant phyllodes tumors (MPTs) have high-grade spindled stromal cells lined by epithelium and subepithelial stromal condensation, creating a classic "leaf-like" architecture with varying amounts of heterologous elements; *MED12* and *TERT* mutations are common.

- Spindle cell carcinomas (SpCCs) and matrix-producing metaplastic breast carcinomas (MP-MBCs) are both high-grade metaplastic breast carcinomas (MBCs). SpCCs are composed of pure spindle cells and foci of benign-appearing epithelioid or squamoid areas with no distinct architecture and growth pattern, whereas MP-MBCs are predominantly composed of malignant heterologous elements with no or focal spindle cells.

- Primary breast sarcomas (PBSs) and metastases to the breast are extremely rare; MPTs, SpCCs, and MP-MBCs must be ruled out with an inclusive immunohistochemical panel and clinical history.

- MPTs are usually positive for CD34, CD117, and BCL-2, and metaplastic carcinomas are positive for epithelial markers; P63 can be seen in both MPTs and MBCs.

- Surgery, sentinel lymph node biopsy, adjuvant radiation therapy, and chemotherapy are standards of care for MBCs, whereas MPTs and PBSs are treated with surgery with negative margins and the use of radiation therapy is more controversial.

ABSTRACT

Most of the high-grade spindle cell lesions of the breast are malignant phyllodes tumors (MPTs), spindle cell carcinomas (SpCCs), and matrix-producing metaplastic breast carcinomas (MP-MBCs). MPTs have neoplastic spindle stromal cells and a classic leaf-like architecture with subepithelial stromal condensation. MPTs are often positive for CD34, CD117, and bcl-2 and are associated with MED12, TERT, and RARA mutations. SpCCs and MP-MBCs are high-grade metaplastic carcinomas, whereas neoplastic epithelial cells become spindled or

show heterologous mesenchymal differentiation, respectively. The expression of epithelial markers must be evaluated to make a diagnosis. SAS, or rare metastatic spindle cell tumors, are seen in the breast, and clinical history is the best supporting evidence. Surgical resection is the standard of care.

OVERVIEW

Spindle cell lesions of the breast include a wide spectrum of entities, from reactive processes to benign neoplasms to high-grade malignant neoplasms. High-grade spindle cell lesions include

---

[a] Department of Anatomical Pathology, The University of Texas MD Anderson Cancer Center, 1515 Holcombe Blvd, Houston TX 77030-4009, USA; [b] Department of Breast Surgical Oncology, The University of Texas MD Anderson Cancer Center, 1515 Holcombe Boulevard, Unit 85, Room G1.3565C, Houston, TX 77030-4009, USA
* Corresponding author.
E-mail address: ecyoon@mdanderson.org

Surgical Pathology 15 (2022) 77–93
https://doi.org/10.1016/j.path.2021.11.005
1875-9181/22/Published by Elsevier Inc.

Abbreviations	
IBC	invasive breast carcinoma
MBC	metaplastic breast carcinoma
MP-MBC	matrix-producing metaplastic breast carcinoma
MPT	malignant phyllodes tumor
PBS	primary breast sarcoma
PT	phyllodes tumor
SpCC	spindle cell carcinoma

malignant phyllodes tumors (MPTs), spindle cell carcinomas (SpCCs), matrix-producing metastatic breast carcinomas (MP-MBCs), primary breast sarcomas (PBSs), and rare metastases. In this article, we focus on MPTs, SpCCs, and MP-MBCs and discuss their relevant differentials (PBSs and metastatic carcinomas), with an emphasis on morphologic characteristics, advancements in molecular data, and differences in prognosis and treatment.

MALIGNANT PHYLLODES TUMOR (MPT)

Phyllodes tumors (PTs) are uncommon fibroepithelial lesions, accounting for less than 1% of breast tumors. The patients are usually 40 to 50 years old, with MPTs occurring 2 to 5 years later than benign PTs.[1] PTs are seen in higher incidences among Asian women, and MPTs are more frequent among Hispanics in Central and South America.[1,2] PTs grow rapidly, and the patients present with a painless, palpable mass, with or without bloody nipple discharge. Unfortunately, imaging modalities do not reliably distinguish MPTs from benign PTs.

GROSS FEATURES

PTs are firm, round, and relatively well-circumscribed multinodular tumors. The mean size of PTs is 4 to 5 cm; MPTs are usually larger than benign PTs. Multifocal and bilateral PTs are rare, and skin changes are uncommon. However, as the tumor grows, it can stretch and even ulcerate the overlying skin, regardless of the histologic

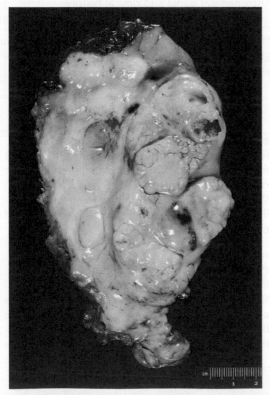

Fig. 1. *Phyllodes tumor (PT).* The cut surface shows a lobulated tumor with a fleshy variegated appearance and hemorrhage composed of solid and cystic components with clefts. Microscopic examination revealed a malignant phyllodes tumor.

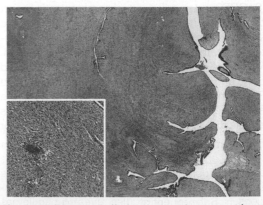

Fig. 2. *Malignant phyllodes tumor.* The tumor shows leaf-like architecture and stromal expansion at low power. *Inset* shows stromal hypercellularity and spindle cell proliferation.

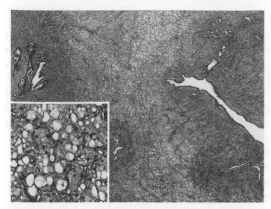

Fig. 3. Malignant phyllodes tumor. Prominent subepithelial condensation and heterologous element. *Inset* shows malignant liposarcomatous differentiation.

grade. The cut surface is typically solid, gray-white, and fibrous. Cleft-like spaces may be seen in large tumors. The flesh-like, myxoid cut surface is often associated with areas of necrosis, cystic degeneration, and hemorrhage (**Fig. 1**).

MICROSCOPIC FEATURES

Stromal hypercellularity with an associated benign epithelial component, resulting in "leaf-like" architecture, is the hallmark of PTs (**Fig. 2**). The neoplastic spindle-shaped fibroblasts and myofibroblasts expand the stroma and exaggerate the intracanalicular growth pattern. A distinct hypercellular stromal layer immediately beneath the ducts and clefts, called subepithelial stromal condensation, is also characteristic (**Fig. 3**). The epithelial cells may undergo apocrine or squamous metaplasia, or hyperplasia with some cytologic atypia; rarely, they undergo malignant transformation. MPTs demonstrate permeative tumor borders with marked and diffused stromal hypercellularity, marked stromal cell atypia, stromal overgrowth (defined by the absence of epithelial elements in one low-power microscopic field), high mitotic count ($\geq$5 mitoses/mm^2), and the presence of malignant heterologous elements such as liposarcoma, chondrosarcoma, or osteosarcoma. PTs containing a well-differentiated liposarcomatous component have a favorable course compared with other malignant heterologous elements, with no recurrence or distant metastases, and do not have *MDM2* reactivity or amplification, making them distinct from liposarcomas of soft tissue.[3] The 5th edition of the WHO's *Breast Tumors* states that the presence of well-differentiated liposarcoma does not characterize a tumor as an MPT (see Fig. 3).[1]

DIFFERENTIAL DIAGNOSIS

In the absence of "leaf-like" architecture and heterologous elements, the main diagnostic considerations are periductal stromal tumors, SpCCs, and sarcomas with fibroblastic differentiation. The differential diagnoses for MPTs with heterologous elements include MP-MBCs and sarcomas of specific mesenchymal differentiation, either primary tumors or metastases.

Periductal stromal tumors are also biphasic tumors in which spindle cells can exhibit varying degrees of atypia and mitosis. They lack the classic "leaf-like" architecture of PTs, but because of some morphologic overlap, some believe that periductal stromal tumors are a subtype of PT.

DIAGNOSIS

In the presence of classic histologic features such as "leaf-like" architecture, subepithelial stromal condensation, and a benign epithelial component, the diagnosis of MPTs can be straightforward. Immunohistochemical (IHC) stains, such as CD34, CD117, BCL-2, actin, and desmin, can support the diagnosis of PT in challenging cases. However, the expression depends on whether the tumor is benign, borderline, or malignant. CD34 is consistently positive in benign PTs, but the positivity decreases to less than 50% in MPTs.[4–7] On the other hand, the expression of CD117 and BCL-2 increases in higher grade PTs.[4,6,8,9] The broad-spectrum cytokeratins (CKs) and high-molecular-weight CKs are negative in MPTs, and their expression supports the diagnosis of SpCCs and MP-MBCs instead. P63 expression is frequently seen across MPTs, SpCCs, and MP-MBCs and is therefore not helpful alone.

MED12, *TERT*, and *RARA* mutations are the 3 most common mutations seen in MPT. Recurrent mediator complex subunit (*MED12*) mutations in exon 2 are common mutations shared by PTs, fibroadenomas, and uterine leiomyomas.[10–22] The reported frequency of *MED12* mutation in MPTs ranges from 8% to 45.8%[15,23,24]; some studies report a decreasing frequency of *MED12* mutations with an increasing histologic grade in PTs,[23,25–27] while other studies do not.[16,20] Telomerase reverse transcriptase (*TERT*) promoter mutations are seen in 52%–70% of all PTs, with higher rates seen in borderline PTs and MPTs.[15,16,25,28–31] *TERT* gene alterations are observed much less commonly in FAs and are found almost exclusively in tumors with *MED12* mutation.[29] Lastly, RARalpha is a part of the ER transcription complex, and the *RARA* mutation is found in 14%–32% of all fibroepithelial lesions, although it is more frequent in PTs than in FAs and is observed in less than 10% of MPTs.[10,13,23] Similar to *TERT* mutation, the coexpression of *MED12* and *RARA* mutations is also statistically significant.[10,27]

PROGNOSIS

PTs are treated with surgical excision with negative margins, and breast-conserving surgery and mastectomies have similar outcomes.[32–39] PTs rarely metastasize to lymph nodes[5]; therefore, sentinel lymph node biopsy and axillary lymph node dissection are not indicated. Local recurrence is common, usually occurring within 2 to 3 years of diagnosis.[1,40] The reported local recurrence rates for benign PTs, borderline PTs, and MPTs are 8%–17%, 13%–25%, and 18%–30%, respectively.[1,41] The recurrent PT can be of the original or a higher grade, and each subsequent event increases the risk of malignant transformation.[42] A positive surgical margin is the most consistently reported risk factor, but margin width less than 1 cm, younger age, large tumor size, necrosis, stromal cellularity, and high histologic grade all have been associated with a higher rate of recurrence.[41–44] In cases of recurrent or metastatic disease, the management approach follows the principles of those for soft tissue sarcoma.

The role and administration of adjuvant radiotherapy (RT) or chemotherapy are still controversial. The utilization of RT in patients with MPT has increased over time,[45] but the data are mixed, and the long-term benefits are unclear. The role of chemotherapy in MPTs is even more limited, and only 2%–3% of patients reported undergoing chemotherapy.[45–47] Chemotherapy may be an option for selected patients with unresectable tumors, and a soft tissue sarcoma regimen may be beneficial in these patients.[48]

Patients with MPTs usually have a dismal prognosis. Stromal atypia, mitoses, overgrowth, and surgical margins (AMOS criteria) are independently significant for predicting clinical behavior, with the surgical margin status being the most important.[49] Metastases develop in about 3%–10% of all patients with PT, usually within 3 to 8 years.[1,2] The metastatic rate ranges from 10% to 50% in MPTs.[32,34,35,39,46] Large tumor size and malignant heterologous elements are also associated with an increased likelihood of metastasis. The most frequent sites of distant metastases are the lungs and bones, and most metastases consist of only stromal elements.[1,5] The survival rate of patients with MPT is approximately 60%–80% at 5 years.[32,50]

SPINDLE CELL CARCINOMA (SpCC)

Spindle cell carcinomas (SpCCs) were previously classified as "squamous cell carcinoma with pseudosarcomatous stroma" because of the presence of benign-appearing squamous epithelium scattered throughout the spindled area.[51] SpCCs belong to the pure monophasic sarcomatoid carcinoma subtype of metaplastic breast carcinomas (MBCs). SpCCs account for 0.02%–0.5% of all invasive breast cancers (IBCs).[52,53] The median patient age ranges from 60 to 68 years old.[53–55] On imaging, SpCCs may seem relatively benign, more similar to fibromyxoid stroma than other aggressive IBCs, with possible calcifications and solid and cystic components.[56,57]

GROSS FEATURES

SpCC is a relatively large firm mass in the breast parenchyma with no associated skin changes or nipple discharge. The macroscopic features are not specific; SpCCs can be nodular, infiltrative, or well circumscribed. The cut surface reveals a white to gray to pink to tan tumor with possible cystic and necrotic areas.

MICROSCOPIC FEATURES

There is no required percentage of spindle cell component for a diagnosis of SpCC, but the tumor is moderately to markedly cellular and spindle cells comprise at least half and, in most cases, more than 80% of the tumor.[54,55,58] SpCCs are typically Nottingham histologic grade 3 with no tubule formation, moderate to severe nuclear pleomorphism, and a high mitotic rate (**Fig. 4**). The spindle cells grow long or short fascicles, making herringbone, interwoven, or storiform patterns, mimicking fibrosarcoma, and often obliterating the normal breast architecture. Foci of epithelioid or squamoid cells, which tend to be located in the tumor periphery, strongly support the diagnosis of SpCC. Generous sampling may reveal such foci and, infrequently, conventional IBC, or an in situ component.

DIFFERENTIAL DIAGNOSIS

The main differential diagnosis for high-grade SpCC includes MPTs and PBS or metastatic sarcoma. However, because of SpCC's pure spindle cell morphologic characteristics, low-grade spindle cell lesions, such as desmoid fibromatosis, fibromatosis-like metaplastic carcinoma, and dermatofibrosarcoma protuberans, may be under diagnostic consideration.

Desmoid fibromatosis lacks squamous or epithelioid foci; the spindle cells are positive for nuclear β-catenin but negative for CKs. Fibromatosis-like MBCs are composed of relatively monomorphic bland spindle cells with pale

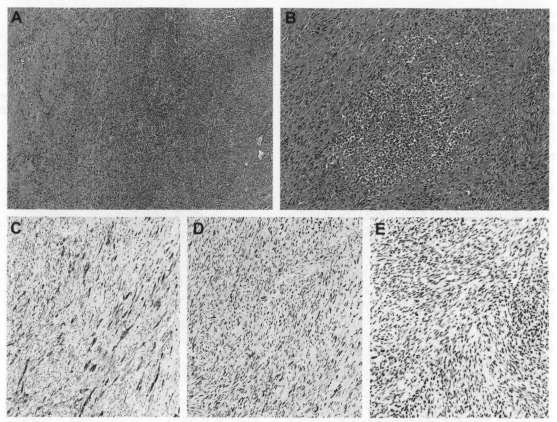

Fig. 4. *Spindle cell carcinoma (SpCC)* (*A*) Spindle cell proliferation intervening through hyalinized stroma. (*B*) Closer inspection reveals a focus of epithelioid cells in the tumor. SpCCs are positive for (*C*) CK5/6, (*D*) p63, and (*E*) TRPS1 stains.

eosinophilic cytoplasm and mild to moderate nuclear atypia. The tumors show varying degrees of collagenization and tend to be less cellular than SpCCs, with fewer mitoses. These tumors are easily distinguished from high-grade spindle cell carcinomas by their benign appearance and have a relatively favorable outcome. Dermatofibrosarcoma protuberance arises in the dermal skin and may extend to the breast parenchyma, and it can mimic primary breast spindle cell lesions. Dermatofibrosarcoma protuberances are hypercellular and composed of spindle cells with hyperchromatic nuclei and scattered mitoses. They are classically arranged in short, storiform, and intersecting fascicles and stain positive for CD34.

DIAGNOSIS

The use of a combination of epithelial and myoepithelial markers is recommended, and the panel usually includes broad-spectrum CKs (AE1/AE3 and MNKF115), high-molecular-weight CKs (34βE12, CK5/6, CK14, and CK17), low-molecular-weight CKs (CK8/18, CAM5.2, CK7, and CK19), EMA and myoepithelial markers, p63, S-100, and smooth muscle actin. Trichorhinophalangeal syndrome 1 (TRPS1) was recently recognized as a highly specific and sensitive breast marker, and its expression is retained even in high-grade tumors, whereby GATA3 is frequently lost.[59] CD34 and β-catenin are often included in the panel to rule out PTs and fibromatosis, respectively. The most sensitive epithelial marker is broad-spectrum CKs, followed by high-molecular-weight CKs and low-molecular-weight CKs.[58,60,61] SpCCs are more likely to be positive for p63, CD10, and CK14 but much less likely to be positive for CK7.[60,61]

In general, MBCs harbor more mutations in the PI3K pathway (*PIK3CA*, *PIK3R1*, and *PTEN*), MAPK pathway (*NF1*, *KRAS*, and *NRAS*), and Wnt pathway (*FAT1* and *CCN6* [*WISP3*]).[62–65] SpCCs do not harbor *TP53* and *RB1* gene mutations as frequently as do other subtypes of MBCs and triple-negative breast carcinomas (TNBCs).[62–64] However, molecular data on the different subtypes of MBC are still somewhat primitive and limited because of the rarity of these tumors and the mutational complexity and diversity in each subtype.

PROGNOSIS

For the most part, SpCCs and other subtypes of MBC are treated the same as high-grade IBCs. Surgery, RT, and chemotherapy are the mainstays of treatment, and there is no difference in OS rate between mastectomy or breast-conserving surgery. Sentinel lymph node biopsy should be part of the surgical planning.[66] The role of endocrine therapy and HER2-targeted therapy is limited, although it has been reported that 5.2% and 23.0% of MBCs are HER2-positive and HER2-negative/hormone receptor-positive, respectively.[67]

Large population-based studies have reported the use of RT and chemotherapy in 38.6%–76% and 65%–79% of patients with MBCs, respectively.[68–71] Improved survival is associated with RT and chemotherapy, especially in the early stages of the disease.[66,68–73] Nevertheless, RT and chemotherapy are still underutilized than conventional IBC.

The survival data on different subtypes of MBC are limited and somewhat confusing in the medical literature. Compared with other IBCs and TNBCs, high-grade MBCs have a more aggressive clinical course and carry a worse prognosis, with a higher risk of local recurrence and shorter disease-free survival (DFS) and overall survival (OS) durations.[68,74–78] The 5-year OS rate of patients with MBC is approximately 54%–69%, compared with 89% for IBC and 73% for patients with TNBC.[79,80] MBCs metastasize hematogeneously; the most common sites of distant metastasis are the lungs and brain.[74]

MATRIX-PRODUCING METAPLASTIC BREAST CARCINOMA (MP-MBC)

Matrix-producing metaplastic breast carcinomas (MP-MBCs) belong to a group of MBCs with heterologous mesenchymal differentiation. MP-MBCs show an abrupt transition from the epithelial to mesenchymal component, usually without the intervening spindle cell component, although a focal presence of intervening spindle cells should not exclude the diagnosis of MP-MBC.[1] Usually patients are diagnosed in their 50s. Imaging usually correlates with the mesenchymal component; for example, ossification can be seen in tumors with osteoid differentiation. MP-MBCs frequently show posterior acoustic enhancement on ultrasound[81,82] and marginal (ring-like) enhancement following IV contrast on MRI.[82–84]

GROSS FEATURES

The tumors are somewhat circumscribed and round to oval and less frequently have infiltrating borders. The mean size is 2.5 to 3.0 cm.[85–87] The appearance of cut surfaces depends on their heterologous mesenchymal component and can be mucoid or glistening and white to gray or pink to

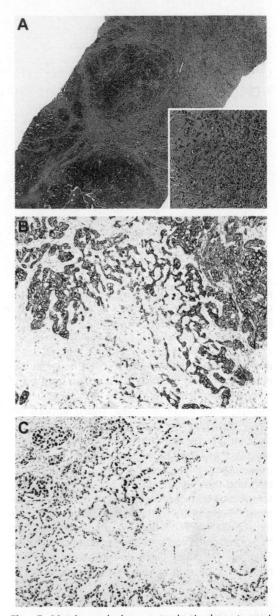

Fig. 5. Matrix-producing metaplastic breast carcinoma (MP-MBC) (A) Core biopsy shows foci of chondroid matrix surrounded by a rim of poorly differentiated carcinoma. *Inset* shows abrupt transition from poorly differentiated carcinoma in a chondroid matrix. Epithelioid cells are positive for (B) AE1/AE3 and (C) TRPS1 stains.

tan. Many have central softening, corresponding to tumor necrosis.

MICROSCOPIC FEATURES

The percentage of epithelial and mesenchymal components varies. Approximately 15%–20% of MP-MBCs lack histologic evidence of an epithelial component, and the diagnosis is based on IHC or ultrastructural findings.[85] The carcinomatous component is usually moderately to poorly differentiated and of the ductal phenotype. Most often, the heterologous mesenchymal elements are chondroid or osseous, but rhabdomyoid, lipomatous, and even neural elements have been reported.[1] The appearance of the matrix can range from mucoid to overt osteoid or cartilaginous with hyalinization. The heterologous components also vary in histologic grade, ranging from benign or low-grade to malignant, resembling their sarcomatous counterpart (**Fig. 5**).

DIFFERENTIAL DIAGNOSIS

The differential diagnosis of MP-MBCs largely depends on the heterologous mesenchymal component and includes a specific subtype of sarcomas, MPTs with heterologous elements, or metastasis, including but not limited to melanoma.

DIAGNOSIS

The presence of an in situ or invasive epithelioid component is highly supportive of MP-MBCs, and the expression of epithelial markers in the heterologous mesenchymal component is required to make a diagnosis. A recently published breast marker, TRPS1, is positive in 86% of MBCs, and more than half of cases demonstrated strong diffuse expression, supporting mammary epithelial cell differentiation in the heterologous elements.[59] Higher proportions of EMA, S100, Bcl-2, and SOX10 are positive in MP-MBCs than in other subtypes of MBC.[61,88] CD34 is consistently negative and helps to differentiate MBCs from MPTs. Clinical history is important in establishing the history of prior malignancy and diagnosis of metastasis. No unique or highly specific molecular alteration has been reliably reported in MP-MBCs.

PROGNOSIS

Treatment is similar to that for other subtypes of MBCs and high-grade IBCs, with most of the patients with MP-MBC undergoing surgical excision and receiving RT and chemotherapy. Lymph node metastasis is relatively uncommon, occurring in 18% of cases in a large review.[85] Distant metastasis occurs in between 8% and 31% of cases, and the lungs and pleura are the most common sites.

PRIMARY BREAST SARCOMA (PBS)

Primary breast sarcomas (PBSs) account for less than 1% of all breast malignancies and are extremely rare.[89,90] Exposure to RT is the most significant risk factor; patients who have been exposed to RT have a 9- to 16-fold increase in the relative risk of developing a secondary sarcoma.[91,92] PBS can also develop de novo, associated with some inherited syndromes, or in the setting of long-standing lymphedema of the arm or breast after lymphadenectomy. The most common PBS is radiation associated or secondary angiosarcoma (SAS).[93,94] SAS occurs in approximately 0.05%–0.2% of patients treated with RT,[2,95] with a mean latency period of 5 to 6 years.[96,97] Fibrosarcomas, undifferentiated pleomorphic sarcoma (UPS, formerly known as malignant fibrous histiocytoma), leiomyosarcoma (LMS), rhabdomyosarcoma (RMS), liposarcoma, osteosarcoma, chondrosarcoma, hemangiopericytoma (solitary fibrous tumor), and sarcomas of peripheral nerves have all been reported in the breast.[2,94,98] The American Joint Committee on Cancer staging system for soft tissue sarcoma is used to stage PBS.

The mean age of patients with PBS is 45 to 50 years, and patients with SASs are usually older than are patients with PBSs. In contrast, RMSs of the breast are almost exclusively reported in adolescents and young adults.[99–101] On imaging, PBSs appear as nonspecific hyperdense masses with indistinct borders.[98]

GROSS FEATURES

PBS is usually a relatively large, rapidly growing, firm, and well-circumscribed tumor located in the deep parenchyma. Nipple discharge and skin

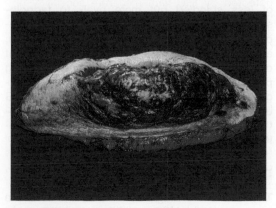

Fig. 6. Angiosarcoma.

changes are uncommon. SASs are dermal-based, with variable infiltration into the subcutaneous tissue, and can present with skin thickening, erythema, or multiple bluish discolorations (**Fig. 6**). LMSs mostly arise in superficial dermis around the nipple–areolar complex. The cut surface of the tumor varies by the type of sarcoma, but for the most part, it seems as an ill-defined mass with a gray, white, or tan fleshy cut surface. Hemorrhage and necrosis are often seen in high-grade sarcomas.

Angiosarcomas can vary from hemangioma-like to solid masses with a hemorrhagic and necrotic center, with more vascular spongy areas toward the periphery of the lesion. Osteosarcomas and chondrosarcomas usually have a variegated appearance, with areas of softening or gelatinous degeneration admixed with foci of necrosis in firm gray to white tissue. Infrequently, a gritty sensation, corresponding to ossification or calcifications, can be appreciated.

MICROSCOPIC FEATURES

For the most part, different PBS subtypes are identical to their counterparts in other parts of the body, with the breast epithelium showing benign changes, including varying degrees of cytologic atypia. However, breast epithelium is nonneoplastic.

SAS and primary angiosarcomas show varying degrees of vasoformative growth patterns, with varying degrees of cellular atypia and mitosis depending on the histologic grade. High-grade angiosarcomas often show a solid growth pattern, with rare slit-like spaces composed of sheets of markedly pleomorphic epithelioid or spindle cells, a high mitotic rate, necrosis, and frequent blood lakes (**Fig. 7**). LMSs and fibrosarcomas are composed of highly pleomorphic spindle cells in fascicles. Most RMSs of the breast are of the alveolar subtype and composed of less spindled but more oval- to tadpole-shaped arranged in fibrous septa encasing "alveolar" nests. Osteosarcomas, chondrosarcomas, and pleomorphic liposarcomas have malignant osteoid, myxochondroid, and bizarre-appearing pleomorphic lipoblasts, respectively. High-grade or poorly differentiated tumors or UPS usually do not have any discernible differentiation seen on histologic examination, IHC, or molecular tests.

DIFFERENTIAL DIAGNOSIS

The differential diagnosis of PBS includes the aforementioned MPTs, SpCCs, MP-MBCs, and

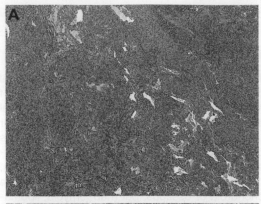
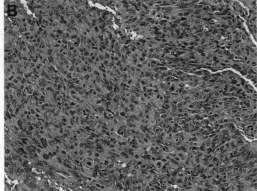
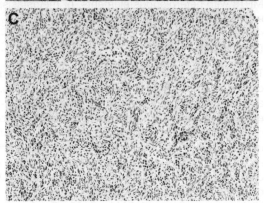

Fig. 7. Angiosarcoma (*A*) Solid neoplasm without a particular growth pattern, with channels and spaces filled with blood and lined by neoplastic endothelial cells. (*B*) High magnification shows markedly pleomorphic spindle cells with a high mitotic rate (*yellow circles*). (*C*) Post-RT angiosarcomas are positive for C-MYC.

metastasis, including melanoma. SpCCs and MP-MBCs contain spindle cells that express epithelial or myoepithelial markers by IHC, whereas MPTs often express CD34, CD117, and BCL-2. Melanoma will stain for melanoma markers (HMB-45, MART-1/Melan-A, tyrosinase, MITF, SOX10, and S-100). Clinical history and body imaging are also important in ruling out metastasis.

DIAGNOSIS

PBSs are extremely rare, and MPTs, MBCs, and metastases should be excluded before making a diagnosis of PBS. IHC analyses are important for confirming the cell lineage, and a panel of negative CKs generally rules out carcinomas. However, focal positivity can be seen in epithelioid areas and should be interpreted with caution.

Angiosarcomas show diffuse and strong immunoreactivity with CD31 and ERG with variable expression of CD34, FL1, and D2-40.[102] Strong nuclear expression of MYC seen in SASs is very helpful for distinguishing between atypical vascular lesions and primary angiosarcomas.[103] Smooth muscle actin and caldesmon are positive in LMSs; myogenin, and myoD1 are positive in RMSs; and desmin is positive in LMSs and RMSs. S-100 can highlight areas of cartilaginous differentiation and help support chondrosarcoma or osteosarcoma. Generally, IHC analysis is of limited use in high-grade sarcomas; generous sampling and meticulous microscopic examination are more useful.

Specific molecular alterations can further support the diagnosis of certain PBSs. For instance, greater than 90% of SASs are associated with high-level amplification of *MYC* at 8q24,[104] and other vascular-specific receptor tyrosine kinases, including TIE1, KDR, TEK, and FLT4, are also characteristically upregulated in angiosarcomas.[102,104] Other diagnostic molecular alterations of sarcoma include PAX3-FHKR (FOXO1) and PAX7-FKHR (FOXO1) fusions (t(21;13) (q35;q14) and t(1;13) (p13;q14)) in RMSs,[101] *MDM2/CDK4* amplification or overexpression in atypical lipomatous tumors/well-differentiated liposarcomas, and *DDIT3* genetic rearrangements or specific *FUS-DDIT3* or *EWSR1-DDIT3* gene fusion in myxoid or round cell liposarcomas. These characteristic molecular alterations are not seen in MPTs or MBCs with heterologous mesenchymal differentiation.

PROGNOSIS

Because of the rarity of PBS, no prospective randomized trials exist to guide therapy, and the treatment principles have been largely extrapolated from nonbreast soft tissue sarcoma treatments. Surgical resection with negative margins is the primary treatment. Although the type of surgical resection does not affect the OS or recurrence rate, the tumors are often large (>5 cm) at presentation, and mastectomy is usually required to achieve a wide negative margin.[90,105] Mastectomy is preferred in primary and secondary angiosarcomas because it affects a much larger area, with multicentricity and a high risk of recurrence.[106] Lymph node metastases are rare, and lymph node dissection is not recommended. Breast sarcomas tend to spread by direct local invasion or hematogenously; the most common sites are the lungs, pleura, and to a lesser extent, the liver and bones.

The roles of RT and chemotherapy in PBS are still unclear; according to the results of 2 large studies, approximately 30% and less than 20% of patients with PBS undergo RT and chemotherapy, respectively.[94,107] There is no consensus, and given that some improved outcomes are associated with RT or chemotherapy, adjuvant RT or chemotherapy could be a reasonable option for selected patients considering the patient's functional status. RT is not generally recommended in those patients with radiation-associated sarcomas. Discussion in a multidisciplinary tumor board is recommended before initiating treatment.

Patients with PBSs generally have a poorer prognosis compared with doing those with IBCs. The prognosis highly depends on the histologic type, tumor size, and disease stage. Some unfavorable prognostic factors are older age,[94,107] tumor size greater than 5 cm[107,108], and the presence of tumor spread or metastasis.[93,109] The 5-year DFS rates and OS rates for PBS range from 44% to 66% and 49% to 67%, respectively.[89,93,105,108,110] Most studies of PBS have had small numbers of patients; thus, comparison outcome data are somewhat limited.

METASTASES TO THE BREAST, INCLUDING MELANOMA

The breast is rarely the site of metastasis unless the disease is widely disseminated. The incidence of metastatic tumors in the breast is approximately 0.2%–3%.[111,112] Most metastases are from the contralateral breast, but metastases from the skin, lungs, stomach, ovaries, kidneys, and soft tissue have been reported.[111–115] RMS alveolar type has a predilection for spreading to the breast in young women.[99–101] Most of the patients have a history of cancer, but in one study, 30% of patients had no history and no metastatic disease elsewhere.[113] Most patients present with a palpable solitary mass involving the unilateral breast.[113,114] Patients can also present with multiple nodules involving the breast or skin, inflammatory skin changes, or completely normal breast tissue. Imaging reveals an ill-defined mass or multiple solitary well-circumscribed nodules. Microcalcifications are not typical of metastasis, and they can be seen in rare incidences.[116]

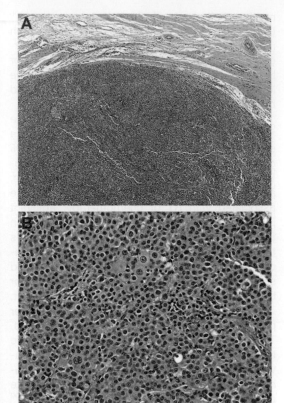

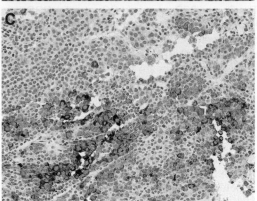

Fig. 8. Metastatic melanoma in the breast. (*A*) Well-circumscribed tumor surrounded by benign breast (*top right arrow*). (*B*) Epithelioid tumor cells with eosinophilic cytoplasm and macronucleoli, resembling melanoma. (*C*) Tumor cells are positive for MART-1, confirming metastatic melanoma.

GROSS FEATURES

Metastatic tumors have no specific macroscopic features; sometimes, they are indistinguishable from the primary breast tumor. Malignant melanoma may show brownish discoloration on the cut surface.

MICROSCOPIC FEATURES

The metastatic tumor presents as a well-circumscribed nodule and is usually sharply demarcated from the surrounding breast tissue. A clue to recognizing metastatic tumors is the absence of in situ carcinoma in the adjacent breast tissue. The histologic characteristics of the original tumor are also helpful. High-grade spindled cells are more commonly associated with metastatic melanomas and sarcomas. Some of the classic features of melanoma include cell discohesion; eosinophilic cytoplasm with fine, dust-like, or coarse granular pigments; and vesicular nuclei with inclusion-like macronucleoli (**Fig. 8**). Metastasis of other sarcomas is extremely rare in the breast; their microscopic features are identical to those found elsewhere in the body.

DIFFERENTIAL DIAGNOSIS

With no prior history of malignancy elsewhere, primary breast carcinomas, including IBCs, MBCs, and MPTs, are included in the main differential diagnosis.

DIAGNOSIS

Investigating a metastasis of unknown primary in the breast can be challenging. A broad panel of organ- or tumor-specific IHC analyses can help, but no marker is 100% specific. TRPS1 is specific for mammary epithelium, and negative expression supports metastasis from nonmammary sites. At least one melanoma marker (HMB-45, MART-1/Melan-A, tyrosinase, MITF, SOX10, and S-100) should be included. However, SOX10 can be positive in MBCs, so it is less helpful than other melanoma markers. The combination of markers and a review of the clinical history, including imaging, can help differentiate between primary breast cancer and a metastatic tumor to the breast.

PROGNOSIS

Resection of metastatic tumors to the breast may be indicated[113] but overall, the prognosis of these patients is extremely poor, with a median survival duration between 10 and 15 months.[113,114]

APPROACH TO CORE NEEDLE BIOPSIES OF HIGH-GRADE SPINDLE CELL LESIONS OF THE BREAST

Core needle biopsy is the most common sampling technique for any breast abnormality, but the technique is not without inherent limitations. All of the aforementioned entities can display marked

Table 1
Useful histomorphologic clues and IHC markers in each entity

High-Grade Spindle Cell Lesions	Histomorphologic Clues	IHC markers[a]	Other Consideration
MPTs	• Leaf-like cellular stromal proliferation • Stromal fronds lined by epithelial cells • Subepithelial stromal condensation	CD34 CD117 CD10	• *MED12* mutation *TERT* mutation *RARα* mutation
SpCCs	• Predominantly spindle or sarcomatoid cells • Epithelioid or squamoid focus may be present • Fascicular, vaguely storiform, or without a discernible pattern • Stromal hyalinization or myxoid changes	CKs p63 TRPS1 SOX10	Test for ER, PR, and HER2 status
MP-MBCs	• Conventional invasive or in situ carcinoma • Abrupt transition to chondroid or osteoid matrix resembling chondrosarcoma or osteosarcoma • Focal spindle cell component may be present	CKs p63 TRPS1 SOX10	Test for ER, PR, and HER2 status
Angiosarcomas	• Vasoformative growth pattern • Hyperchromatic cells lining blood-filled spaces	ERG CD31 c-MYC	*MYC* amplification Clinical history of radiation therapy
Primary or metastatic sarcomas	• Identical to their counterparts • No atypia or carcinoma in situ in surrounding breast parenchyma • In cases of metastatic tumors, well-circumscribed, sharply demarcated nodules, often multiple	Based on morphologic features and history	Clinical history of radiation therapy or sarcoma Translocation and mutation associated with sarcomas elsewhere in the body

[a] The listed IHC markers represent the more commonly used and expressed markers in each entity. Expression may be rare to focal, and overlapping expression may occur.

lesional heterogeneity, and it is sometimes not possible to definitively diagnose high-grade spindle cell lesions. Some classic features can guide and favor one lesion over another, but often, these features are not seen on core needle biopsy. For example, stromal expansion that creates an enhanced intracanalicular growth pattern and clefts that are lined by epithelial and myoepithelial cells favor PT, while the presence of conventional invasive or in situ carcinoma mixed with a malignant mesenchymal component favor SpCCs or

MP-MBCs. IHC stains (CKs, p63, CD34, SOX10, and TRPS1) are helpful, but no one marker is specific, and unexpected staining patterns have been reported, causing a potential diagnostic pitfall. Therefore, when the sample is limited and the histomorphologic characteristics and IHC pattern are ambiguous, it is best to diagnose the tumor as a "high-grade spindle cell neoplasm" and recommend complete excision for final classification. **Table 1** summarizes the useful histomorphologic features and frequently positive IHC markers that can be helpful in the diagnostic workup of spindle cell lesions of the breast.

SUMMARY

High-grade spindle cell lesions in the breast are uncommon, and MPTs, SpCCs, and MP-MBCs account for most of the cases. These lesions can be of pure spindle cells or mixed spindle cells and heterologous elements. MPTs have neoplastic spindle stromal cells lined by benign epithelial cells, creating a leaf-like architecture with subepithelial stromal condensation. The spindle cells are frequently positive for CD34, CD117, and BCL-2 and are associated with *MED12*, *TERT*, and *RARA* mutations. SpCCs and MP-MBCs are high-grade MBC subtypes in which neoplastic epithelial cells become spindled or show heterologous mesenchymal differentiation, respectively. The expression of epithelial markers is strongly desired to make a diagnosis. Occasional PBSs, most commonly SAS or rare metastatic spindle cell tumors, are seen in the breast. A history of prior RT or malignancy is the best supporting evidence in these cases. Surgical resection with negative margins is the standard of care, and the long-term survival benefit of RT and chemotherapy is still under investigation.

Distinguishing epithelial-based tumors from those of mesenchymal origin is important as different treatment algorithms are used for each category of tumors. While the surgical resection may not differ, the decision to perform nodal staging and use neoadjuvant or adjuvant systemic therapy is highly dependent on whether the tumor is of epithelial or mesenchymal origin. The systemic therapy regimens used for tumors of epithelial origin are similar to other invasive breast cancers and depend on biomarker status (estrogen receptor, progesterone receptor, and HER2). Systemic therapy regimens for primary breast sarcomas are similar to those used for soft tissue tumors at other anatomic sites. The use of radiation therapy is standard in the setting of breast-conserving surgery for epithelial-based neoplasm. For mesenchymal-based neoplasms, it is not currently the standard of practice, although radiation therapy is used increasingly. The use of radiation therapy for patients with epithelial-based neoplasms undergoing mastectomy is based on the presence of nodal involvement and other biological factors. RT is rarely used for patients with primary breast sarcoma undergoing mastectomy. Multidisciplinary treatment planning is critical for these patients to achieve the best outcomes.

CLINICS CARE POINTS

MPTs

- Look for leaf-like architecture lined by epithelium and subepithelial stromal condensation.

- Varying amounts of heterologous elements such as chondrosarcoma, liposarcoma (except for well-differentiated liposarcoma), osteosarcoma, rhabdomyosarcoma, angiosarcoma, or leiomyosarcoma are often present in MPTs.

- *MED12* mutation is common in all fibroepithelial lesions, whereas *TERT* mutation is more common in MPTs. *TERT* and *RARA* mutations occur frequently with *MED12* mutations.

- Usually, CD34, CD117, and BCL-2 are positive and CKs are negative.

- P63 can be seen in both MPTs and MBCs.

- Surgery with negative margins is most important. The utility of adjuvant RT and chemotherapy is increasing.

- MPTs often recur, metastasize to the lung and have a poor prognosis.

SpCCs and MP-MBCs

- SpCCs are composed of pure spindle cells with no distinct architecture or growth pattern and may have foci of benign-appearing epithelioid or squamoid areas.

- MP-MBCs are MBCs with heterologous mesenchymal differentiation and are predominantly composed of malignant heterologous elements with no or focal spindle cells.

- Epithelial marker expression is strongly desired to make the diagnosis. TRPS1 is a breast-specific marker that is usually positive in MBCs.

- SpCCs and MP-MBCs are treated with surgery with sentinel lymph node biopsy. Adjuvant RT and chemotherapy are commonly used. SpCCs are associated with a worse prognosis.

PBSs and Metastases

- PBSs are extremely rare; MPTs, SpCCs, and MP-MBCs should be ruled out with a large IHC panel and clinical history.

- Specific molecular alterations are helpful in diagnosing PBSs.

- PBSs are treated with surgical resection of the tumor with negative margins. Patients may undergo adjuvant RT and chemotherapy depending on the type of sarcoma. Prognosis is very poor.

ACKNOWLEDGMENTS

The authors thank Ann Sutton in the Editing Services, Research Medical Library, and Kim-Anh Vu in the Department of Anatomic Pathology at The University of Texas MD Anderson Cancer Center for editing the article and the figures, respectively.

DISCLOSURE

The authors have nothing to disclose.

REFERENCES

1. WHO classification of tumours Editorial Board. Breast tumours. 5th editionVol 2. Lyon (France): International Agency for Research on Cancer; 2019.

2. Hoda SA, Rosen PP, Brogi E, Koerner FC. Rosen's breast Pathology. . Rosen's breast pathology. 5th edition. Philadelphia, PA (USA): Lippincott Williams & Wilkins; 2021.

3. Bacchi CE, Wludarski SC, Lamovec J, et al. Lipophyllodes of the breast. A reappraisal of fat-rich tumors of the breast based on 22 cases integrated by immunohistochemical study, molecular pathology insights, and clinical follow-up. Ann Diagn Pathol 2016;21:1–6.

4. Chia Y, Thike AA, Cheok PY, et al. Stromal keratin expression in phyllodes tumours of the breast: a comparison with other spindle cell breast lesions. J Clin Pathol 2012;65(4):339–47.

5. Tan BY, Acs G, Apple SK, et al. Phyllodes tumours of the breast: a consensus review. Histopathology 2016;68(1):5–21.

6. Dunne B, Lee AH, Pinder SE, et al. An immunohistochemical study of metaplastic spindle cell carcinoma, phyllodes tumor and fibromatosis of the breast. Hum Pathol 2003;34(10):1009–15.

7. Noronha Y, Raza A, Hutchins B, et al. CD34, CD117, and Ki-67 expression in phyllodes tumor of the breast: an immunohistochemical study of 33 cases. Int J Surg Pathol 2011;19(2):152–8.

8. Moore T, Lee AH. Expression of CD34 and BCL-2 in phyllodes tumours, fibroadenomas and spindle cell lesions of the breast. Histopathology 2001;38(1): 62–7.

9. Tan PH, Jayabaskar T, Yip G, et al. p53 and c-kit (CD117) protein expression as prognostic indicators in breast phyllodes tumors: a tissue microarray study. Mod Pathol 2005;18(12):1527–34.

10. Tan J, Ong CK, Lim WK, et al. Genomic landscapes of breast fibroepithelial tumors. Nat Genet 2015; 47(11):1341–5.

11. Pareja F, Geyer FC, Kumar R, et al. Phyllodes tumors with and without fibroadenoma-like areas display distinct genomic features and may evolve through distinct pathways. NPJ Breast Cancer 2017;3:40.

12. Krings G, Bean GR, Chen YY. Fibroepithelial lesions; the WHO spectrum. Semin Diagn Pathol 2017;34(5):438–52.

13. Chang HY, Koh VCY, Md Nasir ND, et al. MED12, TERT and RARA in fibroepithelial tumours of the breast. J Clin Pathol 2020;73(1):51–6.

14. Loke BN, Md Nasir ND, Thike AA, et al. Genetics and genomics of breast fibroadenomas. J Clin Pathol 2018;71(5):381–7.

15. Nozad S, Sheehan CE, Gay LM, et al. Comprehensive genomic profiling of malignant phyllodes tumors of the breast. Breast Cancer Res Treat 2017;162(3):597–602.

16. Cani AK, Hovelson DH, McDaniel AS, et al. Next-gen sequencing exposes frequent MED12 mutations and actionable therapeutic targets in phyllodes tumors. Mol Cancer Res 2015;13(4):613–9.

17. Piscuoglio S, Geyer FC, Burke KA, et al. Massively parallel sequencing analysis of synchronous fibroepithelial lesions supports the concept of progression from fibroadenoma to phyllodes tumor. NPJ Breast Cancer 2016;2:16035.

18. Lim SZ, Ng CCY, Rajasegaran V, et al. Genomic profile of breast sarcomas: a comparison with malignant phyllodes tumours. Breast Cancer Res Treat 2019;174(2):365–73.

19. Lim WK, Ong CK, Tan J, et al. Exome sequencing identifies highly recurrent MED12 somatic mutations in breast fibroadenoma. Nat Genet 2014; 46(8):877–80.

20. Yoshida M, Sekine S, Ogawa R, et al. Frequent MED12 mutations in phyllodes tumours of the breast. Br J Cancer 2015;112(10):1703–8.

21. Croce S, Chibon F. MED12 and uterine smooth muscle oncogenesis: State of the art and perspectives. Eur J Cancer 2015;51(12):1603–10.

22. Je EM, Kim MR, Min KO, et al. Mutational analysis of MED12 exon 2 in uterine leiomyoma and other common tumors. Int J Cancer 2012;131(6): E1044–7.

23. Md Nasir ND, Ng CCY, Rajasegaran V, et al. Genomic characterisation of breast fibroepithelial lesions in an international cohort. J Pathol 2019; 249(4):447–60.

24. Piscuoglio S, Murray M, Fusco N, et al. MED12 somatic mutations in fibroadenomas and phyllodes tumours of the breast. Histopathology 2015;67(5): 719–29.

25. Piscuoglio S, Ng CK, Murray M, et al. Massively parallel sequencing of phyllodes tumours of the breast reveals actionable mutations, and TERT promoter hotspot mutations and TERT gene amplification as likely drivers of progression. J Pathol 2016; 238(4):508–18.

26. Yoon N, Bae GE, Kang SY, et al. Frequency of MED12 mutations in phyllodes tumors: inverse correlation with histologic grade. Genes Chromosomes Cancer 2016;55(6):495–504.

27. Ng CC, Tan J, Ong CK, et al. MED12 is frequently mutated in breast phyllodes tumours: a study of 112 cases. J Clin Pathol 2015;68(9):685–91.

28. Tsang JYS, Hui YK, Lee MA, et al. Association of clinicopathological features and prognosis of TERT alterations in phyllodes tumor of breast. Sci Rep 2018;8(1):3881.

29. Yoshida M, Ogawa R, Yoshida H, et al. TERT promoter mutations are frequent and show association with MED12 mutations in phyllodes tumors of the breast. Br J Cancer 2015;113(8):1244–8.

30. Kim JY, Yu JH, Nam SJ, et al. Genetic and clinical characteristics of phyllodes tumors of the breast. Transl Oncol 2018;11(1):18–23.

31. Liu SY, Joseph NM, Ravindranathan A, et al. Genomic profiling of malignant phyllodes tumors reveals aberrations in FGFR1 and PI-3 kinase/RAS signaling pathways and provides insights into intratumoral heterogeneity. Mod Pathol 2016; 29(9):1012–27.

32. Macdonald OK, Lee CM, Tward JD, et al. Malignant phyllodes tumor of the female breast: association of primary therapy with cause-specific survival from the Surveillance, Epidemiology, and End Results (SEER) program. Cancer 2006;107(9):2127–33.

33. Adesoye T, Neuman HB, Wilke LG, et al. Current trends in the management of phyllodes tumors of the breast. Ann Surg Oncol 2016;23(10):3199–205.

34. Chaney AW, Pollack A, McNeese MD, et al. Primary treatment of cystosarcoma phyllodes of the breast. Cancer 2000;89(7):1502–11.

35. Reinfuss M, Mitus J, Duda K, et al. The treatment and prognosis of patients with phyllodes tumor of the breast: an analysis of 170 cases. Cancer 1996;77(5):910–6.

36. Onkendi EO, Jimenez RE, Spears GM, et al. Surgical treatment of borderline and malignant phyllodes tumors: the effect of the extent of resection and tumor characteristics on patient outcome. Ann Surg Oncol 2014;21(10):3304–9.

37. Yom CK, Han W, Kim SW, et al. Reappraisal of conventional risk stratification for local recurrence based on clinical outcomes in 285 resected phyllodes tumors of the breast. Ann Surg Oncol 2015; 22(9):2912–8.

38. Lin CC, Chang HW, Lin CY, et al. The clinical features and prognosis of phyllodes tumors: a single institution experience in Taiwan. Int J Clin Oncol 2013;18(4):614–20.

39. Jang JH, Choi MY, Lee SK, et al. Clinicopathologic risk factors for the local recurrence of phyllodes tumors of the breast. Ann Surg Oncol 2012;19(8): 2612–7.

40. Barth RJ Jr, Wells WA, Mitchell SE, et al. A prospective, multi-institutional study of adjuvant radiotherapy after resection of malignant phyllodes tumors. Ann Surg Oncol 2009;16(8):2288–94.

41. Lu Y, Chen Y, Zhu L, et al. Local recurrence of benign, borderline, and malignant phyllodes tumors of the breast: a systematic review and meta-analysis. Ann Surg Oncol 2019;26(5): 1263–75.

42. Choi N, Kim K, Shin KH, et al. The characteristics of local recurrence after breast-conserving surgery alone for malignant and borderline phyllodes tumors of the breast (KROG 16-08). Clin Breast Cancer 2019;19(5):345–53.e2.

43. Kim S, Kim JY, Kim DH, et al. Analysis of phyllodes tumor recurrence according to the histologic grade. Breast Cancer Res Treat 2013;141(3): 353–63.

44. Choi N, Kim K, Shin KH, et al. Malignant and borderline phyllodes tumors of the breast: a multicenter study of 362 patients (KROG 16-08). Breast Cancer Res Treat 2018;171(2):335–44.

45. Gnerlich JL, Williams RT, Yao K, et al. Utilization of radiotherapy for malignant phyllodes tumors: analysis of the National Cancer Data Base, 1998-2009. Ann Surg Oncol 2014;21(4):1222–30.

46. Belkacemi Y, Bousquet G, Marsiglia H, et al. Phyllodes tumor of the breast. Int J Radiat Oncol Biol Phys 2008;70(2):492–500.

47. Guillot E, Couturaud B, Reyal F, et al. Management of phyllodes breast tumors. Breast J 2011;17(2): 129–37.

48. Parkes A, Wang WL, Patel S, et al. Outcomes of systemic therapy in metastatic phyllodes tumor of the breast. 3rd186. Breast Cancer Res Treat; 2021. p. 871–82.

49. Tan PH, Thike AA, Tan WJ, et al. Predicting clinical behaviour of breast phyllodes tumours: a nomogram based on histological criteria and surgical margins. J Clin Pathol 2012;65(1):69–76.

50. Kapiris I, Nasiri N, A'Hern R, et al. Outcome and predictive factors of local recurrence and distant metastases following primary surgical treatment of high-grade malignant phyllodes tumours of the breast. Eur J Surg Oncol 2001;27(8):723–30.

51. Gersell DJ, Katzenstein AL. Spindle cell carcinoma of the breast. A clinocopathologic and ultrastructural study. Hum Pathol 1981;12(6):550–61.

52. Moten AS, Jayarajan SN, Willis AI. Spindle cell carcinoma of the breast: a comprehensive analysis. Am J Surg 2016;211(4):716–21.

53. Khan HN, Wyld L, Dunne B, et al. Spindle cell carcinoma of the breast: a case series of a rare histological subtype. Eur J Surg Oncol 2003;29(7): 600–3.

54. Vranic S, Stafford P, Palazzo J, et al. Molecular profiling of the metaplastic spindle cell carcinoma

of the breast reveals potentially targetable bio-markers. Clin Breast Cancer 2020;20(4):326–31.e1.

55. Wargotz ES, Deos PH, Norris HJ. Metaplastic carcinomas of the breast. II. Spindle cell carcinoma. Hum Pathol 1989;20(8):732–40.

56. Raj SD, Sweetwood K, Kapoor MM, et al. Spindle cell lesions of the breast: Multimodality imaging and clinical differentiation of pathologically similar neoplasms. Eur J Radiol 2017;90:60–72.

57. Isomoto I, Sakashita A, Abe K, et al. Spindle cell carcinoma of the breast: MR findings correlated with histopathology. Magn Reson Med Sci 2011;10(2):133–7.

58. Carter MR, Hornick JL, Lester S, et al. Spindle cell (sarcomatoid) carcinoma of the breast: a clinicopathologic and immunohistochemical analysis of 29 cases. Am J Surg Pathol 2006;30(3):300–9.

59. Ai D, Yao J, Yang F, et al. TRPS1: a highly sensitive and specific marker for breast carcinoma, especially for triple-negative breast cancer. Mod Pathol 2020;34(4):710–9.

60. Han M, Zhang H, Dabbs DJ. Best practice (efficient) immunohistologic panel for diagnosing metaplastic breast carcinoma. Appl Immunohistochem Mol Morphol 2020;29(4):265–9.

61. Rakha EA, Coimbra ND, Hodi Z, et al. Immunoprofile of metaplastic carcinomas of the breast. Histopathology 2017;70(6):975–85.

62. McCart Reed AE, Kalaw E, Nones K, et al. Phenotypic and molecular dissection of metaplastic breast cancer and the prognostic implications. J Pathol 2019;247(2):214–27.

63. Ng CKY, Piscuoglio S, Geyer FC, et al. The landscape of somatic genetic alterations in metaplastic breast carcinomas. Clin Cancer Res 2017;23(14):3859–70.

64. Krings G, Chen YY. Genomic profiling of metaplastic breast carcinomas reveals genetic heterogeneity and relationship to ductal carcinoma. Mod Pathol 2018;31(11):1661–74.

65. Zhai J, Giannini G, Ewalt MD, et al. Molecular characterization of metaplastic breast carcinoma via next-generation sequencing. Hum Pathol 2019;86:85–92.

66. Abouharb S, Moulder S. Metaplastic breast cancer: clinical overview and molecular aberrations for potential targeted therapy. Curr Oncol Rep 2015;17(3):431.

67. Schroeder MC, Rastogi P, Geyer CE Jr, et al. Early and locally advanced metaplastic breast cancer: presentation and survival by receptor status in surveillance, epidemiology, and end results (SEER) 2010-2014. Oncologist 2018;23(4):481–8.

68. He X, Ji J, Dong R, et al. Prognosis in different subtypes of metaplastic breast cancer: a population-based analysis. Breast Cancer Res Treat 2019;173(2):329–41.

69. Tseng WH, Martinez SR. Metaplastic breast cancer: to radiate or not to radiate? Ann Surg Oncol 2011;18(1):94–103.

70. Rakha EA, Tan PH, Varga Z, et al. Prognostic factors in metaplastic carcinoma of the breast: a multi-institutional study. Br J Cancer 2015;112(2):283–9.

71. Haque W, Verma V, Naik N, et al. Metaplastic breast cancer: practice patterns, outcomes, and the role of radiotherapy. Ann Surg Oncol 2018;25(4):928–36.

72. Corso G, Frassoni S, Girardi A, et al. Metaplastic breast cancer: prognostic and therapeutic considerations. J Surg Oncol 2021;123(1):61–70.

73. Cimino-Mathews A, Verma S, Figueroa-Magalhaes MC, et al. A clinicopathologic analysis of 45 Patients with metaplastic breast carcinoma. Am J Clin Pathol 2016;145(3):365–72.

74. El Zein D, Hughes M, Kumar S, et al. Metaplastic carcinoma of the breast is more aggressive than triple-negative breast cancer: a study from a single institution and review of literature. Clin Breast Cancer 2017;17(5):382–91.

75. Nelson RA, Guye ML, Luu T, et al. Survival outcomes of metaplastic breast cancer patients: results from a US population-based analysis. Ann Surg Oncol 2015;22(1):24–31.

76. Lee H, Jung SY, Ro JY, et al. Metaplastic breast cancer: clinicopathological features and its prognosis. J Clin Pathol 2012;65(5):441–6.

77. Zhang Y, Lv F, Yang Y, et al. Clinicopathological features and prognosis of metaplastic breast carcinoma: experience of a major Chinese Cancer Center. PLoS One 2015;10(6):e0131409.

78. Schwartz TL, Mogal H, Papageorgiou C, et al. Metaplastic breast cancer: histologic characteristics, prognostic factors and systemic treatment strategies. Exp Hematol Oncol 2013;2(1):31.

79. Song Y, Liu X, Zhang G, et al. Unique clinicopathological features of metaplastic breast carcinoma compared with invasive ductal carcinoma and poor prognostic indicators. World J Surg Oncol 2013;11:129.

80. Leyrer CM, Berriochoa CA, Agrawal S, et al. Predictive factors on outcomes in metaplastic breast cancer. Breast Cancer Res Treat 2017;165(3):499–504.

81. Yang WT, Hennessy B, Broglio K, et al. Imaging differences in metaplastic and invasive ductal carcinomas of the breast. AJR Am J Roentgenol 2007;189(6):1288–93.

82. Shin HJ, Kim HH, Kim SM, et al. Imaging features of metaplastic carcinoma with chondroid differentiation of the breast. AJR Am J Roentgenol 2007;188(3):691–6.

83. Leddy R, Irshad A, Rumboldt T, et al. Review of metaplastic carcinoma of the breast: imaging findings and pathologic features. J Clin Imaging Sci 2012;2:21.

84. Langlands F, Cornford E, Rakha E, et al. Imaging overview of metaplastic carcinomas of the breast: a large study of 71 cases. Br J Radiol 2016; 89(1064):20140644.

85. Rakha EA, Tan PH, Shaaban A, et al. Do primary mammary osteosarcoma and chondrosarcoma exist? A review of a large multi-institutional series of malignant matrix-producing breast tumours. Breast 2013;22(1):13–8.

86. Downs-Kelly E, Nayeemuddin KM, Albarracin C, et al. Matrix-producing carcinoma of the breast: an aggressive subtype of metaplastic carcinoma. Am J Surg Pathol 2009;33(4):534–41.

87. Shimada K, Ishikawa T, Yamada A, et al. Matrix-producing carcinoma as an aggressive triple-negative breast cancer: clinicopathological features and response to neoadjuvant chemotherapy. Anticancer Res 2019;39(7):3863–9.

88. Cimino-Mathews A, Subhawong AP, Elwood H, et al. Neural crest transcription factor Sox10 is preferentially expressed in triple-negative and metaplastic breast carcinomas. Hum Pathol 2013; 44(6):959–65.

89. McGowan TS, Cummings BJ, O'Sullivan B, et al. An analysis of 78 breast sarcoma patients without distant metastases at presentation. Int J Radiat Oncol Biol Phys 2000;46(2):383–90.

90. Blanchard DK, Reynolds CA, Grant CS, et al. Primary nonphylloides breast sarcomas. Am J Surg 2003;186(4):359–61.

91. Huang J, Mackillop WJ. Increased risk of soft tissue sarcoma after radiotherapy in women with breast carcinoma. Cancer 2001;92(1):172–80.

92. Yap J, Chuba PJ, Thomas R, et al. Sarcoma as a second malignancy after treatment for breast cancer. Int J Radiat Oncol Biol Phys 2002;52(5): 1231–7.

93. Bousquet G, Confavreux C, Magne N, et al. Outcome and prognostic factors in breast sarcoma: a multicenter study from the rare cancer network. Radiother Oncol 2007;85(3):355–61.

94. Lee JS, Yoon K, Onyshchenko M. Sarcoma of the breast: clinical characteristics and outcomes of 991 patients from the national cancer database. Sarcoma 2021;2021:8828158.

95. Pierce SM, Recht A, Lingos TI, et al. Long-term radiation complications following conservative surgery (CS) and radiation therapy (RT) in patients with early stage breast cancer. Int J Radiat Oncol Biol Phys 1992;23(5):915–23.

96. Karlsson F, Granath F, Smedby KE, et al. Sarcoma of the breast: breast cancer history as etiologic and prognostic factor-A population-based case-control study. Breast Cancer Res Treat 2020;183(3):669–75.

97. Hodgson NC, Bowen-Wells C, Moffat F, et al. Angiosarcomas of the breast: a review of 70 cases. Am J Clin Oncol 2007;30(6):570–3.

98. Lim SZ, Ong KW, Tan BK, et al. Sarcoma of the breast: an update on a rare entity. J Clin Pathol 2016;69(5):373–81.

99. Hays DM, Donaldson SS, Shimada H, et al. Primary and metastatic rhabdomyosarcoma in the breast: neoplasms of adolescent females, a report from the Intergroup Rhabdomyosarcoma Study. Med Pediatr Oncol 1997;29(3):181–9.

100. Audino AN, Setty BA, Yeager ND. Rhabdomyosarcoma of the breast in adolescent and young adult (AYA) women. J Pediatr Hematol Oncol 2017; 39(1):62–6.

101. Shin J, Kim HJ, Kim DY, et al. Primary rhabdomyosarcoma of the breast: Study of Three Cases at One Institution with a Review of Primary Breast Sarcomas. J Pathol Transl Med 2019;53(5): 308–16.

102. Antonescu C. Malignant vascular tumors–an update. Mod Pathol 2014;27(Suppl 1):S30–8.

103. Fraga-Guedes C, Andre S, Mastropasqua MG, et al. Angiosarcoma and atypical vascular lesions of the breast: diagnostic and prognostic role of MYC gene amplification and protein expression. Breast Cancer Res Treat 2015;151(1):131–40.

104. Guo T, Zhang L, Chang NE, et al. Consistent MYC and FLT4 gene amplification in radiation-induced angiosarcoma but not in other radiation-associated atypical vascular lesions. Genes Chromosomes Cancer 2011;50(1):25–33.

105. Ciatto S, Bonardi R, Cataliotti L, et al. Sarcomas of the breast: a multicenter series of 70 cases. Neoplasma 1992;39(6):375–9.

106. Scow JS, Reynolds CA, Degnim AC, et al. Primary and secondary angiosarcoma of the breast: the Mayo Clinic experience. J Surg Oncol 2010; 101(5):401–7.

107. Yin M, Mackley HB, Drabick JJ, et al. Primary female breast sarcoma: clinicopathological features, treatment and prognosis. Sci Rep 2016;6:31497.

108. Adem C, Reynolds C, Ingle JN, et al. Primary breast sarcoma: clinicopathologic series from the Mayo Clinic and review of the literature. Br J Cancer 2004;91(2):237–41.

109. Moore MP, Kinne DW. Breast sarcoma. Surg Clin North Am 1996;76(2):383–92.

110. Zelek L, Llombart-Cussac A, Terrier P, et al. Prognostic factors in primary breast sarcomas: a series of patients with long-term follow-up. J Clin Oncol 2003;21(13):2583–8.

111. Georgiannos SN, Chin J, Goode AW, et al. Secondary neoplasms of the breast: a survey of the 20th Century. Cancer 2001;92(9):2259–66.

112. Alvarado Cabrero I, Carrera Alvarez M, Perez Montiel D, et al. Metastases to the breast. Eur J Surg Oncol 2003;29(10):854–5.

113. Williams SA, Ehlers RA 2nd, Hunt KK, et al. Metastases to the breast from nonbreast solid

neoplasms: presentation and determinants of survival. Cancer 2007;110(4):731–7.

114. DeLair DF, Corben AD, Catalano JP, et al. Non-mammary metastases to the breast and axilla: a study of 85 cases. Mod Pathol 2013;26(3):343–9.

115. Kaviratna M, Jayawardena T, Dissanayake D, et al. Population screening detected non-lymphomatous non-mammary metastases to the breast. A radiology multi-modality pictorial essay. Clin Imaging 2021;74:156–62.

116. Lee SH, Park JM, Kook SH, et al. Metastatic tumors to the breast: mammographic and ultrasonographic findings. J Ultrasound Med 2000;19(4): 257–62.

Atypical Ductal Hyperplasia-Ductal Carcinoma In Situ Spectrum: Diagnostic Considerations and Treatment Impact in the Era of Deescalation

Melinda E. Sanders, MD*, Mirna B. Podoll, MD

KEYWORDS

- Ductal carcinoma in situ • Atypical ductal hyperplasia • Deescalation

Key points

- Pathologists have the potential to play a critical role in refining appropriate therapy for lesions in the atypical ductal hyperplasia-ductal carcinoma in situ (ADH-DCIS) spectrum by conservatively approaching the diagnosis of lesions limited in size on core needle biopsy.

- Appropriate efforts to deescalate DCIS diagnosis will further promote breast-conserving surgery, sparing women the morbidity of mastectomy, and sentinel node biopsy.

- Patients with lesions at the borderline of ADH-DCIS are the patients most likely to be identified as among "low risk" women who may successfully forgo even limited breast-conserving surgery by clinical trials of active surveillance.

ABSTRACT

As the first node in treatment algorithms for breast disease, pathologists have the potential to play a critical role in refining appropriate therapy for lesions in the atypical ducal hyperplasia-ductal carcinoma in situ (ADH-DCIS) spectrum by conservatively approaching diagnosis of lesions limited in size on core needle biopsy. Appropriate efforts to downgrade the diagnosis of lesions at the borderline of ADH and DCIS will certainly lead to more breast conservation and avoid the common morbidities of mastectomy, sentinel node biopsy, and radiation therapy. Whether results of clinical trials of active surveillance will successfully identify a subset of women who may successfully forgo even limited breast-conserving surgery is eagerly anticipated. Given the increasing concern that a significant number of women with DCIS are overtreated, identification of patients at very low risk for progression who may forgo surgery and radiation therapy safely is of significant interest.

INTRODUCTION

Pathologists have the potential to play a critical role in refining appropriate therapy for lesions in the atypical ducal hyperplasia-ductal carcinoma

Vanderbilt University Medical Center, 1301 Medical Center Drive, 4918A TVC Blg, Nashville, TN 37215
* Corresponding author.
E-mail address: Melinda.sanders@vumc.org

Surgical Pathology 15 (2022) 95–103
https://doi.org/10.1016/j.path.2021.11.006
1875-9181/22/© 2021 Elsevier Inc. All rights reserved.

Abbreviations	
ADH	atypical ductal hyperplasia
DCIS	ductal carcinoma in situ

in situ (ADH-DCIS) spectrum by conservatively approaching diagnosis of lesions of limited size on core needle biopsy. Currently DCIS represents 20% to 25% of newly diagnosed breast cancers per year, accounting for more than 48,000 breast cancer diagnoses in 2019.[1] In current clinical practice, these patients are typically asymptomatic, and a core needle biopsy performed to investigate mammographic calcifications brings lesions in the ADH-DCIS spectrum to clinical attention. The number of newly diagnosed DCIS cases has remained relatively stable over the past 2 decades but represents a nearly 10-fold increased incidence from the decades preceding mammographic screening program implementation.[2] The stable incidence rate of invasive cancer during this time, implies that at least a subset of mammographically detected DCIS cases represents over diagnosis. Some authors interpret natural history studies of DCIS [3–7] as meaning some examples of DCIS will not progress to invasive cancer, even if untreated.[8–11] The results of retrospective and a few prospective studies identify older age, mammographic detection, small pathologic size, low and intermediate histologic grade, and negative surgical margins as features which most consistently characterize "low risk DCIS," as DCIS with lesser risk of local recurrence and/or progression to invasive cancer.[12,13]

Breast-conserving surgery followed by radiation therapy with or without hormonal therapy has become the most frequent treatment modality for patients with DCIS today, a paradigm shift beginning in the early 1990s from universal mastectomy. In addition, multiple studies have shown limited, if any value in the reexcision for margin widths greater than 2 mm for most women, which has been incorporated into current clinical practice.[14] Interestingly, the very low 1% to 3% mortality rate and freedom from distant metastasis for DCIS has remained the same despite the use of radiation therapy, hormone therapy, and significant surgical deescalation.[15] Patients who receive radiation therapy and hormone therapy have a small but real risk of side effects including angiosarcoma, breast edema, telangiectasia, breast shrinkage, chronic pain, arm lymphedema, and dissatisfaction with cosmesis. Efforts to limit the number of patients experiencing these morbidities compromising their quality of life despite eradication of breast disease are warranted. Collectively,

these data suggest further deescalation of treatment of lesions in the ADH-DCIS spectrum is should be investigated. Whether the outcome of active surveillance trials identifies "low-risk" patients in this group for whom surgical excision is unnecessary has yet to be determined. Regardless, these data may permit the refinement of reporting strategies for borderline atypical ductal proliferative lesions of the breast and the pathologic criteria used to determine the lower limit of DCIS diagnosis.

NATURAL HISTORY STUDIES OF ATYPICAL DUCTAL HYPERPLASIA AND DUCTAL CARCINOMA IN SITU

Knowledge of the natural history studies and epidemiology of ADH and DCIS is important when deciding the extent to which each diagnosis impacts treatment algorithms for patients diagnosed with these lesions today. The current disease spectrum encompassed by the diagnosis "DCIS" of the breast is wide. All examples of DCIS are neoplastic proliferations of mammary epithelial cells confined to the ductal-lobular unit system. Without the transgression of the basement membrane, DCIS does not present a threat to life, and therefore the goal of treatment is prophylaxis against progression to invasive carcinoma. However, the disease entity "DCIS" demonstrates considerable heterogeneity with respect to presentation, size, histologic grade, and immunohistochemical and molecular phenotypes.[16] Despite this heterogeneity, all DCIS are regarded as nonobligate precursors to invasive breast cancer. Studies of the natural history of DCIS have shown that some, but not all DCIS will progress to invasive cancer at a frequency of 20% to 50%, with the rate of progression depending on the grade and to some extent the size of the lesion.[3,5–7] The posed risk is to the ipsilateral breast and typically to the same quadrant as the index DCIS lesion.[7] ADH, diagnosed based on epidemiologically verified criteria established by Page[17] and subsequently validated by others,[18–22] is associated with a 3- to 5-fold increased relative risk, an approximately 1% absolute risk per year for at least 25 years, and a 10% to 20% absolute lifetime risk of subsequent invasive carcinoma. The average latency period is 10 years.[23,24] This risk has been conceptualized as a generalized risk, posing a roughly equal risk to either breast. However, results of multiple studies have found the risk for the ipsilateral breast is greater.[17–21]

The natural history studies of both ADH and DCIS are based on lesions initially interpreted as benign which were retrospectively diagnosed as ADH or DCIS during larger reviews of over 10,000 excision specimens with long-term follow-up. By default, these patients received no treatment beyond the diagnostic surgical excision. The goal of these reviews was to identify lesions posing subsequent increased breast cancer risk and establish criteria that would reproducibly allow their distinction from lesions carrying no risk. In the years preceding these studies, thousands of women underwent lumpectomy for a palpable abnormality. The rendered diagnoses were typically either "carcinoma" or "fibrocystic changes". It was recognized that a small subset of these women without "carcinoma" was at risk for subsequent breast cancer; however, the histologic lesions responsible for this risk were unknown. ADH and low-grade DCIS were not formally recognized entities.

Page's original criteria for separating the lesser lesion of ADH from DCIS were conceived after the recognition that a neoplastic population of atypical cells forming a cribriform pattern and completely replacing at least 2 contiguous spaces was linked to a 20% to 50% risk of subsequent invasive carcinoma in the ipsilateral breast.[17,25] Women with lesions composed of the same cells but not meeting these criteria also demonstrated an increased risk of subsequent carcinoma but of lesser magnitude (3-5X) and generalized to both breasts.[17] The degree to which these results can be applied to lesions sampled by core biopsy today has been called into question. Grossing practices at the time, a nonstandardized sampling of the specimen, did not allow for the more precise size measurements and margin evaluation provided by the methods used today.[26] Thus, the size and adequacy of excision of these lesions are unknown. For these reasons, it must be acknowledged that the threshold for separating low-grade DCIS from ADH, 2 completely involved spaces and at least 2 mm in contiguous extent, is less precise than implied by the traditional criteria of Page[17] and of Tavasolli and Norris.[27] Although endorsed in the recently published 5th edition of the WHO Classification of tumors, The WHO Classification of Tumors Editorial Board emphasizes that these criteria should serve as "general guidelines" and should be "applied with caution when lesions of limited extent are identified in core needle biopsies, in which the entire lesion may not be visualized."[12]

The current standard of care treatment for ADH is excision while options for DCIS are mastectomy, breast-conserving surgery followed by radiation therapy, and breast-conserving surgery alone.[28] Any of these treatments maybe followed by endocrine therapy.[29] Although most examples of DCIS can be adequately removed by breast-conserving surgery, many women still choose mastectomy, and even bilateral mastectomy for combined eradication and prophylaxis against secondary events. This means in some cases, a bilateral mastectomy may be performed for a lesion measuring only several millimeters in size, an approach most would view as over treatment. The conservative approach endorsed by the WHO[30] and practiced by the authors, supports diagnosing lesions at the borderline of ADH and DCIS as "well-developed atypical ductal hyperplasia bordering on DCIS" (or similar), driving a lumpectomy rather than mastectomy to delimit the process. Even if upgraded to DCIS on subsequent excision, lumpectomy would be the preferred surgical treatment and importantly avoid the morbidity of mastectomy and sentinel lymph node biopsy.

The use of genomic assays to predict chemotherapy benefit and prognosis, such as Oncotype DX and MammaPrint, has been developed and successfully integrated into treatment planning for patients with invasive breast cancer.[31,32] Until recently, efforts by numerous clinical researchers to identify genomic changes consistently found in DCIS associated with invasive progression or local recurrence risk have been inconsistent and of little clinical utility.[33,34] The Oncotype DX DCIS score[35] predicts the benefit of adjuvant radiation for women receiving breast conservation therapy in reducing local recurrence risk. The assay stratifies women diagnosed with DCIS into low, intermediate, and high-risk groups based on their gene expression profiles as determined by a 12 gene PCR-based assay. However, among women from ECOG E5194 (a prospective study of women treated by breast conservation alone) and the Ontario DCIS cohort, the 10-year local recurrence rates were 12% to 13%, rates at which most clinicians would still recommend radiation.[36,37] A subsequent combined analysis of the Oncotype DX data from both cohorts combined with select clinicopathologic features identified a low-risk group for whom the local recurrence rate was 7.2%.[38] Women in this group were $\geq$ 50 years old, had DCIS measuring less than 10 mm and had a low risk Oncotype DX DCIS score.[38] Most recently, the DCISionRT assay which combines the results of several immunohistochemical biomarkers and clinicopathologic factors, identified a group of

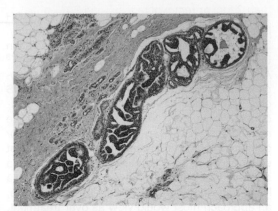

Fig. 1. Well-developed atypical ductal hyperplasia on core biopsy measuring 3 mm present in a single core at the time of core biopsy. No residual lesion remained at the time of excision.

women treated with breast conservation surgery alone with an 8% ipsilateral risk of recurrence at 10 years,[35] and a 10% 10-year ipsilateral risk in the validation study.[39] Collectively, these studies suggest a combination of molecular and clinicopathologic features will a better predictor of women with "low risk DCIS" who may be eligible for active surveillance. However, it must be recognized that the tests discussed above predict the benefit of subsequent radiation assuming negative margins. The thus ability of "low-risk" scores by existing assays to accurately predict women with DCIS who may safely choose active surveillance is unknown and may be meaningless if the disease has been left behind. Thus at present, there are no validated molecular tests that can be used to assist decision-making for women considering active surveillance.

COMPLEXITIES IN THE DIAGNOSIS OF ATYPICAL DUCTAL HYPERPLASIA VERSUS DUCTAL CARCINOMA IN SITU

The concept of deescalation of the diagnosis of DCIS by pathologists is most easily understood

for cribriform lesions meeting or measuring slightly greater than the 2 space and 2 mm traditional criteria used to separate atypical ductal hyperplasia (ADH) from low-grade DCIS. In such instances, rendering a diagnosis that acknowledges the presence of a borderline lesion (eg, well-developed atypical ductal hyperplasia, severely atypical ductal hyperplasia, etc.) would result in a lumpectomy for full characterization of the lesion under the current standard of care.[28] Features such as involvement of a single core, lesions confined to a single lobular unit, or lesions present in several lobular units without the involvement of a contiguous intervening duct, suggest that despite measuring slightly more than 2 mm, the process is likely of limited extent, and raises the possibility that the lesion was removed in its entirety by the biopsy (**Fig. 1**). Mammographic features suggestive of limited extent include presentation as a single cluster of calcifications, calcifications measuring less than 5 mm in extent, and lack of an associated mass lesion.[40–44]

A similar approach can be used with solid pattern atypical ductal hyperplasia, with the caveat that pure solid pattern atypical ductal hyperplasia is uncommon and must be distinguished from atypical lobular hyperplasia (ALH) and classic lobular carcinoma in situ (cLCIS). ALH and cLCIS may be extensive and yet associated with few if any calcifications. In addition, the greater the distension and distortion of the spaces occupied by lobular neoplasia cells (eg, cLCIS), the more likely that the characteristic intracytoplasmic lumina of lobular neoplasia may no longer be evident. Demonstration of loss of E-cadherin expression by immunohistochemistry can be helpful in confirming the H&E impression of a lobular versus ductal process, and avoiding the overdiagnosis of coexistent ALH and atypical ductal hyperplasia as low-grade DCIS.

Patients with cribriform and solid pattern DCIS lesions discussed above are the more obvious candidates for the consideration of deescalation of therapy. However, micropapillary pattern atypia

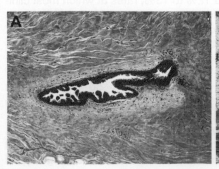 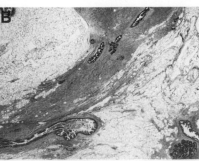

Fig. 2. (A) Micropapillary ductal carcinoma in situ. (B) Single duct with micropapillary atypia and normally polarized cells between micropapillae.

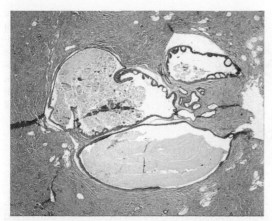

Fig. 3. Atypical ductal hyperplasia involving acini markedly distended by mucin. Although the entire lesion measures 5 mm, the extent and development of the atypia are insufficient to warrant a diagnosis of ductal carcinoma in situ.

and atypia associated with papillary lesions on core biopsy are diagnostically more complex and may be less appropriate for deescalation. When micropapillary pattern atypia is limited in extent in a core biopsy sampling, it may be difficult if not impossible to separate examples of ADH from DCIS . Low-grade micropapillary pattern atypia may show normally polarized cells between micropapillae, violating the commonly relied upon "contiguous extent" rule for diagnosing

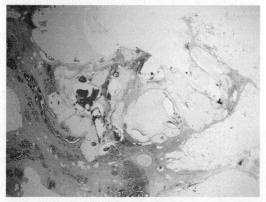

Fig. 4. Large mucocele-like lesion associated with atypical ductal hyperplasia. Multiple disrupted, mucin-filled acini extrude mucin into the adjacent breast tissue. Several curvilinear strips of epithelium with arcades and micropapillae have separated from the basement membrane of the spaces. Although the dimensions of the entire process are greater than 9 mm, the portion occupied by atypical epithelium is insufficient for a diagnosis of ductal carcinoma in situ.

DCIS (**Fig. 2**A). Only when a larger volume of surgically excised tissue can be examined, revealing a more extensive process involving several true ducts, is a diagnosis of micropapillary DCIS confidently rendered (**Fig. 2**B). Micropapillary DCIS is typically more extensive than other patterns[45] and at greatest risk for local recurrence after breast-conserving therapy.[46] However, pathologists should remain cautious when rendering a diagnosis of micropapillary DCIS in the face of borderline findings on core biopsy. The pathologist must be careful not to be overly reliant on the mammographic findings when the histologic findings do not clearly support the diagnosis of DCIS. In fact, micropapillary atypia may be seen in a background of extensive sclerosing adenosis, micropapillomas and other fibrocystic changes which could also account for extensive mammographic calcifications. Micropapillary atypia may also be associated with significant lobular unit distension by mucin, resulting in a lesion 3 to 5 mm or more, yet without evident involvement of ducts (**Fig. 3**). In these examples, the density of micropapillae is typically limited and they may be associated with a mucocele-like lesion (**Fig. 4**). In such cases, diagnosis of a borderline lesion is also preferable. Features most consistent with a diagnosis of micropapillary DCIS are micropapillae in multiple true ducts and involvement of 3 or more cores by the process.[47] Although apocrine atypia is less common, the distinction of low-grade apocrine ADH versus DCIS is complicated by close resemblance to papillary apocrine change, less nuclear uniformity, and variable cytoplasmic volume (**Fig. 5**).

Core needle biopsy of papillary lesions not uncommonly identifies the presence of atypia at the borderline of ADH and DCIS. It has been recommended that foci $\geq$ 3 mm or occupying greater than 30% of the papilloma be diagnosed as DCIS and those that are smaller, be classified as ADH.[48–50] However, similar to the "2 mm and 2 space rules" for separating ADH from DCIS not involving papillomas, data to support this cut off are even more limited.[48,50] Immunohistochemistry showing the loss of cytokeratin 5/6 expression in combination with strong diffuse nuclear estrogen receptor expression can be used to confirm the presence of low-grade ductal neoplasia cells within a papilloma. Caution should be used when using these stains to measure the extent of the lesion as the cells of lobular neoplasia cells and flat epithelial atypia show an identical staining pattern. When abundant, the presence of myoepithelial cells as evidenced by the presence of p63 expression in the uninvolved portion of the papilloma is helpful in excluding an encapsulated

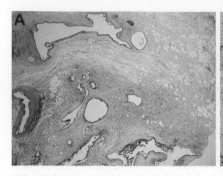
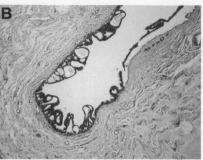

Fig. 5. Low-grade apocrine ductal carcinoma at (*A*) low power showing involvement of several true ducts by arcades of apocrine cells when viewed at higher magnification (*B*) are monotonous with small round nuclei.

papillary carcinoma. When the radiologic studies prompting biopsy demonstrate a mass less than 5 mm or especially the absence of a mass, diagnosis of a papillary lesion with "well-developed ADH bordering on DCIS" will be more prudent than rendering a diagnosis of papillary DCIS or encapsulated papillary carcinoma in a limited sampling (**Fig. 6**), even in the face of patchy or absent p63 expression. Such a diagnosis under current practice would result in an excision/lumpectomy for full characterization of the process.

CLINICAL TRIALS OF ACTIVE SURVEILLANCE AND RISKS OF DEESCALATION

Efforts to downgrade the diagnosis of DCIS to ADH in some contexts will certainly lead to more breast conservation but it is unclear to what degree surgery could or should be completely avoided.[15] Will the data from clinical trials of active surveillance identify a subset of women who may successfully forgo even limited breast-conserving surgery? Although several groups initiated randomized clinical trials to compare active surveillance to the standard of care therapy for women with low-risk DCIS,[8,10,51] only the Comparison of Operative to Monitoring and Endocrine Therapy (COMET) trial continues to accrue patients.[51] The

2 European clinical trials, LORIS (LOw RISk DCIS) and LORD (LOw Risk DCIS), were converted to registry trials due to low accrual and the Japanese LORETTA trial, although prospective, is a single-arm trial of active surveillance and endocrine therapy.[51] Women 40 years of age and older with estrogen receptor and progesterone receptor positive, low or intermediate grade DCIS meet inclusion criteria for the COMET trial. Patients with a history of DCIS and invasive carcinoma are excluded as are patients who have received tamoxifen, an aromatase inhibitor, or raloxifene treatments in the preceding 6 months.[51] Recently, the COMET trial has also opened enrollment to women with positive margins after surgical excision for DCIS who otherwise meet enrollment criteria and women with lesions at the borderline of ADH-DCIS. This important amendment will test whether efforts to deescalate the diagnosis of DCIS successfully identify women who may forgo even limited breast-conserving surgery.

Of greatest concern for women enrolled in active surveillance trials is the small but real risk of concurrent invasion not detected in the core biopsy. This is supported by studies showing not inconsequential rates of upgrade at the time of excision of 6% to 24% for DCIS and 10% to 20% for ADH.[30,51–54] In addition, a recent study by Pilewskie and colleagues identifying patients

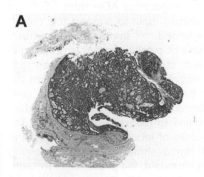
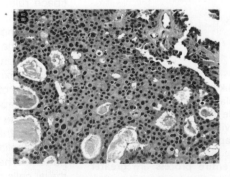

Fig. 6. Intraductal papilloma with well-developed atypical ductal hyperplasia. (A) Low power view of an intraductal papilloma with prominent epithelial hyperplasia. (B) Focally, evenly placed atypical cells with uniform nuclei are present, some of which are polarized around the glandular spaces. The limited extent of involvement by the atypical ductal cells is insufficient to qualify as DCIS.

eligible for the active surveillance trials based on the LORIS criteria who underwent excision, found 20% of patients to have invasive carcinomas at the time of surgery.[54] However, it is important to note that among cases upgraded to invasive carcinoma, the grade of DCIS on the preceding core biopsy was intermediate in 93% of cases and low for 7% of cases. The COMET trial's primary endpoint of no ipsilateral invasive cancer at 2 years seems premature. The planned examination of risk at 5, 7, and 10 years will likely be more informative given the fact that subsequent cancer risk is prolonged in patients with low-grade DCIS.[7]

The possibility that more women will experience in situ and invasive local recurrences as a consequence of DCIS left behind by forgoing surgery is also a likely outcome. Three prospective studies have examined whether patients with low-risk DCIS based on routine clinical and pathologic features can be safely treated with breast conservation without subsequent radiation therapy.[55–57] Local recurrence rates for patients enrolled in these studies ranged from 11.4% to 15.6% after 10 to 12-years follow-up, rates too high to ultimately characterize these patients as "low risk." If these women had been managed without excision even higher recurrence rates would be expected. The applicability of these results to lesions at the lower threshold of diagnosis for DCIS (borderline for ADH vs DCIS) is unknown as this was not a planned subset analysis, but hopefully can be addressed by the results of the COMET trial.

SUMMARY

Although frequently under emphasized, pathologists play a critical role in shaping the direction of care for patients diagnosed with DCIS of the breast. Given increasing concern that a significant number of women with DCIS may be overtreated, identification of patients at very low risk for progression who may forgo surgery and radiation therapy safely is of significant interest. Efforts by pathologists to downgrade the diagnosis of lesions at the borderline of ADH-DCIS to "well-developed ADH" or "severely atypical ductal hyperplasia bordering on DCIS" will certainly lead to more breast conservation in the short run and avoid the common morbidities of mastectomy, sentinel node biopsy, and radiation therapy for many patients. Whether the results of clinical trials of active surveillance will successfully identify a subset of "low risk" women who may successfully forgo even limited breast-conserving surgery, is eagerly anticipated.

DISCLOSURE

The author has nothing to disclose.

REFERENCES

1. DeSantis CE, Ma J, Gaudet MM, et al. Breast cancer statistics, 2019. CA Cancer J Clin 2019;69(6): 438–51.
2. Punglia RS, Schnitt SJ, Weeks JC. Treatment of ductal carcinoma in situ after excision: would a prophylactic paradigm be more appropriate? J Natl Cancer Inst 2013;105(20):1527–33.
3. Collins LC, Tamimi RM, Baer HJ, et al. Outcome of patients with ductal carcinoma in situ untreated after diagnostic biopsy: results from the Nurses' Health Study. Cancer 2005;103(9):1778–84.
4. Erbas B, Provenzano E, Armes J, et al. The natural history of ductal carcinoma in situ of the breast: a review. Breast Cancer Res Treat 2006;97(2):135–44.
5. Eusebi V, Feudale E, Foschini MP, et al. Long-term follow-up of in situ carcinoma of the breast. Semin Diagn Pathol 1994;11(3):223–35. https://www.ncbi.nlm.nih.gov/pubmed/7831534.
6. Rosen PP, Braun DW Jr, Kinne DE. The clinical significance of pre-invasive breast carcinoma. Cancer 1980;46(4 Suppl):919–25.
7. Sanders ME, Schuyler PA, Simpson JF, et al. Continued observation of the natural history of low-grade ductal carcinoma in situ reaffirms proclivity for local recurrence even after more than 30 years of follow-up. Mod Pathol 2015;28(5):662–9.
8. Hwang ES, Solin L. De-Escalation of Locoregional Therapy in Low-Risk Disease for DCIS and Early-Stage Invasive Cancer. J Clin Oncol 2020;38(20): 2230–9.
9. Lazzeroni M, DeCensi A. De-Escalating Treatment of Low-Risk Breast Ductal Carcinoma In Situ. J Clin Oncol 2020;38(12):1252–4.
10. van Seijen M, Lips EH, Thompson AM, et al. Ductal carcinoma in situ: to treat or not to treat, that is the question. Br J Cancer 2019;121(4):285–92.
11. Welch HG. The heterogeneity of cancer. J Natl Cancer Inst 2010;102:605–13.
12. Pinder SE, Collins LC, Fox SB, et al. Ductal carcinoma in situ. WHO Classification of Tumours. Lyon: IARC Press; 2019. p. 76–81.
13. Schnitt SJ. Diagnosis of ductal carcinoma in situ in an era of de-escalation of therapy. Mod Pathol 2021;34(Suppl 1):1–7.
14. Morrow M. De-escalating and escalating surgery in the management of early breast cancer. Breast 2017;34(Suppl 1):S1–4.
15. Morrow M, Winer E. De-Escalating Breast Cancer Surgery for Low-Risk Ductal Carcinoma in Situ-Reply. JAMA Oncol 2020;6(7):1118.

16. Tamimi RM, Baer HJ, Marotti J, et al. Comparison of molecular phenotypes of ductal carcinoma in situ and invasive breast cancer. Breast Cancer Res 2008;10(4):R67.

17. Page DL, Dupont WD, Rogers LW, et al. Atypical hyperplastic lesions of the female breast. A long-term follow-up study. Cancer 1985;55(11):2698–708.

18. Collins LC, Baer HJ, Tamimi RM, et al. Magnitude and laterality of breast cancer risk according to histologic type of atypical hyperplasia: results from the Nurses' Health Study. Cancer 2007;109(2):180–7.

19. Degnim AC, Visscher DW, Berman HK, et al. Stratification of breast cancer risk in women with atypia: a Mayo cohort study. J Clin Oncol 2007;25(19):2671–7.

20. Fitzgibbons PL, Henson DE, Hutter RV. Benign breast changes and the risk for subsequent breast cancer: an update of the 1985 consensus statement. Cancer Committee of the College of American Pathologists. Arch Pathol Lab Med 1998;122(12):1053–5. https://www.ncbi.nlm.nih.gov/pubmed/9870852.

21. Hartmann LC, Sellers TA, Frost MH, et al. Benign breast disease and the risk of breast cancer. N Engl J Med 2005;353(3):229–37.

22. London SJ, Connolly JL, Schnitt SJ, et al. A prospective study of benign breast disease and the risk of breast cancer. JAMA 1992;267(7):941–4. https://www.ncbi.nlm.nih.gov/pubmed/1734106.

23. Hartmann LC, Degnim AC, Santen RJ, et al. Atypical hyperplasia of the breast–risk assessment and management options. N Engl J Med 2015;372(1):78–89.

24. Hartmann LC, Radisky DC, Frost MH, et al. Understanding the premalignant potential of atypical hyperplasia through its natural history: a longitudinal cohort study. Cancer Prev Res (Phila) 2014;7(2):211–7.

25. Page DL, Dupont WD, Rogers LW, et al. Intraductal carcinoma of the breast: follow-up after biopsy only. Cancer 1982;49(4):751–8.

26. Fitzgibbons PL, Connolly JL. Protocol for the examination of biopsy specimens from patients with invasive carcinoma of the breast. College of American Pathologists; 2019.

27. Tavassoli FA, Norris HJ. A comparison of the results of long-term follow-up for atypical intraductal hyperplasia and intraductal hyperplasia of the breast. Cancer 1990;65(3):518–29.

28. Gradishar WJ, Moran MS, Abraham J, et al. NCCN Guidelines(R) Insights: Breast Cancer, Version 4.2021. J Natl Compr Canc Netw 2021;19(5):484–93.

29. Solin LJ. Management of Ductal Carcinoma In Situ (DCIS) of the Breast: Present Approaches and Future Directions. Curr Oncol Rep 2019;21(4):33.

30. Allison KH, Collins LC, Moriya T, et al. Atypical ductal hyperplasia. In: Tumours EBB, editor. WHO Classification of Tumours. Lyon: IARC press; 2019. p. 18–21.

31. Syed YY. Oncotype DX Breast Recurrence Score((R)): A Review of its Use in Early-Stage Breast Cancer. Mol Diagn Ther 2020;24(5):621–32.

32. Sanchez-Forgach ER, Carpinteyro-Espin U, Aleman-Aviles JA, et al. [Validation and clinical application of MammaPrint((R)) in patients with breast cancer]. Cir Cir 2017;85(4):320–4.

33. Pang JM, Gorringe KL, Wong SQ, et al. Appraisal of the technologies and review of the genomic landscape of ductal carcinoma in situ of the breast. Breast Cancer Res 2015;17:80.

34. Thompson AM, Clements K, Cheung S, et al. Management and 5-year outcomes in 9938 women with screen-detected ductal carcinoma in situ: the UK Sloane Project. Eur J Cancer 2018;101:210–9.

35. Bremer T, Whitworth PW, Patel R, et al. A Biological Signature for Breast Ductal Carcinoma In Situ to Predict Radiotherapy Benefit and Assess Recurrence Risk. Clin Cancer Res 2018;24(23):5895–901.

36. Rakovitch E, Nofech-Mozes S, Hanna W, et al. A population-based validation study of the DCIS Score predicting recurrence risk in individuals treated by breast-conserving surgery alone. Breast Cancer Res Treat 2015;152(2):389–98.

37. Solin LJ, Gray R, Baehner FL, et al. A multigene expression assay to predict local recurrence risk for ductal carcinoma in situ of the breast. J Natl Cancer Inst 2013;105(10):701–10.

38. Rakovitch E, Gray R, Baehner FL, et al. Refined estimates of local recurrence risks by DCIS score adjusting for clinicopathological features: a combined analysis of ECOG-ACRIN E5194 and Ontario DCIS cohort studies. Breast Cancer Res Treat 2018;169(2):359–69.

39. Weinmann S, Leo MC, Francisco M, et al. Validation of a Ductal Carcinoma In Situ Biomarker Profile for Risk of Recurrence after Breast-Conserving Surgery with and without Radiotherapy. Clin Cancer Res 2020;26(15):4054–63.

40. Mooney KL, Bassett LW, Apple SK. Upgrade rates of high-risk breast lesions diagnosed on core needle biopsy: a single-institution experience and literature review. Mod Pathol 2016;29(12):1471–84.

41. Pena A, Shah SS, Fazzio RT, et al. Multivariate model to identify women at low risk of cancer upgrade after a core needle biopsy diagnosis of atypical ductal hyperplasia. Breast Cancer Res Treat 2017;164(2):295–304.

42. Rageth CJ, Rubenov R, Bronz C, et al. Atypical ductal hyperplasia and the risk of underestimation: tissue sampling method, multifocality, and associated calcification significantly influence the diagnostic upgrade rate based on subsequent surgical specimens. Breast Cancer 2019;26(4):452–8.

43. Vandenbussche CJ, Khouri N, Sbaity E, et al. Borderline atypical ductal hyperplasia/low-grade

ductal carcinoma in situ on breast needle core biopsy should be managed conservatively. Am J Surg Pathol 2013;37(6):913–23.

44. Williams KE, Amin A, Hill J, et al. Radiologic and Pathologic Features Associated With Upgrade of Atypical Ductal Hyperplasia at Surgical Excision. Acad Radiol 2019;26(7):893–9.

45. Schwartz GF, Patchefsky AS, Finklestein SD, et al. Nonpalpable in situ ductal carcinoma of the breast. Predictors of multicentricity and microinvasion and implications for treatment. Arch Surg 1989;124(1): 29–32.

46. Castellano I, Marchio C, Tomatis M, et al. Micropapillary ductal carcinoma in situ of the breast: an inter-institutional study. Mod Pathol 2010;23(2):260–9.

47. Ely KA, Carter BA, Jensen RA, et al. Core biopsy of the breast with atypical ductal hyperplasia: a probabilistic approach to reporting. Am J Surg Pathol 2001;25(8):1017–21.

48. Lewis JT, Hartmann LC, Vierkant RA, et al. An analysis of breast cancer risk in women with single, multiple, and atypical papilloma. Am J Surg Pathol 2006;30(6):665–72.

49. MacGrogan G, Tavassoli FA. Central atypical papillomas of the breast: a clinicopathological study of 119 cases. Virchows Arch 2003;443(5):609–17.

50. Page DL, Salhany KE, Jensen RA, et al. Subsequent breast carcinoma risk after biopsy with atypia in a breast papilloma. Cancer 1996;78(2):258–66.

51. Grimm LJ, Shelley Hwang E. Active Surveillance for DCIS: The Importance of Selection Criteria and Monitoring. Ann Surg Oncol 2016;23(13):4134–6.

52. Jakub JW, Murphy BL, Gonzalez AB, et al. A Validated Nomogram to Predict Upstaging of Ductal Carcinoma in Situ to Invasive Disease. Ann Surg Oncol 2017;24(10):2915–24.

53. Patel GV, Van Sant EP, Taback B, et al. Patient Selection for Ductal Carcinoma In Situ Observation Trials: Are the Lesions Truly Low Risk? AJR Am J Roentgenol 2018;211(3):712–3.

54. Pilewskie M, Stempel M, Rosenfeld H, et al. Do LORIS Trial Eligibility Criteria Identify a Ductal Carcinoma In Situ Patient Population at Low Risk of Upgrade to Invasive Carcinoma? Ann Surg Oncol 2016;23(11):3487–93.

55. McCormick B, Winter K, Hudis C, et al. RTOG 9804: a prospective randomized trial for good-risk ductal carcinoma in situ comparing radiotherapy with observation. J Clin Oncol 2015;33(7):709–15.

56. Solin LJ, Gray R, Hughes LL, et al. Surgical Excision Without Radiation for Ductal Carcinoma in Situ of the Breast: 12-Year Results From the ECOG-ACRIN E5194 Study. J Clin Oncol 2015;33(33):3938–44.

57. Wong JS, Chen YH, Gadd MA, et al. Eight-year update of a prospective study of wide excision alone for small low- or intermediate-grade ductal carcinoma in situ (DCIS). Breast Cancer Res Treat 2014;143(2):343–50.

A New Landscape of Testing and Therapeutics in Metastatic Breast Cancer

Geetha Jagannathan, MBBS[1], Marissa J. White, MD[1],
Rena R. Xian, MD[1,2], Leisha A. Emens, MD, PhD[3],
Ashley Cimino-Mathews, MD[1,2],*

KEYWORDS

- Biomarkers • Metastasis • Breast cancer • PD-L1 • Tumor mutation burden
- Companion diagnostic

Key points

- Biomarker testing on metastatic breast carcinoma enables selection of targeted therapies, and companion diagnostics are required assays coupled to an associated therapy.

- The National Comprehensive Cancer Network (NCCN) recommends biomarker assessment of hormone receptor status, HER2, and *BRCA1/2* on all metastatic breast carcinomas, and suggests second-line biomarker assessment of *PIK3CA* on metastatic hormone receptor positive, HER2 negative carcinomas.

- The NCCN recommends biomarker assessment of PD-L1 on metastatic triple negative carcinomas, with assessment of tumor mutation burden, mismatch repair protein status/microsatellite instability, and *NTRK* status in select circumstances.

ABSTRACT

Predictive biomarker testing on metastatic breast cancer is essential for determining patient eligibility for targeted therapeutics. The National Comprehensive Cancer Network currently recommends assessment of specific biomarkers on metastatic tumor subtypes, including hormone receptors, HER2, and *BRCA1/2* mutations, on all newly metastatic breast cancers subtypes; programmed death-ligand 1 on metastatic triple-negative carcinomas; and *PIK3CA* mutation status on estrogen receptor-positive carcinomas. In select circumstances mismatch repair protein deficiency and/or microsatellite insufficiency, tumor mutation burden, and *NTRK* translocation status are also testing options. Novel biomarker testing, such as detecting *PIK3CA* mutations in circulating tumor DNA, is expanding in this rapidly evolving arena.

OVERVIEW

Metastatic breast cancer remains an incurable disease, with significantly lower 5-year survival (28%) compared with localized cancer (99%) and cancers with nodal involvement (86%).[1] The therapeutic options for patients with metastatic breast cancer were historically limited; however, research has generated new and promising targeted therapies for patients with metastatic breast cancer. Targeted therapies typically require unique biomarker testing to determine eligibility for treatment, many of which must be performed with one particular assay.

[1] Department of Pathology, The Johns Hopkins University School of Medicine, 401 N Broadway, Weinberg 2242, Baltimore, MD 21287, USA; [2] Department of Oncology, The Johns Hopkins University School of Medicine, 401 N Broadway, Weinberg 2242, Baltimore, MD 21287, USA; [3] Department of Oncology, UPMC Hillman Cancer Center/Magee Women's Hospital, 5117 Centre Avenue, Room 1.46e, Pittsburgh, PA 15213, USA
* Corresponding author. 401 N Broadway, Weinberg 2242, Baltimore, MD 21287.
E-mail address: acimino1@jhmi.edu

Surgical Pathology 15 (2022) 105–120
https://doi.org/10.1016/j.path.2021.11.007
1875-9181/22/© 2021 Elsevier Inc. All rights reserved.

The National Comprehensive Cancer Network (NCCN) clinical practice guidelines recommend assessment of the following biomarkers in metastatic breast cancer: hormone receptors, human epidermal growth factor receptor-2 (HER2), programmed death-ligand 1 (PD-L1) (in triple negative), and germline *BRCA1* and *BRCA2* status, with the option to test for *PIK3CA* as a second line in estrogen receptor (ER)-positive, HER2-negative cancers, and in select circumstances to test for mismatch repair protein status and tumor mutational burden and/or *NTRK* (**Tables 1–3**).[2] Recommended testing methods include immunohistochemistry (IHC), chromogenic in situ hybridization (CISH), fluorescent in situ hybridization (FISH), targeted gene sequencing, and large-panel next-generation sequencing. Many of these biomarkers must be determined using an assay that is designated by the US Food and Drug Administration (FDA) as a companion diagnostic for its associated targeted therapeutic agent.[3–5] In this review, we cover the recommended biomarker assessment, testing methods, and companion diagnostics for metastatic breast cancer.

Summary Box 1: Recommended biomarker assessment in metastatic breast cancer

1. Hormone receptors: ER and PR (all newly metastatic)

2. HER2 (all newly metastatic)

3. PD-L1 by 22C3 in triple-negative metastatic breast carcinomas

4. MSI or dMMR[a]

5. TMB[a]

6. *BRCA1* and *BRCA2* (germline testing on all newly metastatic patients)

7. *PIK3CA* (as a second-line option in ER-positive, HER2-negative metastatic cancer)

8. *NTRK*[a]

dMMR, mismatch repair protein deficiency; MSI, microsatellite instability; PD-L1, programmed death-ligand 1; PR, progesterone receptor; TMB, tumor mutation burden.

[a]In select circumstances.

HORMONE RECEPTOR AND HUMAN EPIDERMAL GROWTH FACTOR RECEPTOR-2 TESTING

CLINICAL RELEVANCE

ER, progesterone receptor (PR), and HER2 testing are the prototype of predictive and prognostic

biomarker testing in breast cancer. Retesting ER, PR, and HER2 on metastatic breast cancers at first occurrence, each recurrence, and on different sites of disease are standard of care. Based on their expression, breast cancers fall into 3 distinct prognostic and predictive groups: (1) hormone receptor positive and HER2 negative, (2) HER2 positive with or without hormone receptor expression, and (3) triple negative for both hormone receptors and HER2. Most often, metastatic disease has the same hormone receptor and HER2 expression profile as the primary tumor. However, a small but significant subset of the metastatic disease shows discordance in expression of these markers, which can significantly impact treatment decisions. In addition, tumoral heterogeneity and divergent clonal evolution can result in the presence of different hormone receptor or HER2 status in different tumor sites or in regions within one tumor (**Fig. 1**).[6,7]

Two notable independent prospective studies, the Breast Recurrence In Tissues Study (BRITS) and DESTINY studies, evaluated the changes in ER, PR, and HER2 expression in the primary tumor and any subsequent recurrences, both locoregional and distant metastases. A pooled analysis of the 2 studies' data by Amir and colleagues[8] showed that the overall discordance rates for the 3 markers were 12.6%, 31.2%, and 5.5%, respectively. Among the 3 markers, expression of PR was more often discordant than ER and HER2. The trend in the PR expression discordance was often a conversion from a positive to a negative result. This decrease or loss of PR is relevant (**Fig. 2**), because it can signal poorer response to antihormonal therapy.[9]

The discordance is explained by a wide variety of factors, including tumor biology (eg, tumor heterogeneity, clonal evolution), preanalytical variables (eg, tissue fixation, method of staining), and analytical variables (eg, subjectivity of scoring, interobserver variability). The current NCCN and American Society of Clinical Oncology (ASCO) guidelines recommend retesting all new metastatic breast cancers for ER, PR, and HER2 status. Retesting is especially important when the markers were previously unknown, initially negative, or not overexpressed. The conversion of hormone receptors and HER2 from negative to positive expression is the most clinically significant. In the analysis of Amir and colleagues,[8] 13% of hormone receptor-negative and 5% of HER2-negative primary tumors gained expression of the biomarkers in their respective metastatic tumor foci. Biomarker discordances contributed to change in therapy in approximately 14% of the patients enrolled in the 2 studies.[8] Retesting offers a

Table 1

Biomarker characteristics for estrogen receptor, progesterone receptor, and human epidermal growth factor receptor-2

Marker Tested	Breast Cancer Subtype	Test Method Type	Sample Type	Scoring	Companion Diagnostics[5]	Manufacturer	FDA-Approved Drugs
ER and PR	Any	IHC	FFPE	Score intensity and percentage of tumor cells labeling: <1%: Negative ≥1%: Positive 1%–10% ER expression: Low positive	Any FDA-approved antibody platform. No formally designated companion diagnostic		Aromatase inhibitors; tamoxifen; CDK4/6 inhibitors with aromatase inhibitors or fulvestrant
HER2	Any	IHC	FFPE	Score intensity, completeness of membranous labeling and percentage of tumor cells labeling[14]: Negative (score 0 or 1+) Equivocal (2+) Positive (3+)	InSite Her-2/neu KIT	Biogenex Laboratories, Inc	Trastuzumab
					Bond Oracle HER2 IHC System HercepTest	Leica Biosystems Dako Denmark A/S	Trastuzumab Trastuzumab; pertuzumab; T-DM1
					PATHWAY anti-Her2/neu (4B5) Rabbit Monoclonal Primary Antibody	Ventana Medical Systems, Inc	Trastuzumab; T-DM1
		FISH		Score average HER2 copy number and ratio of HER2 to CEP17 in tumor cells[15]	INFORM HER2 Dual ISH DNA Probe Cocktail	Ventana Medical Systems, Inc	Trastuzumab; T-DM1
					INFORM HER-2/neu	Ventana Medical Systems, Inc	Trastuzumab
					HER2 FISH pharmDx Kit	Dako Denmark A/S	Trastuzumab; Pertuzumab; T-DM1
					VENTANA HER2 Dual ISH DNA Probe Cocktail	Ventana Medical Systems, Inc	Trastuzumab
					PathVysion HER-2 DNA Probe Kit	Abbott Molecular Inc	Trastuzumab
		CISH		Score average HER2 copy number in tumor cells	SPOT-Light HER2 CISH Kit	Life Technologies Corporation	Trastuzumab
		NGS			HER2 CISH pharmDx Kit	Dako Denmark A/S	Trastuzumab
					FoundationOne CDx	Foundation Medicine, Inc	Trastuzumab; pertuzumab; T-DM1

Abbreviations: CEP17, chromosome enumeration probe 17; CISH, chromogenic in situ hybridization; F=PE, formalin-fixed paraffin-embedded; FISH, fluorescence in situ hybridization; IHC, immunohistochemistry; NGS, next-generation sequencing; T-DM1, ado-trastuzumab emtansine

Table 2
Biomarker characteristics for immunotherapy: programmed death-ligand 1, tumor mutation burden, and microsatellite instability/mismatch repair protein deficiency

Marker	Breast Cancer Subtype Tested	Test Method	Sample Type	Scoring	Companion Diagnostics	Manufacturer	FDA-Approved Drugs
PD-L1	Advanced HR-negative, HER2-negative	IHC	FFPE	CPS = number of PD-L1$^+$ tumor cells plus the number of PD-L1$^+$ immune cells (lymphocytes and macrophages only), divided by the total number of tumor cells, multiplied by 100	PD-L1 IHC 22C3 Pharm Dx	Dako North America, Inc	Adjuvant pembrolizumab with chemotherapy (nab-paclitaxel, or paclitaxel, or gemcitabine plus carboplatin)
MSI/d-MMR	Any	IHC/PCR	FFPE	MSI testing evaluates for the presence of additional peaks in microsatellites of tumor in comparison to nonneoplastic tissue dMMR is determined by loss of IHC labeling for MMR proteins, MLH1, PMS2, MSH2, MSH6	Any FDA-approved antibody platform. No companion diagnostic is available at present		Pembrolizumab
TMB	Any	NGS	FFPE	High TMB is > 10 mutations/megabase of genome tested	FoundationOne CDx	Foundation Medicine, Inc	Pembrolizumab

Abbreviations: CPS, combined positive score; dMMR, mismatch repair protein deficiency; FFPE, formalin-fixed paraffin-embedded; HR, hormone receptor; MSI, microsatellite instability; NGS, next-generation sequencing; PCR, polymerase chain reaction; PD-L1, programmed death-ligand 1; TMB, tumor mutation burden.

Table 3
Biomarker characteristics for single-gene alterations

Marker	Breast Cancer Subtype Tested	Test Method	Sample Type	Companion Diagnostics	Manufacturer	FDA-Approved Drugs
PIK3CA mutations	HR-positive, HER2-negative	PCR	Blood for circulating tumor DNA or FFPE	therascreen PIK3CA RGQ PCR Kit	QIAGEN GmbH	Alpelisib
		NGS	Blood for circulating tumor DNA	Foundation One Liquid CDx	Foundation Medicine, Inc	
		NGS for somatic and germline detection	FFPE	Foundation One CDx	Foundation Medicine, Inc	Alpelisib
BRCA1/BRCA2 germline and somatic mutations	Any	Germline testing by PCR and Sanger sequencing	Blood	ERACAnalysis CDx	Myriad Genetic Laboratories, Inc	Olaprib Talazoparib
NTRK fusions	Secretory carcinomas	NGS	FFPE	FoundationOne CDx	Foundation Medicine, Inc	Larotrectinib

Abbreviations: FFPE, formalin-fixed paraffin-embedded; HR, hormone receptor; NGS, next-generation sequencing; PCR, polymerase chain reaction.

subset of patients an additional treatment option with endocrine therapy, CDK 4/6 inhibitors, and/or trastuzumab.[10] Patients with discordant ER and HER2 results due to biomarker conversion tend to have worse survival than those with concordant biomarker results.[11]

TESTING TECHNIQUES

ASCO and College of American Pathologists (CAP) jointly developed guidelines for the interpretation and reporting of ER, PR, and HER2 in breast cancer. As of this writing, the most recent updates to the guidelines for ER/PR and HER testing occurred in 2020 and 2018, respectively.[12,13] ER and PR testing are routinely performed by IHC. The latest guidelines recommend classifying tumors with an ER labeling of 1% to 10% as "ER low positive." These tumors more closely resemble basallike breast cancers in histology, molecular profile, and response to neoadjuvant chemotherapy than ER-positive breast cancers. The data on the benefit of endocrine therapy in this group are limited and potentially low. However, these patients are still eligible to receive endocrine therapy.[12] Cases with less than 10% ER labeling and those close to the threshold require a laboratory-specific standard operating procedure such as a

second pathologist to review the score to ensure reproducibility.

HER2 assessment can be performed by IHC, FISH, CISH, or silver in situ hybridization (SISH). Although IHC is commonly used as first line for its quick turnaround time and cost-effectiveness, any approved method of testing may be used for first-line testing. An equivocal result is reflexed to a different testing method to provide a definitive result. The algorithms for the interpretation of hormone receptor and HER2 expression in metastatic tumors are the same as those for primary tumors, and guidelines are available for free online from the CAP.[14,15]

CHALLENGES AND PRACTICAL CONSIDERATIONS

Although specific IHC assays for ER and PR are not formally designated as FDA-approved companion diagnostic tests, in practice they function as companion diagnostics to deem patients as candidates for endocrine therapy. On the other hand, there are specific FDA companion diagnostic tests for HER2, as detailed in **Table 1**.

The most common distant site of breast cancer metastasis is the bone.[16] Biomarker expression

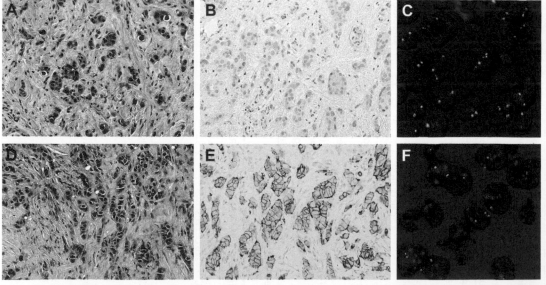

Fig. 1. Tumoral HER2 heterogeneity within a pleomorphic lobular carcinoma. Most of this primary invasive lobular carcinoma displays classic morphology with uniform cells arranged singly and in nests. (*A*, hematoxylin-eosin [H&E], original magnification ×200). This classic component is negative for HER2 protein overexpression by IHC (*B*, original magnification ×200) and is negative for *HER2* amplification by FISH, with a *HER2:-CEP17* ratio of 1.6 and a *HER2* copy number of 2.3 signals per cell (*C*; green = *CEP17*, red = *HER2* locus). However, a subset of this tumor is pleomorphic, with enlarged and variably sized nuclei (*D*, H&E, original magnification ×200). This pleomorphic component is equivocal (IHC 2+) for HER2 overexpression by IHC (*E*, ×200) and is positive for *HER2* amplification by FISH, with a *HER2:CEP17* ratio of 4.4 and a *HER2* copy number of 8.7 signals/cell (*F*; green = *CEP17*, red = *HER2* locus). Tumoral HER2 heterogeneity could result in disparate biomarker profiles in different metastatic sites, or clonal expansion and predominance of biomarker profile.

testing in this setting is particularly challenging due to the confounding effects of decalcification on antigenicity and DNA integrity in bone specimens. Rapidly acting, strong acid buffers such as hydrochloric acid lower the antigenicity of the tumor cells and frequently produce false-negative results in hormone receptor and HER2 expression results by IHC (see **Fig. 2**), as well as false-negative amplification of *HER2* by FISH.[17] Weaker acid buffers containing acetic acid and formic acid and chelating agents such as EDTA[18] are currently more widely used. Although they are slow acting, their use improves antigen preservation and stability. Bone fragments should be separated out from soft tissue in these specimens to minimize the amount of tissue subjected to decalcification. Biomarker testing can also be performed on cytology specimens, which have results comparable to core biopsies.[19]

Key points Box 1: Estrogen receptor, progesterone receptor, and human epidermal growth factor receptor-2 testing in metastatic breast cancer

1. ER, PR, and HER2 should be retested on all new metastases due to the possibility of discordance and potential management changes.

2. ER-low positive is a new category of tumors with 1% to 10% ER labeling; patients are eligible for endocrine therapy but are less likely to benefit from it.

3. Decalcification with strong acid buffers can cause false-negative results for ER, PR, and HER2 expression; this is mitigated but not eliminated with agents containing EDTA and weaker acids.

4. When sampling and grossing metastatic tumors in bone, the soft tissue fragments should be separated out to avoid decalcification of the entire tumor and to improve biomarker assessment.

PROGRAMMED DEATH-LIGAND 1 TESTING FOR IMMUNOTHERAPY

CLINICAL RELEVANCE

Immunotherapy has shown a long-lasting, durable treatment response in various tumor types. Triple-negative breast carcinoma (TNBC) and HER2-positive carcinoma often display brisk tumor-infiltrating lymphocytes (TILs), reflecting a host antitumor immune response.[20] The checkpoint inhibitor pembrolizumab targeting the programmed

death 1 (PD-1) receptor recently gained regular FDA approval for both high-risk early (regardless of programmed death-ligand 1 [PD-L1] status) and locally advanced unresectable or metastatic TNBC (for PD-L1+ disease); this reflects a major advance for an aggressive breast tumor subtype for which few targeted therapies are available. For advanced PD-L1+ TNBC, pembrolizumab in combination with several chemotherapeutic options (nab-paclitaxel, or paclitaxel, or gemcitabine plus carboplatin) is endorsed by the FDA.[21] Notably, the use of atezolizumab in combination with nab-paclitaxel demonstrated clinical activity in randomized phase 3 clinical trials of advanced TNBC[22]; however, the accelerated approval for its use in this setting was voluntarily withdrawn by the sponsor in 2021. Of note, the FDA also granted full approval for the addition of pembrolizumab to standard neoadjuvant chemotherapy, followed by pembrolizumab monotherapy, for high-risk early-stage TNBC regardless of PD-L1 expression.[23]

TESTING TECHNIQUES

IHC for PD-L1 is used to identify patients with metastatic TNBC who are eligible for checkpoint inhibition with pembrolizumab. As of this writing, there is one FDA-approved companion diagnostic assay for the use of pembrolizumab in TNBC (see **Table 2**). To guide the use of pembrolizumab in the advanced disease setting, the PD-L1 status of a tumor is determined by the combined positive score (CPS), which is the number of PD-L1+ tumor cells plus the number of PD-L1+ immune cells (lymphocytes and macrophages only), divided by the total number of tumor cells, multiplied by 100. A tumor is considered PD-L1 positive, and the patient eligible for pembrolizumab, when the CPS score is 10 or more (**Fig. 3**). The only FDA-approved PD-L1 companion diagnostic that uses the CPS scoring system is the PD-L1 IHC 22C3 pharmDx assay ("22C3 assay"). For high-risk early-stage TNBC, the addition of pembrolizumab to standard neoadjuvant chemotherapy is a treatment option regardless of PD-L1 status, so PD-L1 testing to determine eligibility for neoadjuvant immunotherapy is not recommended.[23]

For the clinical trials and during the accelerated approval period for atezolizumab with nab-paclitaxel, the PD-L1 status of a breast tumor was determined by the immune cell (IC) score, which is the percentage of the tumor area occupied by PD-L1+ immune cells (TILs, plasma cells, neutrophils, eosinophils, and macrophages). A tumor was considered PD-L1 positive, and the patient eligible for atezolizumab, when the IC score was 1% or greater (see **Fig. 3**). The PD-L1

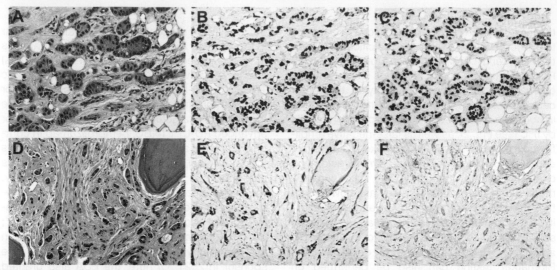

Fig. 2. PR discordance between a primary and metastatic tumor to bone in a decalcified specimen. This primary invasive ductal carcinoma (*A*, H&E, original magnification ×200) is diffusely and strongly positive for estrogen receptor (ER) (*B*, original magnification ×200) and PR (*C*, original magnification ×200). However, although biomarker testing on the patient's metastatic tumor in the iliac crest bone (*D*, H&E, original magnification ×200) shows concordant ER expression (*E*, original magnification ×200), the PR is discordant with negative (0%) labeling (*F*, original magnification ×200). Absence of biomarker labeling in a decalcified specimen could reflect true discordance, or a false-negative result due to the decalcification process.

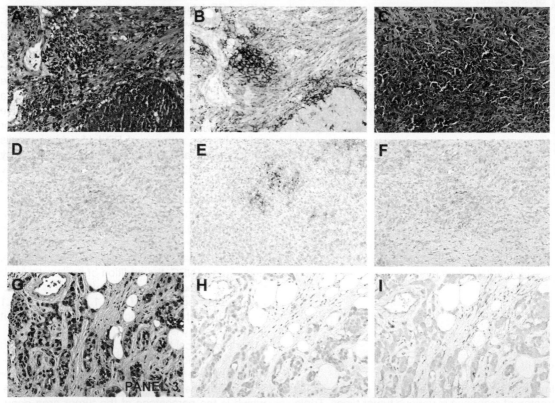

Fig. 3. PD-L1 immunohistochemistry: the PD-L1 IHC 22C3 pharmDx assay. PANEL 1: A locally advanced, primary TNBC (*A*, H&E, original magnification ×200) is PD-L1 positive by the 22C3 assay, with a CPS of 10 or more (*B*, original magnification ×200). This patient is eligible for pembrolizumab plus approved chemotherapy. PANEL 2: The archival primary tumor of a patient with metastatic TNBC (*C*, H&E, original magnification ×200) is PD-L1 negative by the 22C3 assay, with a CPS less than 10 (*F*, original magnification ×200). This patient is not eligible for pembrolizumab.

companion diagnostic that used the IC scoring system was the Ventana PD-L1 (SP142) assay ("SP142 assay"). The indication for atezolizumab in advanced TNBC was voluntarily withdrawn by the sponsor in 2021.

CHALLENGES AND PRACTICAL CONSIDERATIONS

PD-L1 testing currently should only be performed on tumor samples from patients with locally advanced or metastatic TNBC, and only upon request from the oncologist. The PD-L1 22C3 IHC assay can be performed on both newly obtained metastatic tumor samples and archival primary tumors. Exploratory biomarker analyses from patients on clinical trials with atezolizumab showed that the likelihood of a positive PD-L1 result does vary between the primary and metastatic tumor, as well as between different metastasis niche sites. In general, metastases tend to have fewer TILs than primary tumors, decreasing the chances of having immune cells present to express PD-L1. In addition, metastases to the liver and brain tend to have fewer TILs than metastases to other sites such as the lung.[24] It is not known if this extends to PD-L1 expression as determined by the 22C3 assay. Given the totality of the data, it is preferable to avoid PD-L1 testing on liver samples if possible. Of note, the PD-L1 IHC assays are not validated for decalcified bone specimens, cytology cell blocks or smears, or circulating tumor cells.

Unlike chemotherapy, which causes well-recognized cytotoxic side effects, immunotherapy causes a spectrum of immune-related adverse events (irAEs), affecting various organ systems. Pathologists need to be aware of and recognize the histopathology of irAEs across organ types, including dermatitis, thyroiditis, hepatitis, colitis, and potentially fatal pneumonitis.[25]

Key Points Box 2: Programmed death-ligand 1 testing in metastatic breast cancer

1. PD-L1 testing is currently indicated for patients with locally advanced or metastatic TNBC

2. The 22C3 assay uses the CPS scoring system to determine patient eligibility for pembrolizumab plus chemotherapy for advanced TNBC

3. The CPS score is the total number of PD-L1$^+$ cells (tumor cells plus mononuclear immune cells), divided by the total number of tumor

cells, multiplied by 100, with a positivity cut-off in breast cancer of 10 or more.

4. PD-L1 testing can be performed on either new metastatic tumor biopsies or archival primary tumor samples.

MISMATCH REPAIR PROTEIN DEFICIENCY, MICROSATELLITE INSTABILITY, AND TUMOR MUTATION BURDEN TESTING

CLINICAL RELEVANCE

Some tumor types have higher tumor mutation burden (TMB) than others. Mutations accumulate in tumors by various mechanisms, including mutations (germline or somatic) in genes involved in repair of DNA base pair mismatches (mismatch protein [MMR] proteins) or double-strand DNA breaks (*BRCA1/2*). As mutations accumulate, tumor cells express new antigens on the cell surface and can become highly immunogenic and susceptible to immunotherapy.[26]

The prevalence of mismatch repair protein deficiency (dMMR) in breast cancer (~2%) is significantly lower than that in cancers of the colon (~15–20%) and endometrium (~20–30%). dMMR testing and microsatellite instability (MSI) testing have become standard of care in colon and endometrial carcinomas, whereas their use in breast cancers is limited. dMMR breast cancers are frequently high grade, associated with high TILs, and often negative for PR expression.[27] A high TMB is seen in about 5% of breast cancers, which predominantly includes TNBC and metastatic tumors. Among metastatic tumors, high TMB is more frequently seen in metastatic lobular carcinoma than metastatic ductal carcinoma. These tumors are also associated with high TILs and *BRCA1/2* germline mutations (**Fig. 4**).[28]

Single-agent pembrolizumab is now approved for any advanced solid tumor with MSI-high status, dMMR, or high TMB. Pembrolizumab is the first drug to be ever approved based on biomarkers across all tumor types (ie, a "tumor agnostic" approval).[29]

TESTING TECHNIQUES

MMR testing in breast cancer is based on techniques that have been widely used in colorectal and endometrial cancers. The most commonly used testing methods are IHC or polymerase chain reaction (PCR). IHC assays for MMR proteins, namely MLH1, PMS1, MSH2, and MSH6, evaluate for loss of nuclear expression in the tumor cells. MSI is formally assessed by PCR to look for the

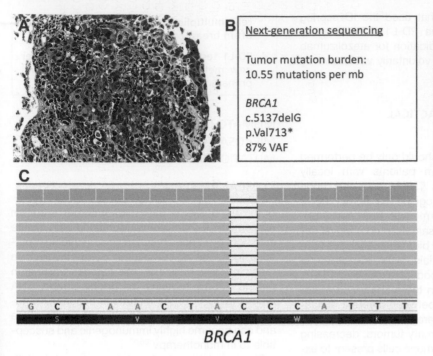

Fig. 4. BRCA1 mutation in a TNBC with high tumor mutation burden. This TNBC metastatic to the brain (*A*, H&E, original magnification ×200) underwent next-generation sequencing (NGS). NGS revealed a high tumor mutation burden of 10.55 mutations per megabase (Mb) (where high TMB is ≥ 10 mutations per Mb) and a pathogenic BRCA1 mutation (*B*, *C*). The BRCA1 mutation was previously identified as a germline change. In the tumor, this mutation has a variant allele frequency (VAF) of 87%, which is consistent with loss of heterozygosity (LOH), and biallelic inactivation of BRCA1 in the tumor. High TMB makes the patient eligible for single-agent pembrolizumab, and the germline BRCA1 mutation (with LOH in the tumor) makes the patient eligible for PARP inhibitors.

presence of additional peaks in microsatellites in the tumor compared with normal nonneoplastic tissue. The tumors that are microsatellite unstable are further classified based on the number of unstable markers as MSI low (1 marker) and MSI high (≥2 markers). In April 2021, the FDA approved the MMR IHC assay VENTANA MMR RxDx (Roche) as companion diagnostic for selecting endometrial cancers for dostarlimab-gxly immunotherapy.[30] At present, there are no MMR or MSI companion diagnostics for breast cancer. Any FDA-cleared assay may be used to determine eligibility for immunotherapy; however, this may change in the future, as new companion diagnostics are developed.[30,31]

TMB is determined either by whole-genome or whole-exome sequencing, or by sequencing targeted regions of the genome. TMB is defined as the total number of somatic mutations in a megabase of the genomic sequence analyzed. Tumors with 10 or more mutations per megabase of the genome are generally accepted as having high TMB. Unlike MSI and MMR testing, TMB testing has a companion diagnostic assay, the FoundationOneCDx assay (Foundation Medicine, Inc) (see **Table 2**), which is often required to determine patient eligibility for single-agent pembrolizumab.

CHALLENGES AND PRACTICAL CONSIDERATIONS

Studies on dMMR and MSI in breast cancer have shown some major drawbacks to MMR IHC in breast cancer: (1) IHC for MMR proteins shows significant heterogeneity within the tumors, which can be particularly problematic in small biopsies, and (2) loss of MMR proteins by IHC does not correlate well with MSI testing by PCR in breast cancer. Thus, the 2 testing methods (IHC and PCR) cannot be used interchangeably in breast cancer, unlike what is done in colon or endometrial cancer. Loss of MMR proteins by IHC is more frequent than MSI.[32] At present, there are no breast cancer-specific testing guidelines for dMMR and MSI testing.

Assessment of TMB can be particularly useful in metastatic TNBC. Testing is largely driven by the oncologist in circumstances in which there are no other satisfactory treatment options available. However, because MSI and TMB are included in most next-generation sequencing assays performed for actionable mutations, this information will be available for any tumor subjected to broad sequencing.

SINGLE-GENE ALTERATION TESTING FOR TARGETED THERAPY

BRCA 1 AND BRCA 2

BRCA1 and *BRCA2* are tumor suppressor genes whose protein products repair double-strand DNA breaks by homologous recombination. Approximately 10% of breast cancers have mutations in one of these genes. About two-thirds of them are germline, whereas the rest are somatic.[33,34] There are some key differences between breast cancers that arise in carriers of *BRCA1* versus *BRCA2* mutations. *BRCA1*-mutated breast cancers are often TNBC, metaplastic carcinomas, or medullary pattern and have high nuclear grade and TILs (see **Fig. 4**). *BRCA2*-mutated cancers are often of luminal immunophenotype and with variable histologic patterns and grades.[35]

Poly(adenosine diphosphate-ribose) polymerase (PARP) inhibitors (olaparib and talazoparib) and platinum-based chemotherapies are effective in patients with *BRCA1/2*-mutated breast cancers. In breast cancer, PARP inhibitors are currently approved only for patients with metastatic breast cancer and *germline* mutation in either gene.[36] In contrast, PARP inhibitors are approved for use in patients with ovarian carcinoma and either *germline or somatic BRCA1/2* mutations. Recent trials have shown that PARP inhibitors are also effective in patients with breast cancer and somatic *BRCA1/2* mutations, which, if approved, would expand the population of eligible patients.[37] *BRCA* testing not only offers a targeted therapeutic option to patients but also helps identify family members who may be at risk, and *BRCA* testing is initiated by the treating oncologist. The companion diagnostic assay is BRACAnalysisCDx (Myriad Genetic Laboratories, Inc), which uses Sanger sequencing and multiplex PCR to detect various *BRCA* mutations (see

Table 3). This assay is currently only intended to detect germline mutations.

PIK3CA

Most (70%) breast cancers are hormone receptor positive and HER2 negative. The first line of treatment of these cancers, whether primary or metastatic, is endocrine therapy to suppress the tumor's estrogen-dependent growth. In the metastatic setting, CDK4/6 inhibitors are also considered first line in ER-positive, HER2-negative cancers (no additional testing except ER positivity required). However, about half of these patients will eventually develop resistance to endocrine therapy. One strategy to overcome the resistance is by inhibiting the PI3K/AKT/mTOR pathway components, which regulate cell functions such as growth, division, and survival. About 40% of hormone receptor-positive and HER2-negative tumors harbor activating mutations in *PIK3CA* (**Fig. 5**). At present, *PIK3CA* inhibitor alpelisib, in combination with selective estrogen receptor downregulator fulvestrant, is a second-line therapy in patients with metastatic breast cancer who have progressed on endocrine therapy with or without CDK4/6 inhibitors.[38] The treating oncologist initiates *PIK3CA* testing. There are 3 companion diagnostic assays available to detect *PIK3CA* mutations: therascreen *PIK3CA* RGQ PCR Kit (PCR test), FoundationOne Liquid CDx assay (NGS test), and FoundationOne CDx assay (NGS test) (see **Table 3**).[39] The first 2 assays can be performed on patients' blood samples using circulating tumor DNA. *PIK3CA* is the only biomarker in breast cancer that has been approved for detection in the blood through circulating tumor DNA.[40–42]

NTRK TESTING

NTRK inhibitors (larotrectinib and entrectinib) are newly developed targeted therapies for solid tumors with fusions involving genes of the *NTRK* family, independent of tumor histology.[43,44] In the breast, secretory carcinomas are a rare tumor type accounting for less than 0.15% of all invasive breast cancers. These tumors are characterized by unique histology with intracellular and extracellular eosinophilic secretions, typically TNBC phenotype, and a pathognomonic *ETV6-NTRK3* gene fusion (**Fig. 6**). These tumors are identical to their counterparts in the salivary gland, thyroid, and skin.[45] Most of these tumors are indolent, whereas a small subset is aggressive with late recurrences and may benefit from *NTRK* inhibitors.

NTRK testing is unique because it is triggered by the pathologist upon histologic diagnosis of

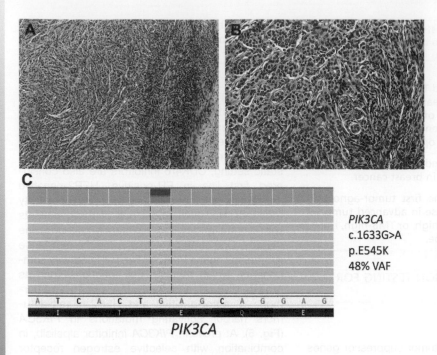

PIK3CA
c.1633G>A
p.E545K
48% VAF

Fig. 5. PIK3CA mutation in an ER[+] breast carcinoma. Sections of an ovarian tumor (*A*, H&E, original magnification ×100) reveal nests of uniform cells (*B*, H&E, X200) that are diffusely ER[+] (not shown), consistent with a metastasis from the patient's known breast primary. Next-gen eration sequencing revealed a pathogenic PIK3CA mutation (*C*) with 48% variant allele frequency (VAF). The p.E545K mutation is one of the most common activating mutations in PIK3CA commonly detected in breast carcinoma. This PIK3CA mutation makes the patient eligible for PIK3CA-targeted therapy.

secretory carcinoma rather than by the treating clinician. Until recently, *NTRK* fusions were detected by molecular methods such as FISH and NGS. Now, a pan-*NTRK* IHC stain is available, and the *ETV6-NTRK* fusion causes a nuclear localization of the fusion protein and nuclear labeling with IHC. Diffuse and/or at least focally strong nuclear labeling with IHC has good sensitivity (83%) and specificity (100%) in detecting the *ETV6-NTRK3* fusion in secretory carcinomas of the breast.[46] IHC may be a valuable and cost-effective screening tool for secretory carcinomas, but it is not an approved companion diagnostic and molecular testing is required to confirm gene rearrangements in tumors in which *NTRK* inhibitors are being considered. The approved companion diagnostic for *NTRK* analysis is the next-generation sequencing platform FoundationOne CDx assay (see **Table 3**).[47] *NTRK* analysis is typically part of large next-generation sequencing platforms and will be assessed in all breast cancer subtypes submitted for sequencing. However, the vast majority of breast cancers known to have *NTRK* alterations are secretory carcinomas.[48]

Key Points Box 4: Single mutation testing in metastatic breast cancer

1. Patients with germline *BRCA1/2* mutations and metastatic breast cancer are eligible for therapy with PARP inhibitors

2. Patients with somatic *PIK3CA* mutations in ER-positive, HER2-negative metastatic breast cancer are eligible for targeted therapy with alpelisib

3. Patients with *NTRK* rearrangement metastatic breast secretory carcinomas are eligible for targeted therapy with larotrectinib and entrectinib

4. Although *NTRK* assessment can be performed on any breast cancer subtype, there is no utility in testing nonsecretory carcinomas.

5. IHC to detect NTRK protein is an effective screening and diagnostic tool in secretory carcinomas, but molecular confirmation is required for treatment with NTRK inhibitors.

FUTURE DIRECTIONS

NOVEL ASSAYS

Liquid biopsies of blood for circulating tumor DNA (ctDNA) is a time- and cost-effective, noninvasive method for obtaining tumor material for testing. Liquid biopsies have a unique advantage of capturing tumor heterogeneity within a single tumor site and across multiple metastases. ctDNA testing can be used to detect new actionable genetic alterations in tumors that progress, to measure tumor burden, and to monitor tumor relapse or metastasis.[49] Two of the most common single-gene alterations detected by testing ctDNA are *PIK3CA* and *ESR1*, both relevant therapeutically.[50] At present, the only FDA-approved

Fig. 6. NTRK-ETV6 translocation in primary secretory carcinoma of the breast. This primary breast carcinoma displays cribriform architecture (*A*, H&E, original magnification ×200), uniform nuclei, and eosinophilic luminal secretions (*B*, H&E, original magnification ×400), suggesting secretory carcinoma. Targeted gene sequencing confirms the presence of a translocation between *ETV6* exons 1 to 5 and *NTRK* exons 15 to 20 (*C*), confirming the diagnosis of secretory carcinoma. If the patient were to develop metastatic disease, the presence of the *NTRK-ETV6* translocation would make the patient eligible for *NTRK*-targeted therapy.

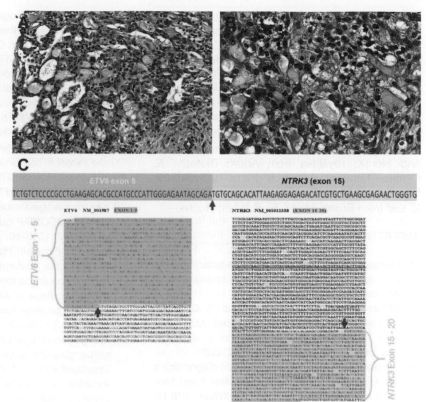

companion diagnostic assay that uses ctDNA in breast cancer is for detecting *PIK3CA* for treatment with alpelisib. All other uses of ctDNA in breast cancer remain experimental at present.

EMERGING BIOMARKERS

The presence of TILs is both a prognostic and predictive biomarker in breast cancer.[51,52] Society-level guidelines for scoring and reporting TILs and clinical guidelines for meaningful use of this information will be required before TILs can be incorporated into clinical practice.

Another big challenge in the interpretation of biomarkers is interobserver and intraobserver variability. Image digitization and image analysis technologies may provide reproducible, objective, and accurate assessment of biomarkers, as platforms are validated and approved for clinical use.[53] Finally, novel anti-HER2 therapeutic agents such as antibody drug conjugates have shown beneficial responses even in HER2 nonamplified breast cancers in clinical trials, leading to a proposed new category of breast tumors, "HER2-low."[54] Future testing algorithms may see inclusion of this category to identify tumors that respond well to emerging anti-HER2 agents.

SUMMARY

Metastatic breast cancers remain a challenge to treat. However, the landscape of testing and therapeutics in these cancers is evolving rapidly. As new targeted therapeutics are developed, corresponding companion diagnostic assays are also being developed to determine which patients will benefit from these therapies Sequencing platforms are a cost-effective tool to comprehensively gather genomic information on multiple biomarkers simultaneously to guide therapy. It is important for the practicing pathologist to be aware of biomarker recommendations and testing platforms to effectively participate in and guide the multidisciplinary care of patients with metastatic breast cancer.

DISCLOSURE

G. Jagannathan: None; M.J. White: None; R.R. Xian: None; L.A. Emens: honoraria from AbbVie, Amgen, Celgene, Chugai, GCPR, Gilead, Gritstone, MedImmune, Peregrine, Shionogi, and Syndax; honoraria and travel support from AstraZeneca, Bayer, MacroGenics, Replimune, and Vaccinex; travel support from Bristol Myers

Squibb, Genentech/Roche, and Novartis; potential future stock from Molecuvax; institutional support from AbbVie, Aduro Biotech, AstraZeneca, the Breast Cancer Research Foundation, Bristol Myers Squibb, Bolt Therapeutics, Compugen, Corvus, CyTomX, the US Department of Defense, EMD Serono, Genentech, Maxcyte, Merck, the National Cancer Institute, the NSABP Foundation, SU2C, Silverback, Roche, the Translational Breast Cancer Research Consortium, Takeda, Tempest, and HeritX; royalties from Aduro Biotech; A. Cimino-Mathews: Research grants to institution from Bristol-Myers Squibb; consultancy/honoraria to self from Bristol-Myers Squibb and Roche.

REFERENCES

1. Female breast cancer — cancer stat facts. Available at: https://seer.cancer.gov/statfacts/html/breast.html. Accessed January 2, 2021.
2. NCCN Clinical Practice Guidelines in Oncology (NCCN Guidelines): Breast Cancer. NCCN.org. 2021. Available at: https://www.nccn.org/guidelines/category_1. Accessed April 26, 2021.
3. Jørgensen JT, Hersom M. Companion diagnostics-a tool to improve pharmacotherapy. Ann Transl Med 2016;4(24). https://doi.org/10.21037/atm.2016.12.26.
4. U.S. FDA. Developing and labeling in vitro companion diagnostic devices for a specific group of oncology therapeutic products guidance for industry. FDA guidance documents. 2020. Available at: https://www.fda.gov/vaccines-blood-biologics/guidance-compliance-regulatory-information-biologics/biologics-guidances. Accessed April 25, 2021.
5. U.S. FDA. List of Cleared or Approved Companion Diagnostic Devices (In Vitro and Imaging Tools). 2021. Available at: https://www.fda.gov/medical-devices/in-vitro-diagnostics/list-cleared-or-approved--companion-diagnostic-devices-in-vitro-and-imaging-tools. Accessed April 28, 2021.
6. Allott EH, Geradts J, Sun X, et al. Intratumoral heterogeneity as a source of discordance in breast cancer biomarker classification. Breast Cancer Res 2016;18(1):1–11.
7. Jabbour MN, Massad CY, Boulos FI. Variability in hormone and growth factor receptor expression in primary versus recurrent, metastatic, and post-neoadjuvant breast carcinoma. Breast Cancer Res Treat 2012;135(1):29–37.
8. Amir E, Clemons M, Purdie CA, et al. Tissue confirmation of disease recurrence in breast cancer patients: pooled analysis of multi-centre, multidisciplinary prospective studies. Cancer Treat Rev 2012;38(6):708–14.
9. Bardou VJ, Arpino G, Elledge RM, et al. Progesterone receptor status significantly improves outcome prediction over estrogen receptor status alone for adjuvant endocrine therapy in two large breast cancer databases. J Clin Oncol 2003;21(10):1973–9.
10. Van Poznak C, Somerfield MR, Bast RC, et al. Use of biomarkers to guide decisions on systemic therapy for women with metastatic breast cancer: American Society of Clinical Oncology clinical practice guideline. J Clin Oncol 2015;33(24):2695–704.
11. Hoefnagel LDC, Moelans CB, Meijer SL, et al. Prognostic value of estrogen receptor α and progesterone receptor conversion in distant breast cancer metastases. Cancer 2012;118(20):4929–35.
12. Allison KH, Hammond MEH, Dowsett M, et al. Estrogen and progesterone receptor testing in breast cancer: ASCO/CAP guideline update. J Clin Oncol 2020;38(12):1346–66.
13. Wolff AC, Elizabeth Hale Hammond M, Allison KH, et al. Human epidermal growth factor receptor 2 testing in breast cancer: American society of clinical oncology/college of American pathologists clinical practice guideline focused update. J Clin Oncol 2018;36(20):2105–22.
14. Estrogen and progesterone receptor testing in breast cancer guideline update. American Society of Clinical Oncology/College of American Pathologists; 2020. Available at: https://www.cap.org/protocols-and-guidelines/cap-guidelines/current-cap-guidelines/guideline-recommendations-for-immunohistochemical-testing-of-estrogen-and-progesterone-receptors-in-breast-cancer. Accessed April 19, 2021.
15. HER2 testing in breast cancer. American Society of Clinical Oncology/College of American Pathologists; 2018. Available at: https://www.cap.org/protocols-and-guidelines/cap-guidelines/current-cap--guidelines/recommendations-for-human-epidermal--growth-factor-2-testing-in-breast-cancer. Accessed April 26, 2021.
16. Chen MT, Sun HF, Zhao Y, et al. Comparison of patterns and prognosis among distant metastatic breast cancer patients by age groups: a SEER population-based analysis. Sci Rep 2017;7(1):1–8.
17. Clark BZ, Yoest JM, Onisko A, et al. Effects of hydrochloric acid and formic acid decalcification on breast tumor biomarkers and HER2 fluorescence in situ hybridization. Appl Immunohistochem Mol Morphol 2019;27(3):223–30.
18. van Es SC, van der Vegt B, Bensch F, et al. Decalcification of breast cancer bone metastases With EDTA does not affect ER, PR, and HER2 results. Am J Surg Pathol 2019;43(10):1355–60.
19. Pareja F, Murray MP, Jean RD, et al. Cytologic assessment of estrogen receptor, progesterone receptor, and HER2 status in metastatic breast carcinoma. J Am Soc Cytopathol 2017;6(1):33–40.
20. Cimino-Mathews A. Tumor-in filtrating lymphocytes and PD-L1 in breast cancer (and, what happened to medullary carcinoma?). Diagn Histopathol 2021;1–7.

21. Cortes J, Cescon DW, Rugo HS, et al. Pembrolizumab plus chemotherapy versus placebo plus chemotherapy for previously untreated locally recurrent inoperable or metastatic triple-negative breast cancer (KEYNOTE-355): a randomised, placebo-controlled, double-blind, phase 3 clinical trial. Lancet 2020;396(10265):1817–28.

22. Schmid P, Adams S, Rugo HS, et al. Atezolizumab and Nab-paclitaxel in advanced triple-negative breast cancer. N Engl J Med 2018;379(22):2108–21.

23. Schmid P, Cortes J, Pusztai L, et al. Pembrolizumab for early triple-negative breast cancer. N Engl J Med 2020;382(9):810–21.

24. Cimino-Mathews A, Ye X, Meeker A, et al. Metastatic triple-negative breast cancers at first relapse have fewer tumor-infiltrating lymphocytes than their matched primary breast tumors: a pilot study. Hum Pathol 2013;44(10):2055–63.

25. Michot JM, Bigenwald C, Champiat S, et al. Immune-related adverse events with immune checkpoint blockade: a comprehensive review. Eur J Cancer 2016;54:139–48.

26. Fusco MJ, West HJ, Walko CM. Tumor mutation burden and cancer treatment. JAMA Oncol 2021;7(2):316.

27. Cheng AS, Leung SCY, Gao D, et al. Mismatch repair protein loss in breast cancer: clinicopathological associations in a large British Columbia cohort. Breast Cancer Res Treat 2020;179(1):3–10.

28. Barroso-Sousa R, Jain E, Cohen O, et al. Prevalence and mutational determinants of high tumor mutation burden in breast cancer. Ann Oncol 2020;31(3):387–94.

29. Marabelle A, Fakih M, Lopez J, et al. Association of tumour mutational burden with outcomes in patients with advanced solid tumours treated with pembrolizumab: prospective biomarker analysis of the multicohort, open-label, phase 2 KEYNOTE-158 study. Lancet Oncol 2020;21(10):1353–65.

30. U.S. FDA. FDA grants accelerated approval to dostarlimab-gxly for dMMR endometrial cancer. Drug approvals and databases. Available at: https://www.fda.gov/drugs/drug-approvals-and-databases/fda-grants-accelerated-approval-dostarlimab-gxly-dmmr-endometrial-cancer. Accessed April 26, 2021.

31. Venetis K, Sajjadi E, Haricharan S, et al. Mismatch repair testing in breast cancer: The path to tumor-specific immuno-oncology biomarkers. Transl Cancer Res 2020;9(7):4060–4.

32. Fusco N, Lopez G, Corti C, et al. Mismatch repair protein loss as a prognostic and predictive biomarker in breast cancers regardless of microsatellite instability. JNCI Cancer Spectr 2018;2(4). https://doi.org/10.1093/jncics/pky056.

33. Winter C, Nilsson MP, Olsson E, et al. Targeted sequencing of BRCA1 and BRCA2 across a large unselected breast cancer cohort suggests that one-third of mutations are somatic. Ann Oncol 2016;27(8):1532–8.

34. Nik-Zainal S, Davies H, Staaf J, et al. Landscape of somatic mutations in 560 breast cancer whole-genome sequences. Nature 2016;534(7605):47–54.

35. Sønderstrup IMH, Jensen MBR, Ejlertsen B, et al. Subtypes in BRCA-mutated breast cancer. Hum Pathol 2019;84:192–201.

36. Robson M, Im S-A, Senkus E, et al. Olaparib for metastatic breast cancer in patients with a Germline BRCA mutation. N Engl J Med 2017;377(6):523–33.

37. Tung NM, Robson ME, Ventz S, et al. TBCRC 048: phase II study of olaparib for metastatic breast cancer and mutations in homologous recombination-related genes. J Clin Oncol 2020;38(36):4274–82.

38. André F, Ciruelos E, Rubovszky G, et al. Alpelisib for PIK3CA-mutated, hormone receptor–positive advanced breast cancer. N Engl J Med 2019;380(20):1929–40.

39. Martínez-Sáez O, Chic N, Pascual T, et al. Frequency and spectrum of PIK3CA somatic mutations in breast cancer. Breast Cancer Res 2020;22(1):1–9.

40. U.S. FDA. FDA approves first PI3K inhibitor for breast cancer. Available at: https://www.fda.gov/news-events/press-announcements/fda-approves-first-pi3-k-inhibitor-breast-cancer. Accessed April 26, 2021.

41. U.S. FDA. FDA approves liquid biopsy NGS companion diagnostic test for multiple cancers and biomarkers. Available at: https://www.fda.gov/drugs/fda-approves-liquid-biopsy-ngs-companion-diagnostic-test-multiple-cancers-and-biomarkers. Accessed April 26, 2021.

42. U.S. FDA. FDA approves alpelisib for metastatic breast cancer. Available at: https://www.fda.gov/drugs/resources-information-approved-drugs/fda-approves-alpelisib-metastatic-breast-cancer. Accessed April 26, 2021.

43. Scott LJ. Larotrectinib: first global approval. Drugs 2019;79(2):201–6.

44. Al-Salama ZT, Keam SJ. Entrectinib: first global approval. Drugs 2019;79(13):1477–83.

45. Diallo R, Schaefer KL, Bankfalvi A, et al. Secretory carcinoma of the breast: a distinct variant of invasive ductal carcinoma assessed by comparative genomic hybridization and immunohistochemistry. Hum Pathol 2003;34(12):1299–305.

46. Harrison BT, Fowler E, Krings G, et al. Pan-TRK immunohistochemistry. Am J Surg Pathol 2019;43(12):1693–700.

47. U.S. FDA. FDA approves companion diagnostic to identify NTRK fusions in solid tumors for Vitrakvi. Available at: https://www.fda.gov/drugs/fda-approves-companion-diagnostic-identify-ntrk-fusions-solid-tumors-vitrakvi. Accessed April 25, 2021.

48. Remoué A, Conan-Charlet V, Bourhis A, et al. Non-secretory breast carcinomas lack NTRK rearrangements and TRK protein expression. Pathol Int 2019;69(2):94–6.

49. Canzoniero JVL, Park BH. Use of cell free DNA in breast oncology. Biochim Biophys Acta 2016;1865(2):266–74.

50. Buono G, Gerratana L, Bulfoni M, et al. Circulating tumor DNA analysis in breast cancer: Is it ready for prime-time? Cancer Treat Rev 2019;73:73–83.

51. Tan PH, Ellis I, Allison K, et al. The 2019 World Health Organization classification of tumours of the breast. Histopathology 2020;77(2):181–5.

52.. Tan PH, Ellis I, Allison K, et al. World Health Organization Classification of Tumours: breast tumors. 5th editionVol 2. Lyon, France: IARC Press; 2019.

53. Dermawan JK, Mukhopadhyay S, Shah AA. Frequency and extent of cytokeratin expression in paraganglioma: an immunohistochemical study of 60 cases from 5 anatomic sites and review of the literature. Hum Pathol 2019;93:16–22.

54. Tarantino P, Hamilton E, Tolaney SM, et al. HER2-low breast cancer: pathological and clinical landscape. J Clin Oncol 2020;38(17):1951–62.

The Critical Role of Breast Specimen Gross Evaluation for Optimal Personalized Cancer Care

Allison S. Cleary, MD, PhD[b], Susan C. Lester, MD, PhD[a],*

KEYWORDS

- Gross evaluation • Pathology • Breast • Lymph nodes • Radiologic-pathologic correlation
- Imaging • Neoadjuvant therapy

Key points

- Gross examination is the foundation for the pathologic evaluation of all surgical specimens.
- Rapid gross identification of cancer to preserve biomolecules and histologic integrity is essential for personalized patient care.
- Multiple features of cancers critically important for treatment and prognosis require information from gross evaluation—these include tumor size, multiple foci of invasion, margin status, and lymph node involvement.
- Optimal gross evaluation is dependent on training, experience, radiography of specimens, and access to key clinical information.
- New techniques for microscopic evaluation of fresh tissues may provide an important bridge between gross and microscopic tissue diagnosis.

Video content accompanies this article at http://www.surgpath.theclinics.com

ABSTRACT

Gross examination is the foundation for the pathologic evaluation of all surgical specimens. The rapid identification of cancers is essential for intraoperative assessment and preservation of biomolecules for molecular assays. Key components of the gross examination include the accurate identification of the lesions of interest, correlation with clinical and radiologic findings, assessment of lesion number and size, relationship to surgical margins, documenting the extent of disease spread to the skin and chest wall, and the identification of axillary lymph nodes. Although the importance of gross evaluation is undeniable, current challenges include the difficulty of teaching grossing well and its possible perceived undervaluation compared with microscopic and molecular studies. In the future, new rapid imaging techniques without the need for tissue processing may provide an ideal melding of gross and microscopic pathologic evaluation.

OVERVIEW

The visual and tactile inspection of surgical specimens yields a wealth of information, including tumor shape, color, density, and spatial location, that is not available after specimens are converted to essentially 2-dimensional pieces of tissue on glass slides. Thorough and accurate gross assessment is paramount for rendering the best diagnosis for the patient and guiding future care

[a] Department of Pathology, Brigham and Women's Hospital, Harvard Medical School, 75 Francis Street, Boston, MA 02115, USA; [b] Department of Pathology, Huntsman Cancer Hospital, 1950 Circle of Hope, Salt Lake City, UT 84112

* Corresponding author.
E-mail address: slester@bwh.harvard.edu

Surgical Pathology 15 (2022) 121–132
https://doi.org/10.1016/j.path.2021.11.008
1875-9181/22/© 2021 Elsevier Inc. All rights reserved.

decisions. The microscopic evaluation alone cannot capture all the important features of breast cancers. In addition, most breast excisions are not entirely evaluated microscopically, and mastectomies are never entirely sampled.[1] Therefore, the value of microscopic diagnosis is highly dependent on the careful selection of the tissue that will be examined and, in addition, the interpretation of microscopic findings must always be informed by the gross findings.

In an important publication, the sources of errors in breast cancer reporting were studied.[2] A large academic medical center conducted a retrospective re-review of 1120 breast surgical specimens over a 3-year period. Major diagnostic discrepancies were identified in 53 (5%) of the specimens after a second gross examination, including 37 cases with missed cancers, 8 cases with additional positive lymph nodes, 4 cancers upstaged due to revised size, and 4 cases with missed tumor invasion of skin. By contrast, re-examination of the histologic slides from 733 cases during the same period discovered major interpretative discrepancies in only 11 cases (1%). Thus suboptimal gross examination was the most common source of errors in this study and the errors identified could have had potentially serious clinical consequences for prognosis and treatment. Unfortunately, such errors can rarely be rectified by second opinions by another pathologist as usually only the slides are available at the time of consultation.

In this review, we will discuss recommendations for best practices in the gross evaluation of breast specimens, current challenges in achieving these practices, and potential future advances.

EVALUATION OF BREAST SPECIMENS

STEP 1: CLINICAL INFORMATION

Ideally, the prosector will approach each case armed with the relevant history that enables the understanding of the significance of the specimen in the context of the care of the patient (Box 1). However, sufficient information for this purpose is rarely provided on specimen requisition forms. Specifically designed requisition forms for breast specimens can assist in informing clinicians about the data important to include and aid in the transfer of this information.[3] An agnostic approach to specimen evaluation divorced from the clinical and radiologic history can lead to significant errors such as missing lesions or misinterpreting lesions that have been altered by iatrogenic changes. Examples of the latter include mistaking reactive spindle cell nodules at biopsy sites for spindle cell malignancies, mistaking pseudopapillary

endothelial hyperplasia in an area of hemorrhage for an angiosarcoma, or failing to find the tumor bed after neoadjuvant therapy and mistaking the absence of tumor for a pathologic complete response. With electronic medical record systems, pathologists may be able to access clinical information and imaging on their own. However, some pathologists lack this access, others may not have been trained in what clinical and imaging information is useful, and some may find the time expenditure in reviewing patient records prohibitive.

STEP 2: SPECIMEN RADIOGRAPHY

In current medical care in which most breast carcinomas are detected by breast imaging, and numerous patients undergo neoadjuvant therapy (with complete or almost complete resolution of the cancers in many cases), the ability to use the "super power" of x-ray vision to see into specimens to identify lesions and markers (clips and localizing devices) has become very important for many breast specimens. The specimen radiograph is an essential map as to what is present in the specimen and occasionally provides critical evidence that something expected to be in the specimen is absent (Fig. 1).

It is important that specimen radiographs are performed before the specimen is sectioned. Sectioning can displace clips and localizing devices (which creates the possibility they will be dislodged from the specimen and lost), can separate clusters of calcifications, and may make it difficult or impossible to identify small masses or more subtle lesions such as architectural distortion. Radiographs of sliced specimens can be useful when the initial radiograph identifies a lesion, which is not then identified on gross examination.

Radiographs are routinely performed and interpreted by radiologists when patients undergo localized excisions. In a study from 1997, a survey of 434 institutions reported that pathologists were provided the radiograph (at that point in time this was a film copy) in 78% of cases, but the radiologist's interpretation was only provided in 45% of cases.[4] Over half of specimens (62%) did not have a grossly evident lesion, whereas only about a third (37%) were completely evaluated microscopically, creating the possibility that important lesions were not sampled. Since the time of this study, additional challenges have arisen for prosectors to obtain specimen radiographs. Now that digital imaging is standard, the prosector may need to search for the specimen radiograph and its interpretation in an electronic medical record.

> **Box 1**
> **Information needed to fully understand the clinical context of a specimen to perform an optimal gross evaluation**
>
> 1. Why has the patient undergone this surgery?
>
>   Examples: palpable mass, nipple inversion or skin involvement (signs and symptoms of inflammatory breast carcinoma or ulceration), finding on breast imaging (mass, calcifications, architectural distortion, other), clip marking biopsy site, risk reduction.
>
> 2. What is the scope of the surgery?
>
>   Examples: incisional biopsy, excision (with or without localization, type of localization device), mastectomy (with or without skin and nipple), chest wall resection, sentinel lymph node biopsy, axillary dissection.
>
> 3. If there has been previous tissue sampling, what was the type and location?
>
>   Examples: core needle biopsy (type of clip marking site), excision, mastectomy.
>
>   Quadrant, distance from nipple, distance from skin or chest wall.
>
> 4. What prior pathologic diagnoses have been made?
>
>   Examples: carcinoma (breast or otherwise), benign tumors, inflammatory lesions, others.
>
> 5. Is there a single or multiple lesions?
>
>   Examples: number of lesions, spatial relationship to each other.
>
> 6. Has the patient received prior treatment for breast cancer?
>
>   Examples: neoadjuvant therapy (chemotherapy, endocrine, other), radiation therapy.
>
> 7. Has a specimen radiograph been performed and interpreted?
>
>   The radiograph and interpretation should be available to the prosector.
>
> 8. Does the patient have other diseases that could involve the breast?
>
>   Examples: nonbreast malignancies, sarcoidosis, diabetes, lupus, elevated prolactin, others.
>
> 9. Is there a history of drug use that could affect the breast?
>
>   Examples: hormones, psychoactive drugs, cyclosporine, coumadin, others.

Ironically, pathologists receive the least assistance in the evaluation of the most challenging specimens—mastectomies. Women not eligible for breast conserving therapy often have multiple cancers (often with multiple biopsies or excisions), extensive cancers (possibly involving skin and chest wall), recurrent cancers, and/or have undergone neoadjuvant therapy. Although mastectomies remove most breast tissue including cancers, in a small percentage of cases, cancers can be left in the patient—particularly when they are located very superficially, peripherally (close to the junction of breast and skin), retroareolar (in the case of nipple-sparing mastectomies), or in the high axilla.[5] When nonpalpable image-detected lesions are present, a radiograph may be the only method of ensuring that important lesions are found and sampled.[6,7] Specimen radiography is not routine in these cases and is rarely performed by radiologists. However, a large specimen often with small, sometimes grossly occult lesions, creates the opportunity for error. This was substantiated in the study previously mentioned as most errors occurred when sampling mastectomies.[2] A few pathology departments can perform their own radiographs but the quality may not be optimal and prosectors may not be trained in the interpretation of such images. However, pathology departments in some centers have successfully used their own performance of specimen radiography to improve practice.[6,7] One strategy institutions could use to address this issue would be to develop a standard practice of requesting that mastectomies removed for clinically nonpalpable imaging findings be radiographed in the radiology department and the radiographs interpreted by radiologists.

STEP 3: EXAMINING THE SPECIMEN

The preliminary external evaluation determines the type of specimen (eg, excision or mastectomy) and examines the outer surface for any abnormal findings (eg, tumors grossly at the margin or skin ulceration). The intact specimen is palpated to locate abnormal masses. Important measurements are taken to record the size of the breast tissue present, as well as of other structures (eg, skin

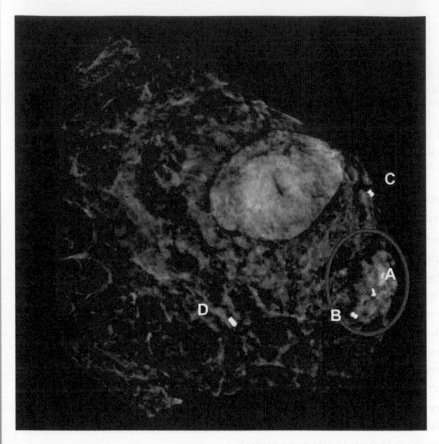

Fig. 1. This radiograph of a mastectomy specimen identifies multiple findings that must be evaluated pathologically. The circle surrounds an area of calcifications suspicious for malignancy. The wing clip (A) within this area identifies the site of a core needle biopsy of a mass that showed invasive carcinoma. An hourglass clip (B) within the same area marks a mass suspicious for an invasive carcinoma that had not been biopsied. A second hourglass clip (C) marks the site of a core needle biopsy that showed invasive carcinoma. This clip is located very superficially. This intraoperative radiograph showed that the clip had been removed but was very close to the subcutaneous tissue of the skin flap. An additional margin was taken in this area. A fourth cylinder clip (D) marks the site of a core biopsy that showed benign changes. This radiograph was very helpful in guiding sampling that showed 2 invasive carcinomas associated with an area of DCIS marked by calcifications, and a third separate invasive carcinoma. It could have been very difficult for a prosector to identify these areas grossly and for the pathologist to interpret the microscopic findings in the absence of the radiologic image. (*Courtesy* of E. Rhei, MD)

and nipple). If received oriented, the surgical margins are then inked in such a manner so that specific margins can be identified.

Several critically important features of breast cancers are best evaluated by gross examination and sometimes can only be evaluated by gross examination (**Box 2**).

Identification of the Lesion

For most breast excisions, identifying a lesion (or lesions) should begin with inspection of the specimen radiograph. The type of lesion can be determined (eg, mass, architectural distortion, or calcifications) and its location within the specimen identified including the relationship to margins. After serial sectioning, the gross appearance can then be correlated with the image. This also allows the prosector to determine if gross lesions are associated with biopsy clips or localizing devices.

Excisions performed without the need for specimen radiography usually contain a palpable mass. Most palpable masses are grossly apparent and can be distinguished from the surrounding fibrous parenchyma. After thinly sectioning the specimen, each slice is carefully palpated as breast lesions are often best appreciated by their dense consistency compared with normal breast tissue (**Fig. 2**). Many breast lesions are white in color and blend into the adjacent white fibrous breast tissue visually. Unlike carcinomas, which are usually very firm to hard, normal fibrous breast parenchyma has a soft to rubbery texture.

Invasive carcinomas usually present as firm, white masses with irregular or stellate borders and have a gritty consistency upon sectioning (like a water chestnut). Some invasive carcinomas such as triple-negative carcinomas or mucinous carcinomas are well-circumscribed and may be firm or soft. Mucinous carcinomas may have a gelatinous

---

Box 2
Features of primary tumors that require information from gross evaluation, especially when the entire specimen is not sampled

1. Identification of the lesion or lesions
2. Size of the lesions
3. Number of lesions and relationship of lesions to each other
4. Relationship of the lesion to margins
5. Identification of lymph nodes and number of lymph nodes
6. Size of the largest lymph node metastasis

---

appearance. Tumors that have undergone neoadjuvant therapy may become soft and difficult to distinguish from the surrounding fibrous tissue.

Fibroepithelial lesions tend to be ovoid masses with a rubbery consistency that appear to bulge outward from the surrounding parenchyma. The cut surface may show cleft-like spaces, hemorrhage, or necrosis. Fibroadenomas are well-circumscribed lesions, whereas phyllodes tumors may have a circumscribed or infiltrative border.

Other lesions may be more difficult to appreciate grossly. For example, ductal carcinoma in situ (DCIS) is often grossly occult, and, its gross identification often depends on the presence of biopsy clips and localization devices or correlation with areas of calcifications seen on specimen radiographs, as discussed earlier. Occasionally DCIS can be grossly apparent, especially comedo-type DCIS. Comedo-type DCIS can be associated with a periductal fibrosis and can have pinpoint areas of necrosis ("comedone-like"), which may extrude from the tissue when it is gently squeezed.

The grossly involved area may be an ill-defined area of firm gray/white tissue with a "gritty" texture.

In current clinical practice, most lesions undergo core needle biopsy before surgical excision. During the biopsy procedure, a metallic biopsy clip is often deployed to mark the biopsy site. Biopsy clips are available in over 30 different shapes. If a patient has had multiple prior biopsies, their surgical specimen may contain multiple biopsy clips, and each biopsy clip/biopsy site must be accounted for within the resection specimen. For localized excisions, additional localizing devices such as radioactive seeds, magnetic seeds, radiofrequency identification (RFID) tags, radar-localization reflectors, or percutaneous localization wires may also be used to guide surgery. These biopsy clips and localization devices can further aid the pathologist in identifying the targeted lesion, particularly in cases in which the lesion may be grossly occult—such as resections for calcifications or architectural distortion. Although biopsy clips and localization

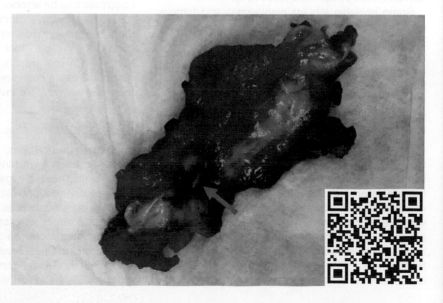

Fig. 2. A clip marking an invasive carcinoma can be seen in this sliced specimen (*arrow*). However, the carcinoma is white in color and blends in with the surrounding fibrous tissue. The edges, and thus the size of the cancer, cannot be determined by visual inspection alone. Tumor size is best evaluated by palpation, as is seen in a video that can be accessed by scanning the QR code with your smartphone or tablet or by using this link. https://doi.org/10.1016/j.path.2021.11.008

devices are helpful tools for identification, it is important to remember that they can sometimes become dislodged and migrate from their original location. If no apparent lesion or biopsy clips can be identified, the possibility that the intended target was not removed within the resection should be considered.

Tumor Size

The size of breast carcinomas is the third most important prognostic factor after distant metastases and regional lymph node involvement and is used for American Joint Committee on Cancer (AJCC) and Union for International Cancer Control (UICC) staging.[8,9] The measurement of tumor size is among the most important elements of the gross examination. As such, great care must be taken to ensure that the measurement is as precise as possible, particularly when measurements approach the threshold values that delineate between pathologic T classifications. For example, an invasive cancer measuring 2.0 cm will be classified as pT1c, whereas one measuring 2.1 cm will be classified as pT2.

Tumor size can often be difficult to determine visually because the stellate borders of invasive carcinomas often blend into the surrounding fibrous tissue. Instead, palpation of the tumor is more effective for determining the size. The edges of a carcinoma usually form a discrete "shelf" that can be pinched between the fingers and defines the extent of the tumor including the surrounding desmoplastic response. Size measurements should be obtained on fresh specimens whenever possible, as the palpable distinction between the firm tumor and soft surrounding tissue becomes less obvious in formalin-fixed specimens (see **Fig 2**).

Some invasive lobular carcinomas and tumors following neoadjuvant treatment have a diffusely infiltrating pattern, and are difficult or impossible to identify grossly. In difficult cases, a best estimate of tumor size for T classification should take into account the size by imaging, the gross size, microscopic findings, and the size on a prior core needle biopsy if larger than that in the excision.[10]

Multiple Invasive Carcinomas

Careful gross evaluation is necessary to document the presence and the relationship of multiple foci of invasion that occur in 10% to 25% of women with breast carcinoma.[11] Multiple foci of invasion are more commonly seen in women with *BRCA1* and *BRCA2* mutations.[12] There are 3 main origins for this finding (**Box 3**). The most common setting is carcinoma in situ involving a ductal system that

has given rise to multiple areas of invasion.[13] In this case, the invasive carcinomas are closely related genomically, but are not identical. The second most common setting is a carcinoma with lymphovascular invasion resulting in intramammary metastases.[13] As in the first case, the carcinomas are closely related but may not be identical. In the study by Desmedt and colleagues, two-thirds of multifocal carcinomas shared mutations, suggesting that they arose from these 2 groups.[11] In these settings, the multiple carcinomas are generally similar in histologic type, grade, and expression of hormone receptors and HER2. The third and less common finding is of multiple completely unrelated carcinomas as was reported in one-third of cases in the Desmedt study.[11] These carcinomas may vary in histologic type, grade, and receptor expression. Ongoing studies continue to evaluate how best to stage these cancers, the need to assess hormone receptors on multiple foci, the impact on local control, and prognosis.[14] Careful gross evaluation to identify multiple foci and to sample each focus and intervening tissue is required to document multiple cancers. This evaluation is also important to determine which foci would yield the most important information if additional tests are performed, such as gene expression profiling or DNA analysis.

There are 3 instances in which a single invasive carcinoma can be mistaken for multiple foci of invasion (see **Box 3**). Carcinomas that invade along fibrovascular bundles, such as lobular carcinomas, can appear to have satellite foci of invasion in 2 dimensions but these foci are actually contiguous with the main carcinoma in 3 dimensions.[10] Secondly, carcinomas that are transected during surgery and removed in more than one specimen can be erroneously interpreted as multiple foci.[15] Finally, carcinomas that undergo a response to neoadjuvant therapy are typically seen as multiple foci scattered in a tumor bed.[16,17] Careful gross evaluation is necessary to recognize these cases and distinguish them from true cases of multiple invasive carcinomas.

Evaluation of the Skin and Chest Wall

In the United States, only rare carcinomas currently present with involvement of the skin or chest wall. These are generally locally advanced carcinomas and the extent of involvement may result in classification as T4 disease. Skin ulceration due to direct invasion by carcinoma is important to document as this results in a T4b classification. Chest wall invasion that would be classified as T4a is rarely seen as the cancer must invade beyond the pectoralis muscles and

---

Box 3
Origins of multiple foci of invasive carcinoma

1. DCIS giving rise to multiple foci of invasion (most common)

2. Invasive carcinoma with lymphovascular invasion giving rise to satellite foci of invasion

3. Biologically separate synchronous invasive carcinomas (least common)

4. Pseudomultifocal cancer: Diffusely infiltrative cancer with long spiculated margins giving the appearance of multiple foci in 2 dimensions

5. Pseudomultifocal cancer: Iatrogenic transection of carcinomas resulting in multiple foci in different specimens

6. Pseudomultifocal cancer: Residual carcinoma after neoadjuvant treatment present as multiple scattered foci over a tumor bed.

---

resection requires removal of ribs. These locally advanced carcinomas often undergo neoadjuvant treatment before excision. Sampling of previously involved areas is important to determine the extent of response to treatment.

Margins

Complete excision of cancers is important to reduce the possibility of local recurrence. For breast conserving excisions, all 6 surgical margins are evaluated: anterior, posterior, superior, inferior, medial, and lateral. These 6 anatomic surfaces can be identified and differentially inked if the surgeon orients the specimen in 2 directions—typically superior and lateral. However, given the amorphous nature of breast excision specimens, the shape of the specimen may flatten between the time of excision and the time it gets to the grossing bench (the so-called "pancake phenomenon"),[18] obscuring the true surface boundaries. Some surgeons prefer to ink specimens in the operating room, before the specimen shape has a chance to settle and because they can best determine the location and extent of each margin with respect to the patient. If multiple colors of ink are used to mark margins, it is helpful to establish an institutional policy for specific ink colors for each margin (eg, black is always used for the posterior margin, blue is always used for the anterior margin, etc). This simplifies the process and reduces the likelihood of errors in reporting.

Ink colors are well seen grossly. However, once specimens are reduced to micron-thick sections, any minor smearing of inks can result in margins that, for example, may be green with flecks of blue, orange, and yellow, creating ambiguity in the identification of the margin. Therefore, it is always helpful to indicate the grossly evident color of the margin placed in each cassette to aid in the microscopic interpretation of the margins.

After serial sectioning, the distance of gross lesions from each margin is measured. For traditional mastectomy specimens, the deep margin is usually the only clinically relevant margin. In the case of skin-sparing or nipple-sparing mastectomy procedures, evaluation of additional anterior and/or nipple margins may also be appropriate.

Intraoperative gross margin evaluation by pathologists is used in some institutions.[19] In one study, this practice prevented the need for later re-excision for 6 of 11 patients.[20]

Alternatively, many surgeons take additional shave margins from within the resection cavity. This practice has been shown to substantially decrease the rates of re-excision.[21–24]

Tissue Allocation

The biomarker profile of a tumor (estrogen receptor, progesterone receptor, and human epidermal growth factor receptor 2 [HER2]) is arguably the most important information the pathologist can provide after a diagnosis of invasive carcinoma to guide clinical management. Additional tests measuring biomarkers are currently used that are critical to personalized patient care and new assays undoubtedly will be developed.

Biomolecules start to deteriorate after the blood supply ceases.[25,26] Rapid degradation is most pronounced for mRNA and phosphorylated proteins, slower (minutes to hours) for other proteins, with the greatest stability observed for DNA. Ideally, cold ischemic time (the time from the cessation of blood flow until the tumor is directly immersed in fixative or frozen) is minimized by rapid transfer of specimens to the pathology department, immediate gross evaluation and specimen processing, and quick fixation.[27] Because fixatives diffuse slowly through tissues, thinly slicing tumors to immediately expose tissues to these solutions is essential to preserve histologic detail as well as integrity of the biomolecules.

It is critically important to choose the best tumor tissue for assays but not compromise pathologic evaluation. The ability to make a primary diagnosis, determine the lesion size, evaluate adjacent tissue for lymphovascular invasion, and evaluate margins must be protected. The ideal sample is a portion of the tumor taken from the periphery of a tumor, but not including the edge of the tumor or adjacent normal tissue (**Fig. 3**A). Carcinomas are often ischemic in the center resulting in the central area being fibrotic or necrotic. Therefore, sampling should avoid this region, particularly for larger masses (**Fig. 3**B). Sampling should also not take sections from the entire side of a carcinoma (eg, bisecting a carcinoma and removing half) as this precludes accurate size evaluation as well as evaluation of the adjacent breast tissue for lymphovascular invasion, and dilutes tumor with normal tissue (**Fig. 3**C). Finally, accurate sampling requires the prosector to identify the cancer because samples taken from normal tissue are useless for these assays and could potentially harm the patient by leading to erroneous results (**Fig. 3**D).

Lymph Nodes

Ideally, all lymph nodes in a specimen will be identified and sampled such that each lymph node can be identified separately. The total number of nodes is important to determine the accuracy of the patient's nodal status and can determine whether

or not additional axillary surgery is required. Nodes are generally best identified grossly by palpation of the tissue and separating all firm nodular masses. Thinly sectioning tissue without palpation is not recommended as it can be very difficult to determine the number of nodes after they are separated into slices. Although special fixatives can help identify a few additional lymph nodes, these nodes are generally very small and rarely harbor metastases.[28] These methods have not been shown to be superior to standard grossing techniques.

Small metastases may not be evident grossly, but larger metastases can be detected as homogeneous firm white masses in a node. In such cases, it is important to determine the size of the metastasis grossly and to submit a representative section. It is not necessary to entirely submit large lymph node metastases.

When extensive extranodal extension is present, multiple nodes may appear as one large irregular mass. The prosector should try to identify separate nodes, but this may not always be possible. In some cases, an accurate node count will not be possible.

Nodes that have undergone needle biopsy may have had a clip placed. In these instances, specimen radiography is important to document the node with the clip and occasionally an accompanying localization device. This is most commonly performed in patients undergoing neoadjuvant

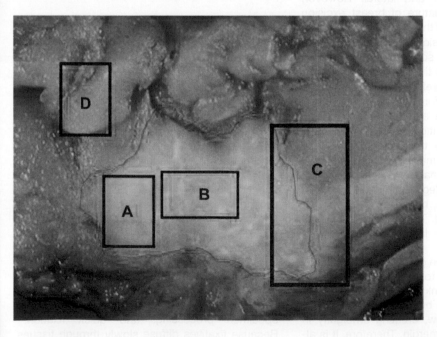

Fig. 3. Gross evaluation is essential for optimal selection of tissue for assays that preclude histologic evaluation. The border of the invasive carcinoma has been outlined for clarity. (A) This is the best tumor sample as it consists entirely of carcinoma and is from the periphery of the carcinoma, which is the regioin most likely to be viable. (B) This is a poor sample because the central portion of carcinomas is often ischemic and fibrotic or necrotic. (C) This is a poor sample because it includes both carcinoma and normal tissue and would interfere with determining the best tumor size and with evaluating peritumoral lymphovascular invasion. (D) This is an unacceptable sample because it consists of normal tissue.

therapy. Identification of the node that previously was involved by metastatic disease is important for patient care and prognosis.

Nodes without evident tumor involvement should never be allocated for studies that preclude microscopic evaluation as small metastases may not be apparent grossly. Nodes that do not have grossly apparent disease should be serially sectioned at 2 mm intervals and entirely submitted, to ensure histologic detection of micrometastases.

Neoadjuvant Specimens

There is a wide range of responses of carcinomas to presurgical treatment ranging from no response (or possibly growth), minimal response (typically a fibrotic rim at the periphery of the mass), marked response (usually multiple foci scattered in a tumor bed), or a pathologic complete response (pCR) with no residual carcinoma.[16,17] The latter 2 types of response

present challenges to gross evaluation as there may be only a subtle area of fibrosis present. In general, carcinomas that are no longer palpable to the clinician after treatment will also not be palpable to the prosector. Carcinomas typically become softer and more pliable after treatment. Careful correlation with the pretreatment imaging is often required to ensure appropriate sampling. Placement of a clip before treatment and identification of the clip after treatment is often essential to document a pCR.

Locally advanced cancers with involvement of the skin or chest wall frequently undergo neoadjuvant treatment as patients with a good response may become candidates for surgery. Areas of prior involvement should be sampled. These areas may need to be marked by the surgeon.

Detailed protocols for the gross examination and sampling of these specimens have been published.[16,17] Megan L. Troxell and Tanya Gupta's article, "Neoadjuvant Therapy In Breast Cancer:

Box 4
Variables influencing the quality of gross evaluation of breast specimens

1. *Training*

    Residency, fellowship, pathology assistant program, on the job

    Grossing often requires tactile examination to identify tumors and lymph nodes. This can only be taught well using real pathologic specimens with person-to-person instruction.

2. *Experience*

    Numbers of cases evaluated with subsequent correlation with microscopic findings

    Note: The least experienced pathologists tend to have the most responsibility for grossing and the most experienced pathologists the least.

3. *Variation in the appearance of breast lesions*

    There is a wide variety of types of breast lesions and each can have multiple appearances.

    Many lesions detected by imaging are not grossly apparent and/or have been altered by core needle biopsy.

    Cancers that have undergone neoadjuvant therapy may not be visible grossly nor palpable.

4. *Access to clinical information*

    Clinical presentation (palpable mass [number and size], involvement of skin or chest wall)

    Radiologic findings (radiograph and interpretation by radiologist)

    Prior biopsies or excisions (types, location, placement of clips, types of clips)

    Type of procedure (excision for a palpable mass, image-guided excision, mastectomy [simple, skin sparing, skin and nipple sparing], oncoplastic resection, sentinel node biopsy, axillary dissection [extent])

    Presurgical treatment (features of pretreatment cancer and changes after treatment)

    Orientation

5. *Access to imaging information*

    Specimen imaging provided and interpreted by the radiology department or available in the pathology department.

Histologic Changes and Clinical Implications," in this issue also provides important information about these specimens.

TRAINING IN GROSS EVALUATION

There are many challenges in teaching gross evaluation (**Box 4**). Detailed published written resources describe gross evaluation and sampling.[15,16,29,30] However, text and illustrations do not completely capture the information conveyed by visual inspection, palpation, and sectioning of organs and tissues. Grossing is taught best in person and using actual surgical specimens. It is challenging to teach these skills using other formats. Videos are a step forward.[31] For example, as previously discussed, for breast specimens, the tactile density of breast tissue is often more important than the visual appearance to determine size, and this is better shown in a video than in a photo (see **Fig. 2**, Video 1 [active link to grossing video]).

Typically, pathology residents are responsible for specimen evaluation during their first and second years of training and perform these duties intermittently after this time. Senior residents and fellows often help train beginning residents. After residency and fellowship, pathologists are not typically primarily responsible for grossing specimens. Faculty may only become involved in gross evaluation when supervising residents or for complex and difficult cases. This hierarchical structure is unfortunate as the most experienced pathologists tend to be the furthest removed from this important task. The absence of senior and expert pathologists in the grossing room has also led to many trainees undervaluing gross examination as an essential technique. Over time, pathology assistants have taken on an increasing role in many important aspects of gross evaluation. They have the advantage of gaining experience with numerous specimens over many years and have outperformed pathology residents in published studies.[32,33] However, the general lack of opportunity to link gross appearances to microscopic diagnoses is a limitation in becoming adept at gross evaluation. Finding ways to maintain pathologist participation in grossing over their careers and developing the means to allow pathology assistants to associate their observations to the final pathologic results would be beneficial steps to improve gross evaluation..

FUTURE DIRECTIONS IN GROSS EVALUATION

Multiple groups are developing imaging techniques to bridge the gap between gross and microscopic evaluation.[34–37] Some techniques apply labels (such as fluorescent dyes) to a cut surface and others use the inherent optical

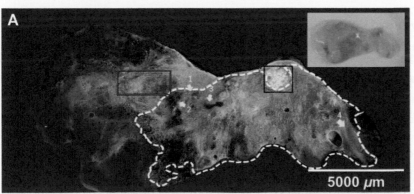

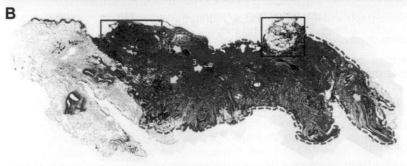

Fig. 4. Several methods for microscopy of unfixed specimens have been developed. In this case, an approximate 1 × 2 cm slice of breast tissue (*box at top right*) was briefly stained with 2 fluorescent dyes and then imaged using a deep-ultraviolet scanning fluorescence microscope (*A*). Invasive lobular carcinoma is indicated by a dotted line, a core needle biopsy site by a black box, adenosis by a red box, and arrows mark foci of DCIS (*A*). The corresponding H&E slide after fixation and processing is shown below (*B*). (*From* Lu T, Jorns JM, Patton M, et al. Rapid assessment of breast tumor margins using deep ultraviolet fluorescence scanning microscopy. J Biomed Opt. 2020;25(12):126501. https://doi.org/10.1117/1.JBO.25.12.126501.)

properties of the tissue. Little or minimal tissue preparation is necessary, in contrast to traditional fixation, paraffin embedding, and sectioning to prepare glass slides. There has been success in identifying minute structures (eg, ducts and lobules) and individual cells.[38] Microscopic diagnoses can be made using some of these techniques (**Fig 4**).[39] Important applications include the evaluation of tissue adequacy at the time of biopsy, intraoperative diagnosis, and the determination of intraoperative margin status.[36] Although none are in general clinical use, the future ability to visualize unfixed surgical specimens at the cellular level would be a significant advance.

SUMMARY

In the age of burgeoning information about the subcellular components of breast lesions, gross evaluation continues to play an important and essential role. Without it, the optimal tissues for these advanced analytical techniques may not be taken or may be taken in such a way that their value is compromised. Numerous features of breast cancers are best, or can only, be determined grossly and are important for determining the best treatment for patients. Pathology faces many challenges in teaching future generations these important skills. New imaging procedures hold out the possibility of reinvigorating interest in grossing and increasing its value by allowing microscopic diagnosis of surgical specimens without the need for tissue processing.

DISCLOSURE

The authors have nothing to disclose.

SUPPLEMENTARY DATA

Supplementary data related to this article can be found online at https://doi.org/10.1016/j.path.2021.11.008.

REFERENCES

1. Apple SK. Variability in gross and microscopic pathology reporting in excisional biopsies of breast cancer tissue. Breast J 2006;12(2):145–9.
2. Wiley EL, Keh P. Diagnostic discrepancies in breast specimens subjected to gross reexamination. Am J Surg Pathol 1999;23(8):876–9.
3. Denison CM, Lester SC. Chapter One: Essential components of a successful breast core needle biopsy program. In: Shin SJ, editor. A Comprehensive guide to core needle biopsies of the breast.

4. Nakhleh RE, Jones B, Zarbo RJ. Mammographically directed breast biopsies: A College of American Pathologists Q-Probes study of clinical physician expectations and of specimen handling and reporting characteristics in 434 institutions. Arch Pathol Lab Med 1997;12(1):11–8.
5. Zeng J, Mercado C, Axelrod D, et al. Missing targets after nipple-sparing mastectomy: a multidisciplinary approach to avoid an undesirable outcome. Breast J 2018;24(4):678–9.
6. Aruda SKC, Garvey LC, Hagemann IS. In-laboratory breast specimen radiography reduces tissue block utilization and improves turnaround time of pathologic examination. BMC Med Imaging 2021;21:59–65.
7. Kallen ME, Sim MS, Radosavcev BL, et al. A quality initiative of postoperative radiographic imaging performed on mastectomy specimens to reduce histology cost and pathology report turnaround time. Ann Diagn Pathol 2015;19(5):353–8.
8. Brierly JD, Gospodarowicz MK, Wittekind C, editors. TNM classification of malignant tumours. 8th edition. Wiley-Blackwell; 2016.
9. Hortobagyi GN, Connolly JL, D'Orsi CJ, et al. In: Amin MB, Edge S, Greene F, et al, editors. For the American Joint Commission on cancer. AJCC cancer staging Manual. New York, (NY): Springer; 2017, (corrected edition published in 2018).
10. Moatamed NA, Apple SK. Extensive sampling changes T-staging of infiltrating lobular carcinoma of breast: a comparative study of gross versus microscopic tumor sizes. Breast J 2006;12(6):511–7.
11. Desmedt C, Fumagalli D, Pietri E, et al. Uncovering the genomic heterogeneity of multifocal breast cancer. J Pathol 2015;236:457–66.
12. McCrorie AD, Ashfield S, Begley A, et al. Multifocal breast cancers are more prevalent in BRCA2 versus BRCA1 carriers. J Pathol Clin Res 2020;6(2):146–53.
13. Alexander M, Gonzalez GA, Malerba S, et al. Multifocal invasive ductal cancer: distinguishing independent tumor foci from multiple satellites. Int J Surg Pathol 2017;25(4):298–303.
14. Salgado R, Aftimos P, Sotiriou C, et al. Evolving paradigms in multifocal breast cancer. Sem Cancer Biol 2015;111–8.
15. Lester SC, Bose S, Chen Y-Y, et al. Protocol for the examination of specimens from patients with invasive carcinoma of the breast 2009;133(10):1515–38.
16. Bossuyt V. Processing and reporting of breast specimens in the neoadjuvant setting. Surg Pathol Clin 2018;11(1):213–30.
17. Troxell M. Neoadjuvant therapy in breast cancer: histologic changes and clinical implications. Surg Pathol Clin, Allison K (ed). 2021

18. Graham RA, Homer MJ, Katz J, et al. The pancake phenomenon contributes to the inaccuracy of margin assessment in patients with breast cancer. Am J Surg 2002;184(2):89–93.

19. Nunez A, Jones V, Schulz-Costello, et al. Accuracy of gross intraoperative margin assessment for breast cancer: experience since the SSO-ASTRO margin consensus guidelines. Sci Rep 2020;10(1): 17344–6.

20. Hoekstra S, Stoller D, Raef H. Does gross margin examination reduce re-excision rate in breast conservation for invasive carcinoma? CALLER review. Eur J Breast Health 2020;16(3):198–200.

21. Dupont E, Tsangaris T, Garcia-Cantu C, et al. Resection of cavity shave margins in stage 0-III breast cancer patients undergoing breast conserving surgery: A prospective multicenter randomized controlled trial. Ann Surg 2019. https://doi.org/10.1097/SLA.0000000000003449.

22. Chagpar AB, Killelea BK, Tsangaris TN, et al. A randomized, controlled trial of cavity shave margins in breast cancer. N Engl J Med 2015;373(6): 503–10.

23. Huston TL, Pigalarga R, Osborne MP, et al. The influence of additional surgical margins on the total specimen volume excised and the reoperative rate after breast-conserving surgery. Am J Surg 2006; 192(4):509–12.

24. Kobbermann A, Unzeitig A, Xie X, et al. Impact of routine cavity shave margins on breast cancer re-excision rates. Ann Surg Oncol 2011;18(5):1349–55.

25. Khoury T. Delay to formalin fixation alters morphology and immunohistochemistry for breast carcinoma. Appl Immunohistochem Mol Morphol 2012;20(6):531–42.

26. Vaught J. Biobanking comes of age: the transition to biospecimen science. Annu Rev Pharmacol Toxicol 2016;56:211–28.

27. Lester SC. Gross examination. In: Lester SC, editor. Diagnostic pathology: intraoperative consultation 2nd. 2nd edition. Salt Lake City, Utah: Elsevier; 2018. p. 34–41.

28. Ghezzi TL, Pereira MP, Corleta OC, et al. Carnoy solution versus GEWF solution for lymph node revealing in colorectal cancer: a randomized control trial 2019;34(12):2189–93.

29. Lester SC. Manual of surgical pathology. 4th edition. Elsevier; 2010.

30. Westra WH, Hruban RH, Phelps TH, et al. Surgical pathology dissection: an illustrated guide. 2nd edition. Springer, Switzerland: Springer; 2003.

31. Harrison BT. Breast: Radioactive seed localization. In: Lester SC, editor. Diagnostic pathology: intraoperative consultation. 2nd edition. Salt Lake City, Utah: Elsevier; 2018. p. 78–81.

32. Bortesi M, Vartino V, Marchetti M, et al. Pathologist's assistant (PathA) and his/her role in the surgical pathology department: a systematic review and a narrative synthesis. Virchows Arch 2018;472(6):1041–54.

33. Galvis CO, Raab SS, D'Amico F, et al. Pathologist's assistants practice: A measurement of performance. Am J Clin Pathol 2001;116(6):816–22.

34. Krishnamurthy S, Brown JQ, Iftimia N, et al. Ex vivo microscopy: a promising next-generation microscopy tool for surgical pathology practice. Arch Pathol Lab Med 2019;143(9):1058–68.

35. Mathur SC, Fitzmaurice M, Reder NP, et al. Development of functional requirements for ex vivo pathology applications of in vivo microscopy systems: a proposal from the in vivo microscopy committee of the College of American Pathologists. Arch Pathol Lab Med 2019;143:1052–7.

36. Scimone MT, Krishnamurthy S, Maguluri G, et al. Assessment of breast cancer surgical margins with multimodal optical microscopy: a feasibility clinical study. PLoS One 2021;16(2):e0245334.

37. Shimao D, Sunaguchi N, Yuasa T, et al. X-ray dark-field imaging (XDFI) – a promising tool for 3D virtual histopathology. Mol Imaging Biol 2021;23(4): 481–94.

38. Schmidt H, Connolly C, Jaffer S, et al. Evaluation of surgically excised breast tissue microstructure using wide-field optical coherence tomography. Breast J 2020;26(5):917–23.

39. Lu T, Jorns JM, Patton M, et al. Rapid assessment of breast tumor margins using deep ultraviolet fluorescence scanning microscopy. J Biomed Opt 2020;25. https://doi.org/10.1117/1.JBO.25.12.126501.

Papillary Neoplasms of the Breast
Diagnostic Features and Molecular Insights

Dara S. Ross, MD[a], Timothy M. D'Alfonso, MD[b],*

KEYWORDS

• Papillary • Breast • Solid-papillary • Papillary carcinoma • *PIK3CA* • Adenomyoepithelioma

Key points

- Tumors of the breast classified as papillary neoplasms by the World Health Organization (WHO) include intraductal papilloma, intraductal papilloma with atypical ductal hyperplasia (ADH)/ductal carcinoma in situ (DCIS), papillary DCIS, encapsulated papillary carcinoma, solid papillary carcinoma (in situ and with invasion), and invasive papillary carcinoma. Adenomyoepitheliomas are biphasic epithelial–myoepithelial tumors that can also display a papillary growth pattern.

- Immunohistochemical stains for myoepithelial cells can aid in the classification of papillary neoplasms of the breast. These markers can also assist in the diagnosis of stromal invasion, however, in situ papillary carcinomas often show loss or diminished myoepithelial staining and should be interpreted with caution to prevent overdiagnosis of invasive carcinoma.

- Activating mutations in the PI3K-AKT1 pathway have been identified in intraductal papillomas with and without atypia, but are not typical for papillary carcinoma. Clonality studies, copy number alterations, and hierarchical clustering suggest that intraductal papillomas, particularly atypical papillomas, may be nonobligate precursors of synchronous ER-positive carcinomas but not papillary carcinomas.

- Papillary carcinomas of the breast, including encapsulated papillary carcinoma, solid papillary carcinoma, and invasive papillary carcinoma, display relatively simple genomic profiles with similar copy number alterations (including 1q gains, 16p gains, and 16q losses); however, significant differences in the transcriptomic profiles may account for their different histologic features.

ABSTRACT

Papillary neoplasms of the breast are a heterogeneous group of tumors characterized by fibrovascular cores lined by epithelium, with or without myoepithelial cells. Papillary neoplasms include benign, atypical, and malignant tumors that show varying histopathologic features and clinical outcomes. Appropriate pathologic classification is crucial to guide clinical treatment. Classification of papillary neoplasms is largely based on morphology, with immunohistochemistry playing an ancillary role to establish diagnoses. Recent molecular studies have provided insight into the genomics of these lesions. This review summarizes the histologic, immunohistochemical, and molecular features of papillary neoplasms of the breast that are important for diagnosis and treatment.

OVERVIEW

Papillary neoplasms of the breast are heterogeneous and include benign, atypical, and malignant tumors. Tumors of the breast classified as papillary

[a] Memorial Sloan Kettering Cancer Center, 1275 York Avenue, S-624, New York, NY 10065, USA; [b] Memorial Sloan Kettering Cancer Center, 1275 York Avenue, A-504, New York, NY 10065, USA
* Corresponding author.
E-mail address: dalfonst@mskcc.org

Surgical Pathology 15 (2022) 133–146
https://doi.org/10.1016/j.path.2021.11.009

neoplasms by the World Health Organization (WHO)[1] include intraductal papilloma, intraductal papilloma with atypical ductal hyperplasia(ADH)/ductal carcinoma in situ (DCIS), papillary DCIS, encapsulated papillary carcinoma, solid papillary carcinoma (SPC) (in situ and with invasion), and invasive papillary carcinoma. Adenomyoepitheliomas (AME) are biphasic epithelial-myoepithelial tumors that can also display a papillary growth pattern. Recognition of the various histologic features is key for accurate classification. Immunohistochemistry, particularly specific epithelial and myoepithelial markers which will be discussed later in discussion, can be used as a helpful diagnostic tool. Molecular studies are not used routinely for diagnosing papillary neoplasms, but have provided insight into the classification, relationship, and features of progression that can aid in the clinical management of these neoplasms. This review summarizes the histologic, immunohistochemical, and molecular characteristics of papillary neoplasms of the breast and how this information is used to facilitate diagnosis and guide clinical management.

INTRADUCTAL PAPILLOMA (INCLUDING PAPILLOMA WITH ATYPICAL DUCTAL HYPERPLASIA/DUCTAL CARCINOMA IN SITU)

INTRODUCTION

Intraductal papilloma is a benign papillary neoplasm that occurs at virtually any age but most commonly in adult women between the ages of 40 and 60 years. Papillomas arising in central ducts may present with unilateral nipple discharge that is clear or bloody. Papillomas can be detected on screening imaging as a circumscribed mass. Larger papillomas (>2 cm) may present as palpable masses.

Papillomas may pose diagnostic challenges for pathologists, particularly when they are involved by hyperplastic or atypical processes or undergo significant sclerosis. Although most papillomas historically underwent excision, the current clinical management for most benign papillomas includes following by imaging, rather than surgery, due to low upgrade rates on excision. Molecular analyses have demonstrated that papillomas are clonal neoplasms with a high prevalence of mutations in the PI3K-AKT1 pathway.

MICROSCOPIC AND IMMUNOHISTOCHEMICAL FEATURES

Intraductal papillomas can be seen within central dilated ducts or in peripheral terminal ductal lobular units (Fig. 1A, B). Typically, papillomas arising within large central ducts are solitary, while peripheral papillomas occur as multiple foci. Central and peripheral papillomas essentially share the same histologic features. Papillomas are characterized by a dual population of ductal epithelial cells and an inner layer of myoepithelial cells lining an arborizing proliferation of fibrovascular cores

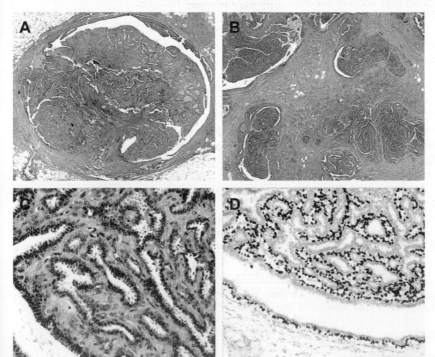

Fig. 1. Intraductal papilloma. (*A*). Central papilloma showing an arborizing proliferation of fibrovascular cores arising within a dilated duct. (*B*) Multiple peripheral papillomas arising in terminal duct lobular units. (*C*) Papilloma shows a dual population of outer ductal cells and inner myoepithelial cells that are easily identified in this case. (*D*) A p63 immunostain highlights a continuous layer of myoepithelial cells lining the fibrovascular cores and duct wall.

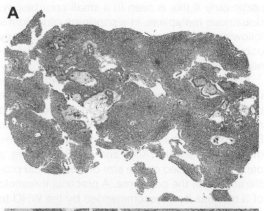

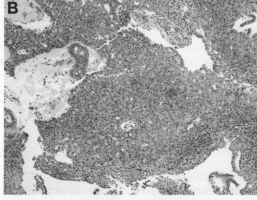

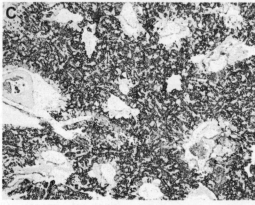

Fig. 2. Intraductal papilloma with usual ductal hyperplasia. (*A*) Core biopsy specimen showing a fragment of tissue with fibrovascular cores and proliferative epithelium with solid growth. (*B*) Higher power shows a streaming pattern of overlapping cells and irregular spaces, indicative of usual ductal hyperplasia. (*C*) A CK5/6 immunostain shows a variable mosaic pattern of staining, confirming the diagnosis.

(**Fig. 1**C). Epithelial cells are cuboidal to columnar without significant cytologic atypia. Myoepithelial cells can be flatted or cuboidal and exhibit clear cell features in some cases. Myoepithelial cells can be demonstrated using immunohistochemical stains such as p63, calponin, and smooth muscle

myosin heavy chain (**Fig. 1**D). The distribution of myoepithelial cells is usually diffuse and continuous within the papilloma.

A variety of benign, atypical, and malignant processes can be seen in papillomas. Common benign proliferations in papillomas include usual ductal hyperplasia, adenosis, and apocrine metaplasia. In papillomas with usual ductal hyperplasia, a CK5/6 immunostain will show a variable "mosaic" pattern of staining within hyperplastic areas, similar to the pattern of CK5/6 staining in hyperplasia outside of a papilloma (**Fig. 2**). One caveat is that CK5/6 may be negative in apocrine metaplasia within an otherwise benign papilloma, and this staining should not be interpreted as atypia. Some papillomas undergo a significant amount of stromal sclerosis ("sclerosing papilloma") resulting in entrapped glands in the peripheral stroma of the papilloma, and such cases often show morphologic overlap with radial scars/complex sclerosing lesions. Squamous metaplasia may be focal or prominent in some cases (**Fig. 3**) and worrisome for squamous cell carcinoma,

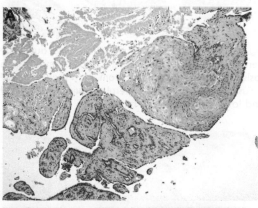

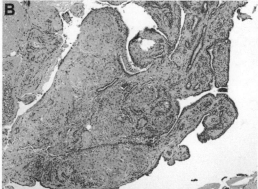

Fig. 3. Squamous metaplasia in intraductal papilloma. (*A, B*) Squamous metaplasia seen as squamous pearls within fibrovascular cores of a papilloma. The papilloma had undergone infarction and necrotic tissue can be seen in the top left of both images.

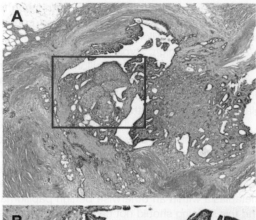

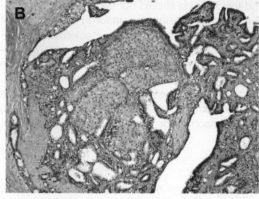

Fig. 4. Intraductal papilloma with atypical ductal hyperplasia (ADH). (A) Intraductal papilloma with sclerosis. (B) Area in red box from "A" shows a small focus of atypical ductal hyperplasia with solid growth and low-grade cytologic features.

particularly if this is seen in a small core biopsy. Squamous metaplasia in a papilloma often forms following infarction of the papilloma, which may occur in the setting or prior core biopsy or fine-needle aspiration.

ADH or DCIS involving a papilloma is characterized by a monotonous population of cells within a papilloma that exhibit low-grade cytologic and architectural atypia, similar to ADH or low-grade DCIS outside the setting of a papilloma. The distinction between ADH and DCIS involving a papilloma is based on the size of the atypical proliferation with the papilloma. A practical threshold of 3 mm has been recommended by the WHO to distinguish ADH versus DCIS in a papilloma whereas papilloma with ADH is diagnosed if the atypical proliferation is less than 3 mm (Fig. 4), and papilloma with DCIS (Fig. 5) is diagnosed if the atypical proliferation is 3 mm or greater in the papilloma. A diagnosis of DCIS in a papilloma is warranted when there are intermediate-high-grade features that are diagnostic of DCIS, regardless of the size of the proliferation.

DIFFERENTIAL DIAGNOSIS

The main consideration in the differential diagnosis of papilloma is papillary carcinoma or papilloma involved by ADH/DCIS. In core biopsy samples, papillary lesions often appear as detached fragments of tissue that may be associated with a dilated duct. Benign papillomas tend to appear as more solid cohesive clusters with complex

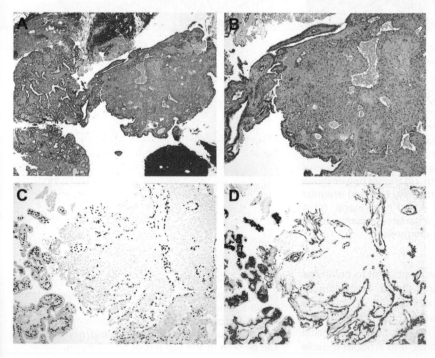

Fig. 5. Intraductal papilloma with ductal carcinoma in situ DCIS. (A) Partially fragmented core biopsy sample shows areas of benign papilloma (left of image) merging with areas that show more solid growth (right of image). (B) Higher power view shows a monotonous population of cells with solid growth within the papilloma. (C, D) The benign-appearing papilloma component on the left of the images shows a continuous layer of myoepithelial cells with p63 (C) and calponin (D), while the area of solid growth, representing DCIS in this case, shows loss of myoepithelial staining.

growth. Papillary carcinomas, in contrast, seem more fragmented with slender fibrovascular cores and exhibit a more basophilic appearance from low power. Immunohistochemical stains for myoepithelial cell markers show a continuous layer of myoepithelial cells in papilloma. In papillomas with ADH/DCIS, myoepithelial cells are diminished or absent in areas of atypia (see **Fig. 5**C, D). In contrast to the mosaic pattern of staining with CK5/6 seen in hyperplasia within a papilloma, ADH/DCIS within a papilloma will show lack of staining, similar to ADH/DCIS outside of a papilloma. ER tends to be diffusely expressed in papillary carcinoma and in ADH/DCIS in a papilloma, while ER will most often show a variable staining pattern in papilloma.

ASSOCIATED GENETIC ALTERATIONS

Early studies using the loss of heterozygosity (LOH) analyses showed that papillomas are clonal neoplasms and show a high frequency of LOH at the 16p and 16q loci in both benign papillomas and those containing DCIS, suggesting that these are early events in the development of these lesions.[2,3] Subsequent studies revealed papillomas show frequent alterations in the PI3K/AKT/mTOR signaling pathway. Troxell and colleagues reported papillomas to harbor *PIK3CA* or *AKT1* mutations in 66% of cases studied, while papillary carcinoma showed mutations in the PI3KCA/AKT pathway in only 30%.[4] The majority (77%) of *PIK3CA* mutations in papillary neoplasms were exon 20 hotspot activating mutations, and these mutations seemed more common in papillomas with moderate to florid epithelial hyperplasia. In a separate study, Jahn and colleagues reported *AKT1* or *PIK3CA* mutations in 57% (4/7) of papillomas containing usual ductal hyperplasia.[5] In a study of 60 papillomas, Mishima and colleagues reported *PIK3CA* mutations in 17 (28%) and *AKT1* mutations in 12 (20%) papillomas, with *PIK3CA* mutations being more common in papillomas with hyperplasia.[6] Recently, Kader and colleagues performed a detailed analysis of benign papillomas, papillomas with ADH/DCIS, and those with synchronous invasive carcinoma/DCIS.[7] 69% of papillomas (both with and without ADH) harbored *PIK3CA* mutations in their analysis. Over half of papillomas with coexisting DCIS or invasive carcinoma were found to be clonally related to carcinoma and clonal-relatedness was more frequently demonstrated with atypical papillomas than benign papillomas, suggesting that a subset of papillomas may serve as a substrate for the development of carcinoma.[7] Further, papillomas clonally related to carcinoma were distinguished from benign papillomas by the lack of *PIK3CA* mutations and copy number alterations including 16q loss, 1q gain, and 11q loss.[7]

MANAGEMENT AND PROGNOSIS

The main management consideration is whether or not to excise a papilloma when it is present in a core biopsy sample. Historically, all papillary lesions, including benign papillomas routinely underwent excision. Currently, papillomas with atypia or DCIS require excision. Recent data support observation, rather than routine excision of benign papillomas, as studies observing strict radiologic-pathologic correlation show upgrade rates to carcinoma less than 5%.[8–14] Based on these low upgrade rates, most benign papillomas will not be excised when diagnosed in a core biopsy. Surgical excision is considered with large and/or symptomatic papillomas, or if the patient is high-risk for developing breast carcinoma.

The risk for developing subsequent breast carcinoma for patients with benign papilloma is approximately twofold the general population, similar to proliferative fibrocystic changes. The risk for papillomas with ADH is similar to that for patients with ADH, conveying a relative risk of approximately 4 to 5.[15,16]

Clinics care points – intraductal papilloma
• Intraductal papilloma shows low upgrade rates to carcinoma on excision and most papillomas do not require excision when diagnosed in a core biopsy sample
• The distinction between ADH and DCIS involving a papilloma is based on a 3 mm size cutoff, which is used as a practical guideline (<3 mm: papilloma with ADH; ≥ 3 mm: papilloma with DCIS)
• Intermediate to high-grade atypical proliferations that would be diagnostic of disease outside of a papilloma should be classified as DCIS when occurring within a papilloma, regardless of the size of the atypical proliferation

PAPILLARY DUCTAL CARCINOMA IN SITU

INTRODUCTION

Papillary DCIS refers to a type of DCIS with carcinoma cells lining fibrovascular cores that lack myoepithelial cells.[1] In contrast to papilloma with DCIS, there is no underlying benign papilloma associated with papillary DCIS. Papillary DCIS is often present in association with other DCIS growth patterns including cribriform and micropapillary types. Papillary DCIS mostly occurs in postmenopausal women and can present as a mass or calcifications on imaging. The outcome for papillary DCIS is similar to other types of DCIS and is staged pTis according to the American Joint Committee on Cancer (AJCC).[17] There are no specific genetic alterations associated with papillary growth in DCIS.

MICROSCOPIC AND IMMUNOHISTOCHEMICAL FEATURES

Papillary DCIS may grow in central ducts and therefore be mass-forming or occur in peripheral terminal duct lobular units and be associated with other types of DCIS. DCIS is graded according to nuclear grade, similar to other growth patterns of DCIS. Carcinoma cells are cuboidal to columnar in shape, monotonous, and are evenly spaced along slender delicate fibrovascular cores (**Fig. 6**A). Comedo-type necrosis may be present in some cases. The nuclear features of papillary DCIS are often deceptively bland with low-grade nuclei. In core biopsy samples, papillary DCIS is less cohesive than papilloma and often appears as multiple basophilic fragments. Myoepithelial cells are not present along fibrovascular cores but may be evident lining the periphery of the involved duct. Immunohistochemical staining for myoepithelial markers can help support an in situ process; however, in many cases of papillary DCIS, staining can be absent at the periphery or markedly attenuated with only rare myoepithelial cells staining (**Fig. 6**B). In cases lacking myoepithelial cell staining, rounded contours of ducts that lack irregular borders support an in situ process. In some cases, a dimorphic appearance can be appreciated with so-called "globoid cells" displaying abundant eosinophilic cytoplasm lining fibrovascular cores (**Fig. 6**C).[18] These cells may mimic myoepithelial cells morphologically but do not stain with myoepithelial markers. Similar to other types of low to intermediate DCIS, papillary DCIS typically shows strong and diffuse staining with ER. CK5/6 will show loss of staining in carcinoma cells in the center of the duct but may highlight myoepithelial cells at the periphery.

Invasive carcinoma occurring in association with papillary DCIS is typically invasive carcinoma, no special type (NST), and does not often show papillary growth. Invasive carcinoma is recognized as irregular growth of carcinoma cells often in perpendicular orientation to the duct. Stromal reaction to the invasive carcinoma may or may not be present. Invasive carcinoma associated with papillary DCIS is staged according to the largest contiguous focus of definitive invasive carcinoma.[17]

SOLID PAPILLARY CARCINOMA

SPC is a clinically and genomically distinct form of ER-positive breast cancer that is characterized by a solid growth pattern with delicate fibrovascular

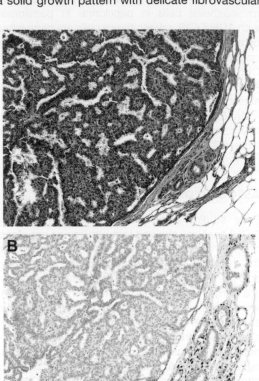

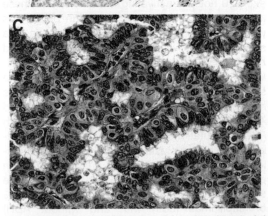

Fig. 6. Papillary ductal carcinoma in situ (DCIS). (*A*) Papillary proliferation with slender fibrovascular cores and circumscribed contour, indicative of a noninvasive process. (*B*) A p63 immunostain shows the absence of myoepithelial cells within fibrovascular cores, and also at the periphery of the lesion in this example. (*C*) Higher power view of the papillary proliferation shows a dimorphic population of cells with one type showing more clear to eosinophilic cytoplasm. These "globoid cells" are negative for p63 in "B."

cores and frequent neuroendocrine differentiation. SPC can be in situ or invasive. It occurs primarily in postmenopausal women and tends to have an overall favorable outcome.[1]

MICROSCOPIC AND IMMUNOHISTOCHEMICAL FEATURES

SPC is so named for its tendency to grow as expansile nodules or sheets of monotonous, round to spindle-shaped epithelial cells in a solid pattern with inconspicuous fibrovascular cores (**Fig. 7**).[1] Nuclear atypia is generally mild to moderate and the mitotic count is variable. Mucin vacuoles or signet-ring cell features may be prominent and extracellular mucin production can also be present. A subset of SPC demonstrates neuroendocrine differentiation[19] which can be appreciated morphologically by the observation of eosinophilic granular cytoplasm and also confirmed with immunohistochemistry (see later in discussion).

Morphologic assessment is key for the distinction between in situ and invasive SPC as immunohistochemical stains for myoepithelial cells can often be noncontributory, particularly for in situ lesions.[20] SPC in situ displays well-circumscribed borders; however, myoepithelial cells may be attenuated and not detectable with immunohistochemistry. SPC with invasion is diagnosed when SPC is associated with small foci or large clusters of neoplastic cells showing clear infiltration of the stroma. The invasive component can exhibit abundant extracellular mucin with solid papillary glands floating in pools of mucin, similar to that seen in mucinous carcinoma. The invasive component associated with SPC may also be a more conventional type, such as invasive ductal NST.[21] "Invasive solid papillary carcinoma" in contrast is characterized by nodules of tumor lacking myoepithelium with ragged contours creating a jigsaw pattern within desmoplastic stroma.[19,22]

SPC populations are characterized by "luminal" cytokeratin staining, in contrast to usual ductal hyperplasia they are cytokeratin 5/6 negative. SPC displays a strong and diffuse expression of ER and does not show overexpression of HER2.

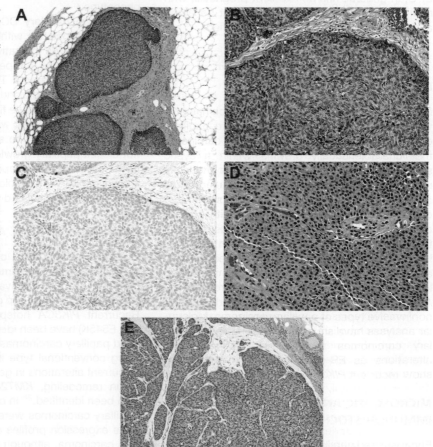

Fig. 7. Solid papillary carcinoma. (*A*) Solid papillary carcinoma is characterized by geographic islands of cells with solid growth. (*B*) The nodule shows a circumscribed contour and contains uniform spindle cells and inconspicuous fibrovascular cores. (*C*) Rare myoepithelial cells at the periphery of the duct are evident by p63 immunostaining. (*D*) Solid papillary carcinoma with uniform ovoid cells with eosinophilic cytoplasm, a feature of solid papillary carcinomas with neuroendocrine differentiation. (*E*) Solid papillary carcinoma with mucinous differentiation. Solid papillary carcinoma is entirely invasive in this image with islands of cells present in extracellular mucin.

Synaptophysin, chromogranin and/or CD56 staining is also common in SPC with neuroendocrine features.

GENETIC ALTERATIONS

SPC displays relatively simple genomic profiles. The genetic landscape includes a low level of copy number alterations, including 1q gains, 16p gains, and 16q losses[23] and the identification of PIK3CA mutations in 43% of cases.[24] A comparison between SPCs and encapsulated papillary carcinomas suggested that, consistent with the reported neuroendocrine morphologic and immunohistochemical phenotype of SPCs, genes related to neuroendocrine differentiation in human cancers including RET, ASCL1, and DOK7, were expressed at significantly higher levels in SPCs than in encapsulated papillary carcinomas.[24]

PROGNOSIS

Outcome data are difficult to assess for patients with SPC owing to small studies, partial follow-up, inconsistent staging, and variable treatment. SPC, in general, has an excellent prognosis, with multiple studies confirming its indolent behavior, and nodal metastases are rarely identified.[1,19]

ENCAPSULATED PAPILLARY CARCINOMA

INTRODUCTION

Encapsulated papillary carcinoma, which has previously been referred to as "intracystic papillary carcinoma," refers to a type of papillary carcinoma that characteristically growths within a cystic space lined by a dense fibrous capsule and lacks myoepithelial cells in both fibrovascular cores and at the periphery.[1] Affected patients are most often postmenopausal that present with a mass on imaging, with or without nipple discharge.[25] Due to the lack of myoepithelial cells in encapsulated papillary carcinoma, there has been debate as to whether this represents an in situ or invasive lesion. It is currently staged as Tis according to the AJCC and is generally managed similarly to other noninvasive types of papillary carcinoma. Molecular analyses have shown that encapsulated papillary carcinomas show similar copy number alterations as ER-positive breast cancers and show recurrent PIK3CA hotspot mutations.

MICROSCOPIC AND IMMUNOHISTOCHEMICAL FEATURES

Encapsulated papillary carcinoma is characterized by a papillary mass within a cystic space lined by a fibrous wall that often contains chronic inflammation and evidence of hemorrhage in the form of hemosiderin-laden macrophages (**Fig. 8**). In some cases, multinodular growth can be seen with multiple cystic spaces. Carcinoma cells line delicate fibrovascular cores and lack myoepithelial cells. Tumor cells are monotonous, typically of low to intermediate nuclear grade, and have a similar appearance to cells of papillary DCIS. Secondary solid and cribriform growth may be seen in addition to papillary growth and conventional DCIS is seen in association with encapsulated papillary carcinoma in about 1/3 of cases. Characteristically, myoepithelial cells are not present along the periphery of the fibrous capsule lining the papillary tumor; however, in some cases, rare myoepithelial staining may be observed. Encapsulated papillary carcinomas are usually hormone receptor-positive and HER2-negative.

Uncommonly (approximately 5%–10% of cases), encapsulated carcinomas exhibit high-grade cytologic features.[26] These tumors show pleomorphic nuclei, high mitotic activity, and often show areas of solid growth. High-grade encapsulated carcinomas often show a triple-negative phenotype.[26,27]

Similar to papillary DCIS, invasive carcinoma arising in association with encapsulated papillary carcinoma shows infiltrative and irregular growth of carcinoma cells that permeate the fibrous wall often perpendicular to it. This should be differentiated from entrapped glands at the periphery which often grow parallel to the fibrous capsule. Invasive carcinomas associated with encapsulated papillary carcinoma show no special features and do not exhibit papillary growth. Metastases reported from encapsulated papillary carcinoma have shown papillary morphologic features, similar to the primary encapsulated papillary carcinoma.

ASSOCIATED GENETIC ALTERATIONS

Encapsulated papillary carcinomas show copy number alterations similar to those grade-matched ER-positive invasive carcinomas, NST, including 16q losses, 16p gains, and 1q gains.[23,24] Recurrent PIK3CA hotspot mutations (H1047R and E545K) have been identified in both encapsulated papillary carcinomas with and without coexisting conventional type invasive carcinoma.[23,28] Recurrent alterations in genes involved with chromatin remodeling, KMT2A and CREBBP, have also been identified.[28] In one study, encapsulated papillary carcinomas were shown to have similar gene expression profiles as the associated invasive carcinoma, although the invasive carcinoma component was found to be enriched in pathways

Fig. 8. Encapsulated papillary carcinoma. (*A*) Multinodular growth of a papillary lesion within cystic spaces lined by fibrous tissue. (*B*) Higher power shows a uniform papillary proliferation with a pushing border surrounded by a fibrous capsule with chronic inflammation. Myoepithelial cell staining for (*C*) calponin and (*D*) p63 show no staining in fibrovascular cores or at the periphery of the tumor. Benign glands in "*C*" show myoepithelial staining (bottom left). (*E*) Invasive carcinoma arising from encapsulated papillary carcinoma shows irregular growth perpendicular to the fibrous capsule. This case was staged as T1mi (microinvasive carcinoma) based on this focus of invasion.

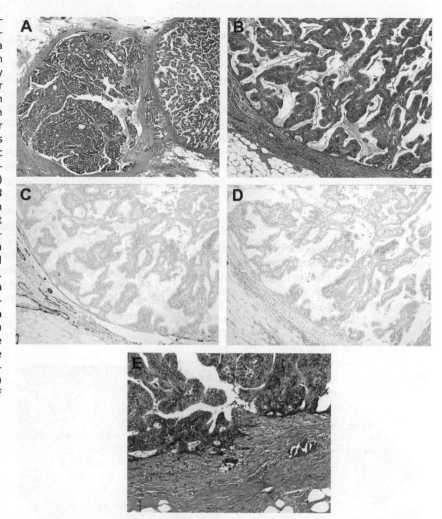

related to invasion, including collagen genes and matrix metalloproteinases.[28]

PROGNOSIS

Encapsulated papillary carcinomas have an excellent prognosis, similar to other types of papillary carcinoma (in situ), although cases of lymph node and distant metastases have been reported.[25] Due to the complete lack of myoepithelial cells and reports of metastases, encapsulated papillary carcinoma is currently regarded as a special low-grade type of invasive carcinoma with a pushing border. However, due to the excellent prognosis, encapsulated papillary carcinoma is staged as an in situ process (Tis) according to the AJCC.[17] When frank invasion is present, the tumor is staged only according to the largest contiguous focus of invasive carcinoma, and should not include the total size of the encapsulated papillary carcinoma. Encapsulated papillary carcinomas

with high-grade features with a triple-negative phenotype should be regarded as invasive carcinoma and treated as such.[1,26]

INVASIVE PAPILLARY CARCINOMA

Invasive papillary carcinoma is an exceedingly rare type of invasive carcinoma in which virtually the entire tumor is composed of glands with papillary architecture that lack myoepithelial cells. The malignant papillary glands show infiltrative growth within a desmoplastic stroma.

Invasive papillary carcinoma should be distinguished from invasive carcinoma arising in association with other types of papillary carcinoma (papillary DCIS, SPC, encapsulated papillary carcinoma), which typically do not show papillary growth. Metastatic carcinoma to the breast should be excluded when a tumor is identified in the breast that shows entirely papillary growth and lacks an in situ component. Specifically, immunohistochemistry should be performed to rule out a metastatic gynecologic serous carcinoma (PAX8+/WT1+) or lung carcinoma (TTF-1+/napsin-A+) with papillary growth.

No specific genetic alterations have been associated with invasive papillary carcinoma. Due to the rarity of this type of papillary carcinoma, there are practically no clinical or outcome data related to the behavior of these tumors. Invasive papillary carcinomas are graded according to the Nottingham system and staged according to AJCC staging.

ADENOMYOEPITHELIOMA

AME is an uncommon biphasic epithelial and myoepithelial tumor that include a spectrum of lesions ranging from benign to malignant with a propensity for recurrence or distant metastasis, and ER-positive and ER-negative cases.[1]

MICROSCOPIC AND IMMUNOHISTOCHEMICAL FEATURES

AME is a mass-forming lesions most commonly consisting of benign glandular structures in close association with a conspicuous myoepithelial cell population. The epithelial component usually forms glands and can occasionally show apocrine, squamous, or sebaceous metaplasia. The myoepithelium often shows glycogen-rich clear cytoplasm and can appear spindle, myoid, or plasmacytoid in appearance. AME show several architectural patterns, including tubular, lobulated, and spindle cell, with variation in the amount of epithelial and myoepithelial components (**Fig. 9**).[1] Some AME also display an intraductal papillary pattern. The tubular growth pattern is characterized by small tubules lined by luminal epithelial cells with prominent and hyperplastic myoepithelial cells. The myoepithelial component often

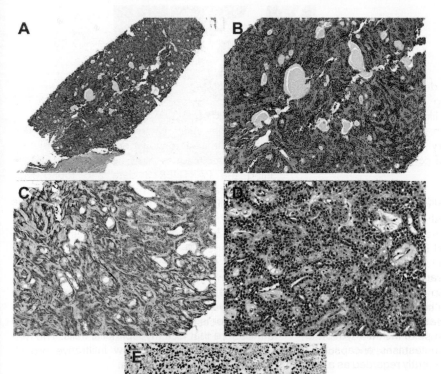

Fig. 9. Adenomyoepithelioma. (*A*) Core biopsy shows a circumscribed cellular proliferation within a dilated duct. (*B*) Higher power reveals uniform spindle cells admixed with glands. (*C*) A calponin immunostain highlights the myoepithelial spindle cells. (*D*) Another example of adenomyoepithelioma with a biphasic appearance and fibrovascular cores. (*E*) A p63 immunostain shows nuclear staining of myoepithelial cells.

Fig. 10. Malignant adenomy-oepithelioma. (*A*) The tumor shows a solid and pushing border from low power with lymphocytic infiltrates at the periphery. (*B, C*) Solid nests of highly atypical glands with an infiltrative appearance and irregular growth are present within a desmoplastic stroma, supporting a diagnosis of malignant adenomyoepithelioma. (*D*) CK7 highlights the epithelial component and (*E*) p63 highlights the myoepithelial component.

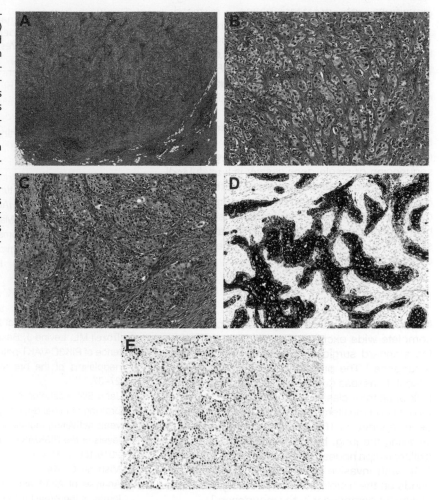

predominates in the lobulated and spindle cell architectural patterns. The lobulated growth pattern is characterized by solid nests of clear, eosinophilic, or plasmacytoid myoepithelial cells that proliferate around epithelial-lined spaces.[29] The spindle cell growth pattern shows a predominance of spindled myoepithelial cells that have few, compressed epithelial lined spaces.[29] Mitoses may be present but should be inconspicuous in benign lesions.

Either the epithelial or myoepithelial component can show malignant transformation in AME and they are characterized by a large spectrum of histologic patterns. Malignant AME show an infiltrative growth pattern, increased mitotic rate, and nuclear enlargement and pleomorphism of the epithelium and/or myoepithelium (**Fig. 10**).[30,31] The malignant transformation of the epithelial component has been reported as showing features of invasive carcinoma of NST in addition to special subtypes, including invasive lobular carcinoma, metaplastic carcinoma, or adenoid cystic carcinoma.[29,32–37] Malignant transformation of the myoepithelial component shows features of myoepithelial carcinoma including the overgrowth of myoepithelial cells, nuclear atypia, and increased mitotic activity.[38,39]

Immunohistochemistry can be helpful in determining the biphasic nature of AME, with the epithelial and myoepithelial cells maintaining their immunophenotype. High-molecular weight cytokeratins show a characteristic staining pattern, with diffuse positivity in the inner epithelial cells and negativity in the outer myoepithelial cells. The myoepithelial component can be confirmed with immunohistochemical stains for p63, S-100, smooth muscle actin, and smooth muscle myosin heavy chain.[40] The epithelial cells can be focally positive for ER and PR. Malignant AME can be ER-positive or ER-negative, but the carcinoma component is most commonly ER-/PR-/HER2-negative.[40]

GENETIC ALTERATIONS

The genetic makeup of AME varies according to the ER status.[41] ER-positive AME are characterized by recurrent mutations affecting *PIK3CA* or *AKT1*, whereas ER-negative tumors harbor recurrent *HRAS* Q61 hotspot mutations, frequently cooccurring with mutations in the PI3K-AKT pathway.[41–43] Given that *HRAS* Q61 hotspot mutations are otherwise extremely rare in breast tumors, their detection by next-generation sequencing or single-gene assays is a useful tool for the diagnosis of these tumors in the breast. *HRAS* Q61R mutations, in particular, may be also detected by IHC with moderate sensitivity and high specificity.[44] Malignant AME displays a similar mutational profile as the benign counterparts.[41,42]

PROGNOSIS

Most of the AME have a benign clinical course and complete wide excision with negative margins is the standard surgical treatment to prevent local recurrence.[1] The prognosis of malignant AME is difficult to assess due to the rarity of these lesions, lack of uniform classification, and short periods of follow-up in the literature. Distant metastases have been reported in 16% to 32% of malignant AME involving the lung, brain, bone, thyroid, liver, and axillary lymph nodes.[40] The prognosis of malignant AME with invasive carcinoma, in particular, depends on the histologic subtype and grade of the malignant component in the recurrence.[1]

Pathologic key features: myoepithelial staining patterns in papillary neoplasms

- Intraductal papilloma: + in fibrovascular cores, + in the periphery of tumor

- Intraductal papilloma with ADH/DCIS: + in fibrovascular cores with diminished staining in areas of ADH/DCIS, + in the periphery of tumor

- Papillary DCIS: Absent in fibrovascular cores, + at the periphery of tumor, often diminished

- SPC: Absent in fibrovascular cores, + or absent in the periphery of tumor

- Encapsulated papillary carcinoma: Absent in fibrovascular cores, absent in the periphery of tumor

- Invasive papillary carcinoma: Absent in fibrovascular cores, absent in the periphery of tumor

---

- Adenomyoepithelioma: Variable depending on the degree of myoepithelial proliferation, + in fibrovascular cores, + in the periphery of tumor

DISCLOSURE

The authors have nothing to disclose.

REFERENCES

1. WHO classification of tumors. Breast tumours. 5th edition. Lyon (France): IARC; 2019.
2. Lininger RA, Park WS, Man YG, et al. LOH at 16p13 is a novel chromosomal alteration detected in benign and malignant microdissected papillary neoplasms of the breast. Hum Pathol 1998;29(10):1113–8.
3. Di Cristofano C, Mrad K, Zavaglia K, et al. Papillary lesions of the breast: a molecular progression? Breast Cancer Res Treat 2005;90(1):71–6.
4. Troxell ML, Levine J, Beadling C, et al. High prevalence of PIK3CA/AKT pathway mutations in papillary neoplasms of the breast. Mod Pathol 2010;23(1):27–37.
5. Jahn SW, Kashofer K, Thuringer A, et al. Mutation profiling of usual ductal hyperplasia of the breast reveals activating mutations predominantly at different levels of the PI3K/AKT/mTOR Pathway. Am J Pathol 2016;186(1):15–23.
6. Mishima C, Kagara N, Ikeda JI, et al. Mutational Analysis of AKT1 and PIK3CA in intraductal papillomas of the breast with special reference to cellular components. Am J Pathol 2018;188(5):1106–12.
7. Kader T, Elder K, Zethoven M, et al. The genetic architecture of breast papillary lesions as a predictor of progression to carcinoma. NPJ Breast Cancer 2020;6:9.
8. Pareja F, Corben AD, Brennan SB, et al. Breast intraductal papillomas without atypia in radiologic-pathologic concordant core-needle biopsies: Rate of upgrade to carcinoma at excision. Cancer 2016;122(18):2819–27.
9. Lee SJ, Wahab RA, Sobel LD, et al. Analysis of 612 benign papillomas diagnosed at core biopsy: rate of upgrade to malignancy, factors associated with upgrade, and a proposal for selective surgical excision. AJR Am J Roentgenol 2021;217(6):1299–311.
10. Kim SY, Kim EK, Lee HS, et al. Asymptomatic benign papilloma without atypia diagnosed at ultrasonography-guided 14-gauge core needle biopsy: which subgroup can be managed by observation? Ann Surg Oncol 2016;23(6):1860–6.
11. Nakhlis F, Baker GM, Pilewskie M, et al. The incidence of adjacent synchronous invasive carcinoma and/or ductal carcinoma in situ in patients with

intraductal papilloma without atypia on core biopsy: results from a prospective multi-institutional registry (TBCRC 034). Ann Surg Oncol 2021;28(5):2573–8.

12. Brogi E, Krystel-Whittemore M. Papillary neoplasms of the breast including upgrade rates and management of intraductal papilloma without atypia diagnosed at core needle biopsy. Mod Pathol 2021; 34(Suppl 1):78–93.

13. Limberg J, Kucher W, Fasano G, et al. Intraductal papilloma of the breast: prevalence of malignancy and natural history under active surveillance. Ann Surg Oncol 2021;28(11):6032–40.

14. Grimm LJ, Bookhout CE, Bentley RC, et al. Concordant, non-atypical breast papillomas do not require surgical excision: A 10-year multi-institution study and review of the literature. Clin Imaging 2018;51: 180–5.

15. Lewis JT, Hartmann LC, Vierkant RA, et al. An analysis of breast cancer risk in women with single, multiple, and atypical papilloma. Am J Surg Pathol 2006;30(6):665–72.

16. Page DL, Salhany KE, Jensen RA, et al. Subsequent breast carcinoma risk after biopsy with atypia in a breast papilloma. Cancer 1996;78(2):258–66.

17. Amin MB, American Joint Committee on Cancer., American Cancer Society. AJCC cancer staging manual. Chicago (IL): American Joint Committee on Cancer, Springer; 2017.

18. Lefkowitz M, Lefkowitz W, Wargotz ES. Intraductal (intracystic) papillary carcinoma of the breast and its variants: a clinicopathological study of 77 cases. Hum Pathol 1994;25(8):802–9.

19. Tan BY, Thike AA, Ellis IO, et al. Clinicopathologic characteristics of solid papillary carcinoma of the breast. Am J Surg Pathol 2016;40(10):1334–42.

20. Nicolas MM, Wu Y, Middleton LP, et al. Loss of myoepithelium is variable in solid papillary carcinoma of the breast. Histopathology 2007;51(5):657–65.

21. Nassar H, Qureshi H, Adsay NV, et al. Clinicopathologic analysis of solid papillary carcinoma of the breast and associated invasive carcinomas. Am J Surg Pathol 2006;30(4):501–7.

22. Tan PH, Schnitt SJ, van de Vijver MJ, et al. Papillary and neuroendocrine breast lesions: the WHO stance. Histopathology 2015;66(6):761–70.

23. Duprez R, Wilkerson PM, Lacroix-Triki M, et al. Immunophenotypic and genomic characterization of papillary carcinomas of the breast. J Pathol 2012; 226(3):427–41.

24. Piscuoglio S, Ng CK, Martelotto LG, et al. Integrative genomic and transcriptomic characterization of papillary carcinomas of the breast. Mol Oncol 2014;8(8):1588–602.

25. Rakha EA, Gandhi N, Climent F, et al. Encapsulated papillary carcinoma of the breast: an invasive tumor with excellent prognosis. Am J Surg Pathol 2011; 35(8):1093–103.

26. Rakha EA, Varga Z, Elsheik S, et al. High-grade encapsulated papillary carcinoma of the breast: an under-recognized entity. Histopathology 2015; 66(5):740–6.

27. Esposito NN, Dabbs DJ, Bhargava R. Are encapsulated papillary carcinomas of the breast in situ or invasive? A basement membrane study of 27 cases. Am J Clin Pathol 2009;131(2):228–42.

28. Schwartz CJ, Boroujeni AM, Khodadadi-Jamayran A, et al. Molecular analysis of encapsulated papillary carcinoma of the breast with and without invasion. Hum Pathol 2021;111:67–74.

29. Moritz AW, Wiedenhoefer JF, Profit AP, et al. Breast adenomyoepithelioma and adenomyoepithelioma with carcinoma (malignant adenomyoepithelioma) with associated breast malignancies: A case series emphasizing histologic, radiologic, and clinical correlation. Breast 2016;29:132–9.

30. Ahmed AA, Heller DS. Malignant adenomyoepithelioma of the breast with malignant proliferation of epithelial and myoepithelial elements: a case report and review of the literature. Arch Pathol Lab Med 2000;124(4):632–6.

31. Loose JH, Patchefsky AS, Hollander IJ, et al. Adenomyoepithelioma of the breast. A spectrum of biologic behavior. Am J Surg Pathol 1992;16(9):868–76.

32. Honda Y, Iyama K. Malignant adenomyoepithelioma of the breast combined with invasive lobular carcinoma. Pathol Int 2009;59(3):179–84.

33. Foschini MP, Pizzicannella G, Peterse JL, et al. Adenomyoepithelioma of the breast associated with low-grade adenosquamous and sarcomatoid carcinomas. Virchows Arch 1995;427(3):243–50.

34. Oka K, Sando N, Moriya T, et al. Malignant adenomyoepithelioma of the breast with matrix production may be compatible with one variant form of matrix-producing carcinoma: a case report. Pathol Res Pract 2007;203(8):599–604.

35. Simpson RH, Cope N, Skalova A, et al. Malignant adenomyoepithelioma of the breast with mixed osteogenic, spindle cell, and carcinomatous differentiation. Am J Surg Pathol 1998;22(5):631–6.

36. Hempenstall LE, Saxena M, Donaldson E. Malignant adenomyoepithelioma with multifocal adenosquamous carcinoma of the breast: A case report. Breast J 2019;25(4):731–2.

37. Yang Y, Wang Y, He J, et al. Malignant adenomyoepithelioma combined with adenoid cystic carcinoma of the breast: a case report and literature review. Diagn Pathol 2014;9:148.

38. Han B, Mori I, Nakamura M, et al. Myoepithelial carcinoma arising in an adenomyoepithelioma of the breast: case report with immunohistochemical and mutational analysis. Pathol Int 2006;56(4):211–6.

39. Fan F, Smith W, Wang X, et al. Myoepithelial carcinoma of the breast arising in an adenomyoepithelioma: mammographic, ultrasound and histologic features. Breast J 2007;13(2):203–4.

40. Rakha E, Hoon Tan P, Ellis I, et al. Adenomyoepithelioma of the breast: A proposal for classification. Histopathology 2021;79(4):465–79.

41. Geyer FC, Li A, Papanastasiou AD, et al. Recurrent hotspot mutations in HRAS Q61 and PI3K-AKT pathway genes as drivers of breast adenomyoepitheliomas. Nat Commun 2018;9(1):1816.

42. Ginter PS, McIntire PJ, Kurtis B, et al. Adenomyoepithelial tumors of the breast: molecular underpinnings of a rare entity. Mod Pathol 2020;33(9):1764–72.

43. Lubin D, Toorens E, Zhang PJ, et al. Adenomyoepitheliomas of the breast frequently harbor recurrent hotspot mutations in pik3-akt pathway-related genes and a subset show genetic similarity to salivary gland epithelial-myoepithelial carcinoma. Am J Surg Pathol 2019;43(7):1005–13.

44. Pareja F, Toss MS, Geyer FC, et al. Immunohistochemical assessment of HRAS Q61R mutations in breast adenomyoepitheliomas. Histopathology 2020;76(6): 865–74.

Risk-Associated Lesions of the Breast in Core Needle Biopsies

Current Approaches to Radiological-Pathological Correlation

Emily B. Ambinder, MD[b], Benjamin C. Calhoun, MD, PhD[a],*

KEYWORDS

- Breast imaging • Breast core needle biopsy • Radiological-pathological correlation
- Atypical lobular hyperplasia • Lobular carcinoma in situ • Lobular neoplasia • Flat epithelial atypia
- Radial scar

Key points

- The clinical management of patients with nonmalignant diagnoses on breast core needle biopsy is evolving.
- Recent studies based on radiologic-pathologic correlation suggest that surveillance may be a safe alternative to surgery for carefully selected patients.
- The lack of standardization in the approach to radiologic-pathologic correlation is an opportunity for improvement in multidisciplinary breast care.

ABSTRACT

Image-guided core needle biopsies (CNBs) of the breast frequently result in a diagnosis of a benign or atypical lesion associated with breast cancer risk. The subsequent clinical management of these patients is variable, reflecting a lack of consensus on criteria for selecting patients for clinical and radiological follow-up versus immediate surgical excision. In this review, the evidence from prospective studies of breast CNB with radiological–pathological correlation is evaluated and summarized. The data support an emerging consensus on the importance of radiologic-pathologic correlation in standardizing the

selection of patients for active surveillance versus surgery.

OVERVIEW: BREAST CORE BIOPSY PATHOLOGY AND RADIOLOGIC-PATHOLOGIC CORRELATION

Image-guided percutaneous core needle biopsy (CNB) has been the standard of care for the evaluation of nonpalpable breast lesions since the 1990s. Over the past few decades, many patients with nonmalignant diagnoses also underwent surgical excision. Surgery was usually recommended to exclude the possibility of an invasive breast cancer or ductal carcinoma in situ (DCIS) in the tissue

a Department of Pathology and Laboratory Medicine, University of North Carolina at Chapel Hill, 160 N. Medical Drive, Campus Box 7525, Chapel Hill, NC 27599, USA; b Breast Imaging Division, The Russell H. Morgan Department of Radiology and Radiological Science, Johns Hopkins Medicine
* Corresponding Author. Department of Pathology and Laboratory Medicine, University of North Carolina at Chapel Hill, 160 N. Medical Drive, Campus Box 7525, Chapel Hill, NC 27599, USA
E-mail address: ben.calhoun@unchealth.unc.edu

Surgical Pathology 15 (2022) 147–157
https://doi.org/10.1016/j.path.2021.11.010
1875-9181/22/© 2021 Elsevier Inc. All rights reserved.

near the biopsy site (ie, the risk of an upgrade). The early CNB literature reported upgrade rates as high as 30% to 50% for many benign and atypical lesions.[1] It should be emphasized that the breast cancer risk associated with many of these lesions was originally defined as the likelihood of developing breast cancer in either breast after several years of follow-up.[2–4] In the CNB era, the word "risk," not otherwise specified, frequently refers to the risk of an upgrade in a surgical specimen.

An important question in current practice is whether we now have sufficient evidence to safely offer surveillance instead of surgery to selected patients with risk-associated lesions diagnosed on CNB. The current literature lends support to the idea of observing many patients with flat epithelial atypia (FEA), atypical lobular hyperplasia (ALH), and classic lobular carcinoma in situ (LCIS) and most with benign and incidental papillomas and radial scars.[5] Atypical ductal hyperplasia (ADH), papillomas with atypia, and variants of LCIS (pleomorphic or florid) should be referred for excision and will not be discussed further in this review.[6] However, recommendations for surgery versus surveillance for many nonmalignant CNB diagnoses vary widely among physicians and institutions.[7–9]

In the contemporary literature based on current imaging modalities, larger sample sizes, and careful radiologic-pathologic correlation, the upgrade rates for many benign and atypical lesions are much lower than those reported in earlier studies. Recent studies of paired CNB and surgical excision specimens have shown very low (ie, <5%) upgrade rates for benign papillomas, FEA, radial scars, papillomas, and classic types of lobular neoplasia.[1,6] These studies included both stereotactic and ultrasound-guided CNB. Similar results have been reported for risk-associated lesions diagnosed on MRI-guided CNB.[10,11] Radial scars are the subject of Chieh-Yu Lin's article, and papillary lesions are the subject of the article by Timothy M. D'Alfonso and Dana S. Ross, elsewhere in this issue. The lower contemporary upgrade rates raise the possibility that it may be safe to offer many patients surveillance as opposed to immediate surgical excision. The goal of developing individualized management recommendations and offering observation to selected patients is similar to the approach being taken in several ongoing clinical trials of active surveillance for DCIS.[12–14] The evolving consensus on the deescalation of surgery for nonmalignant CNB diagnoses is largely based on careful radiologic-pathologic correlation. This article reviews the recent literature and highlights opportunities for evidence-based standardization of radiologic-pathologic correlation.

RADIOLOGIC-PATHOLOGIC CORRELATION: DEFINITION

Radiologic-pathologic correlation is usually defined, at least in part, as an assessment of whether the pathologic findings represent the targeted imaging abnormality and the degree to which the targeted lesion was removed by the CNB procedure. If the CNB pathology does not fully account for the imaging findings, a diagnosis of invasive breast cancer or DCIS on excision should not be regarded a true upgrade. Other exclusion criteria for true upgrades include presentation with a suspicious, palpable mass or a Breast Imaging-Reporting and Data System (BI-RADS) c5 imaging finding. The lower (and probably more accurate) upgrade rates in the recent literature reflect an increased emphasis on radiologic-pathologic correlation and a more rigorous approach to defining true upgrades.

Aspects of radiologic-pathologic correlation that require consideration include whether it is performed prospectively or retrospectively and in a multidisciplinary setting versus being assessed by physicians in a single specialty. In many institutions, radiologic-pathologic concordance, based on the BI-RADS,[15] is determined by physicians in a single specialty, usually radiology. Radiologic considerations for concordance are discussed later in more detail. The radiologic-pathologic correlation performed for many of the studies in the literature was done retrospectively, and follow-up data on lesions that were not excised are often limited. However, there are some informative examples of radiologic-pathologic correlation performed in real time to develop individualized clinical management recommendations.

Most hospitals and cancer centers hold multidisciplinary conferences to discuss the management of patients with newly diagnosed and/or advanced breast cancer. Multidisciplinary conferences for the determination of radiologic-pathologic correlation for nonmalignant CNB diagnoses seem to be less common. The available data indicate that regularly occurring multidisciplinary conferences that include radiology, surgery, and pathology result in fewer patients undergoing immediate surgical excision.[16,17] The publications based on this approach to radiologic-pathologic correlation also provide an important source of follow-up data on lesions that were not excised.[18,19] The management recommendations from these conferences are based on an assessment of clinical, radiological, and pathologic variables.

KEY POINTS

Radiologic-Pathologic Correlation
- Clinical
  - Age
  - Clinical presentation
  - Other breast cancer risk factors
- Radiological
  - Level of suspicion
  - Adequate targeting and sampling
- Pathologic
  - Pathologic diagnosis
  - Targeted versus incidental finding
  - Extent of lesion or number of foci
  - Presence of other risk-associated lesions

The clinical variables include the patient's age, clinical presentation, and other breast cancer risk factors. Correlation of the radiological and pathologic findings is based on whether the pathologic findings explain the imaging findings and represent the targeted lesion versus an incidental finding. The detailed evaluation of targeted lesions incorporates the radiologic finding recommended for the CNB, the modality of biopsy, the extent of the pathologic findings, and the extent to which the lesion was removed by the CNB procedure.[17,20]

RADIOLOGIC-PATHOLOGIC CORRELATION FOR SELECTED SPECIFIC DIAGNOSES

PAPILLOMAS

The criteria for radiologic-pathologic correlation may be tailored to specific pathologic diagnoses. Recent data on intraductal papillomas and classic-type lobular neoplasia provide insights and highlight some unresolved issues that could be addressed in future studies. (Criteria for other risk-associated lesions are discussed later under the heading Radiologic-Pathologic Correlation: Lack of Standardization). Ma and colleagues recently reported results for a series of papillomas evaluated at a biweekly multidisciplinary conference that provides recommendations for patient care in real time.[19] They recommended surveillance for benign papillomas with radiologic-pathologic correlation and at least one-third of the imaging abnormality removed, less than or equal to 2 foci of ADH adjacent to the papilloma, ALH involving the papilloma, and ALH adjacent to the papilloma.[19] In cases of adjacent ADH with intermediate- to high-grade nuclear atypia suspicious for DCIS, patients were referred for surgical excision. The 73 patients who did not have surgery had stable imaging findings and no diagnoses of malignancy after a mean follow-up of 19.1 months (range 6.2–42.6 months).[19] These results are similar to prior retrospective studies of benign papillomas with radiologic-pathologic correlation that were not excised.[21,22] It should be noted that papillomas with risk-associated lesions adjacent to the papilloma were excluded from some series.[21]

LOBULAR NEOPLASIA (CLASSIC TYPE)

Middleton and colleagues reported outcomes for 104 patients with classic-type lobular neoplasia (ALH or LCIS) who were followed clinically and radiologically for a mean of 40.8 months (range 5.3–103.2).[18] Surveillance was recommended for these patients after review at a weekly multidisciplinary conference that included radiology, surgery, and pathology. Variants of LCIS (florid and pleomorphic) were excluded. Cases with coexisting radial scars and papillomas also were excluded.[18] Of the 104 patients who were followed-up, 2 (2%) developed breast cancer near the CNB site (1 DCIS, 1 invasive lobular carcinoma) and 3 developed invasive ductal carcinoma or DCIS at a separate site. The investigators concluded that patients with ALH or classic LCIS in less than 3 terminal duct lobular units (TDLU) and radiologic-pathologic correlation may safely avoid immediate surgical excision (an example of a single focus of incidental ALH is shown in **Fig. 2**).[18] The findings are consistent with those of prior retrospective studies of lobular neoplasia that was not immediately excised.[23,24] Similar to the study reported by Middleton and colleagues, the retrospective studies also excluded variants of LCIS, radial scars, and papillomas. In the study reported by Shah-Khan and colleagues,[23] ALH or classic LCIS was present in less than or equal to 50% of TDLU in 91% of the CNB from patients who were observed.

RECENT PROSPECTIVE STUDIES OF PAPILLOMAS AND LOBULAR NEOPLASIA

The Translational Breast Cancer Research Consortium (TBCRC) recently reported results of multiinstitutional trials for papillomas without

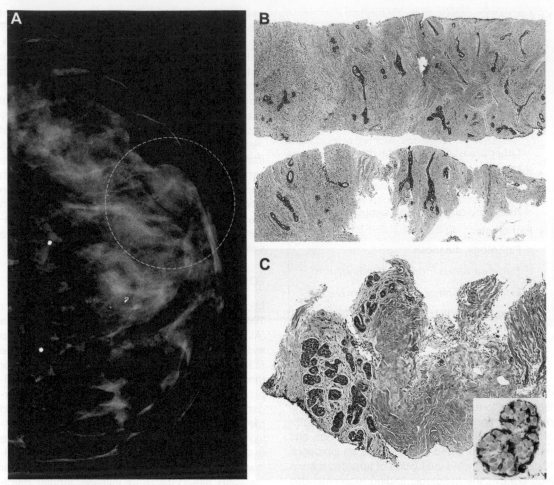

Fig. 1. Mammographic and histologic images from a 44-year-old woman recalled from screening with full-field digital mammography for an obscured 1 cm oval mass in the right upper outer quadrant (*A, lower circle*). Diagnostic mammography with tomosynthesis showed an additional ill-defined 3 cm area of architectural distortion (*A, upper circle*) with no definite ultrasound correlate (BI-RADS 4b). A stereotactic core biopsy showed areas of stromal fibrosis and elastosis (*B*) with entrapped benign glands (*C*), consistent with a radial scar (complex sclerosing lesion) without atypia. The pathologic findings were considered benign but potentially discordant due to the size of the area of architectural distortion. In the absence of definite radiological-pathological concordance and a limited sampling of a large imaging abnormality, this patient may be referred for surgical excision.

atypia (TBCRC 034) and classic-type lobular neoplasia (TCBRC 020) diagnosed on CNB.[25,26] These studies were designed to determine upgrade rates, not to provide follow-up data for lesions that were not excised. However, they may provide a template for future prospective, multi-institutional studies of risk-associated lesions that are not excised. The primary endpoint for TBCRC 034 was a predefined rule that an upgrade rate less than or equal to 3% for benign papillomas diagnosed on CNB would not require surgical excision.[26] Exclusion criteria for the 2 trials were similar. Cases with a palpable mass (or nipple discharge in TBCRC 034), BI-RADS 5 category, concurrent or prior history of breast cancer, or coexisting ADH or LCIS variants were excluded.[25,26] Coexisting radial scars were not listed as an exclusion criterion for TBCRC 034. Radial scars, papillomas, and flat epithelial atypia were not specifically listed as exclusion criteria for TBCRC 020. TBCRC 034 also includes a study of flat epithelial atypia on CNB, and the results were pending when this review was written. The main finding in TBCRC 034 was an upgrade rate of 1.7% for papillomas without atypia based on local pathology review.[26] In TBCRC 020, the upgrade rate for classic-type lobular neoplasia was 3% based on local pathology review and 1% by central pathology review.[25]

The TBCRC trials provide support for an upgrade of less than or equal to 3% as a threshold for offering surveillance versus surgery. They also provide some indirect evidence that it may be reasonable to offer surveillance to patients with coexisting risk-associated lesions that, by themselves, would not warrant immediate surgical excision. Some investigators have advocated surgery for benign, risk-associated lesions based on the likelihood of finding additional risk-associated lesions in the excisions specimen that would warrant high-risk follow-up and discussion of chemoprevention (ie, ADH, ALH, or classic LCIS).[27,28] However, only 4% of patients in TBCRC 034 had ADH, ALH, or classic LCIS in their surgical specimen,[26] indicating that surgery would not change the clinical management of greater than 95% of patients who would meet eligibility criteria for that trial. It is also worth noting the low rates of uptake and adherence to chemoprevention in patients with risk-associated lesions[29,30] and lack of proven survival benefit from chemoprevention.[31]

RADIAL SCARS

The upgrade for radial scars was specifically analyzed in a recent meta-analysis by Farshid and colleagues.[32] A total of 49 studies with 3163 radial scars and surgical outcomes were included. There were 217 upgrades to malignancies (6.7%), most being ductal carcinoma in situ (144/217 = 66.4%).[32] However, on subgroup analysis, they found that radial scars without atypia diagnosed on vacuum-assisted biopsy had 1% upgrade rate to DCIS, suggesting that this group could be safely followed rather than have surgical excision. This contrasts with radial scars with atypia diagnosed with a 14G biopsy device, which had an upgrade rate of 29%.[32]

KEY QUESTIONS

Surveillance versus surgery
- What upgrade rate below which surveillance is a safe alternative surgery?
  - ≤3% based on TBCRC 034 and TBCRC 020
  - More multiinstitutional studies are needed
- Which exclusion criteria have the strongest evidence?
  - Palpable abnormalities
  - BI-RADS 4c and 5 imaging findings
  - Coexisting ADH or LCIS variants
- Which exclusion criteria require further study?
  - Prior history of breast cancer
  - Concurrent diagnosis of breast cancer
  - Coexisting risk-associated lesions other than ADH and LCIS variants

RADIOLOGIC CONCORDANCE AND BREAST CORE BIOPSY PATHOLOGY

The Mammographic Quality and Standards Act (MQSA)[33] states that facilities must have a system in place to correlate imaging and pathology for positive cases. No additional guidance is included. The American College of Radiology (ACR) practice parameter for CNB[34] is more specific stating that it is essential for the physician performing the biopsy to correlate imaging characteristics with histopathologic or cytopathologic results. There is no recommendation for how this should be accomplished. The term concordance is usually used in the context of complying with the requirements of the MQSA and ACR. In practice and in the literature, the terms concordance and correlation are essentially used interchangeably.

The BI-RADS atlas includes assessment categories indicating the level of suspicion and appropriate management.[35] A BI-RADS assessment is included in all breast imaging cases and is an important consideration in determining radiologic-pathologic correlation. For findings assessed as category 4a (low suspicion, chance of malignancy >2% and ≤ 10%), a malignant diagnosis is not expected and a benign diagnosis would typically be considered concordant. An example of a 4a lesion is shown in **Fig. 2**Fig. 1. The biopsy result was benign and concordant. For categories 4c (high suspicion, chance of malignancy >50% and ≤ 95%) and 5 (highly suspicious, chance of malignancy >95%), a benign diagnosis is usually considered discordant. In the BI-RADS atlas, pathologic correlation is specifically described as being a critical step for findings described as category 4b. These cases are considered moderately suspicious with a chance of malignancy greater than 10% and greater than or equal to 50%. This unique category requires careful radiologic-pathologic correlation to confirm that the histologic diagnosis explains the radiologic finding. **Fig. 1**Fig. 2 shows an example of a 4b lesion that was considered discordant from the biopsy result.

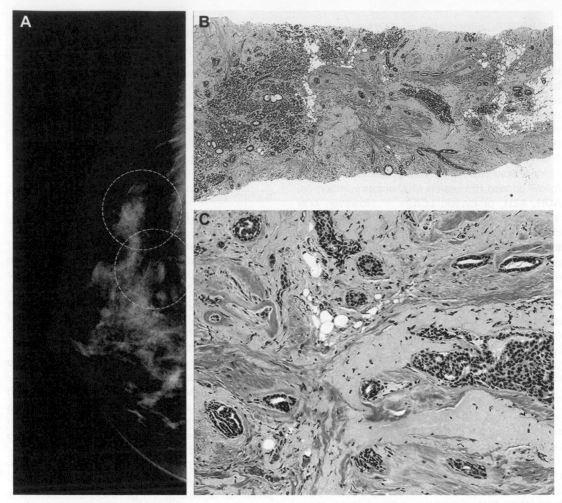

Fig. 2. Mammographic and histologic images from a 48-year-old woman with history of bilateral fibroadenomas who presented with a new left breast mass. A 2.1 cm oval partially circumscribed mass was identified on mammogram (*A*) and ultrasound (BI-RADS 4a). Most of the cores from an ultrasound-guided biopsy showed a fibroadenoma (*B*). A single TDLU partially involved by ALH was present at the end of a core (*C*). An E-cadherin stain showed reduced immunoreactivity (with some staining of myoepithelial cells) in the microscopic focus of ALH that was essentially exhausted in deeper levels (*C*, inset). The diagnosis of fibroadenoma was radiologically concordant. With a single, incidental focus of ALH, this patient could be offered surveillance as an alternative to immediate surgery.

In addition to level of suspicion, the image-guided biopsy targeting and sampling should be assessed when determining radiologic-pathologic correlation.[36] For ultrasound-guided biopsies, the radiologist should confirm adequate positioning of the biopsy needle throughout the procedure. Postfire images should be taken to confirm that the needle passes through the target. Orthogonal images can confirm needle placement, especially for small lesions. The radiologist should also note whether the biopsy is particularly challenging, for example, whether the finding is subtle, deep, or surrounded by dense breast tissue.[37] In stereotactic biopsies for calcifications, a specimen radiograph can confirm the removal of suspicious calcifications.[38] Core samples containing calcifications should be separated from the rest of the specimen to aid the pathologist in interpretation. Clip placement with postbiopsy 2-view mammogram is also important to confirm accurate targeting, especially for stereotactic biopsy of noncalcified findings. When there is suboptimal targeting or sampling, radiologic-pathologic correlation is critical to be sure that the diagnosis fully explains the imaging finding.

Digital breast tomosynthesis (DBT) is a relatively new breast imaging modality but an important consideration for radiologists when doing radiology-pathology correlation. With DBT, a series of images of the breast are acquired and then reconstructed into slices that can be scrolled through. The US Food and Drug Administration

(FDA) approved the use of DBT in combination with diagnostic mammography (DM) for breast cancer screening in 2011. Breast cancer screening programs that incorporate the use of DBT result in fewer false-positive recalls from screening and a higher cancer detection rate when compared with DM alone.[39–41] In some cases, DBT detects suspicious abnormalities that may not be visualized with DM or other imaging modalities.[42–44] Architectural distortion in particular may be detected more often with DBT.[45,46]

The pathologic findings in biopsies of these areas of architectural distortion include invasive carcinoma and DCIS as well as ADH, ALH, and LCIS.[47–50] Radial scars also seem to account for a significant proportion of cases with architectural distortion seen only with DBT (an example of this is shown in **Fig. 1**).[47–50] Most large studies comparing DBT and DM have focused primarily on the cancer detection rate, and the data on risk-associated lesions are more limited.[39,41,51] In one of the larger published series, Bahl and colleagues reported pathologic findings corresponding to architectural distortion in 395 mammographic examinations for 389 patients.[47] In the DBT and DM groups, architectural distortion was detected in 274 (0.14%) and 121 (0.07%) cases, respectively (P<.001).[47] Radial scars were the most common nonmalignant pathologic findings in the DBT and DM groups accounting for 33.2% and 11.6% of cases, respectively (P<.001).[47] Thus, screening with DBT doubled the rate of detection of architectural distortion and tripled the rate of detection of radial scars.

RADIOLOGIC-PATHOLOGIC CORRELATION: LACK OF STANDARDIZATION

Radiologic-pathologic correlation may be performed informally by radiologists and pathologists on a case-by-case basis, by pathologists reviewing the imaging reports or imaging studies concurrently with CNB histology or by radiologists comparing imaging reports and pathology reports for concordance.[52] In a College of American Pathologists (CAP) Q-Probes study of 1399 cases from 48 institutions, the participating pathologists reported radiologic-pathologic correlation in 94.9%.[53] The rate of radiologic-pathologic correlation was higher for cases discussed at a multidisciplinary conference and lower when correlation was based on a central review of documented findings in the imaging and pathology reports.[53] There are examples in the literature of regularly occurring, multidisciplinary radiologic-pathologic correlation conferences that provide clinical

management recommendations for patients in real time.[17,18,54,55] Many more institutions have similar conferences but have not published their criteria for radiologic-pathologic correlation or the follow-up for patients who were offered surveillance or surgery. Multidisciplinary conferences for radiologic pathologic correlation for nonmalignant CNB diagnoses are not specifically required by the CAP, ACR, Commission on Cancer, or the National Accreditation Program for Breast Centers (NAPBC). As discussed earlier, the ACR practice parameter states that is essential to establish concordance for all percutaneous breast CNB, but there is no requirement for a regularly occurring meeting that includes surgery and pathology. The variability and paucity of peer-reviewed data limits our ability to assess the impact of prospective radiologic-pathologic correlation on clinical outcomes. However, reductions in the rates of discordance, false-negative CNB, and unnecessary surgical interventions seem to be consistent findings.[36,54–56]

Prakash and colleagues reported a series of 1387 patients presented at a multidisciplinary breast conference that included radiology, surgery, and pathology.[55] Cases were selected for discordance or questions about clinical management (primarily by radiologists) and accounted for 29.4% of all CNB from a 4-year period. Among the 74 (5.3%) of cases with a change in management, 22 (29.7%) were changed from discordant to concordant, allowing these patients to avoid surgery or short-term interval imaging. There were 23 (31.1%) cases that changed from concordant to discordant, leading to surgery and a diagnosis of breast cancer in 3 (13%) of these patients.[55]

Li and colleagues recently reported a series of 127 high-risk lesions presented at a biweekly multidisciplinary conference that included radiology, surgery, and pathology.[17] For cases of ADH, excision was recommended for greater than 2 foci or removal of less than 90% of associated calcifications. Radial scars without atypia were excised if less than half of the lesion was removed. ALH and LCIS were excised if they were associated with targeted calcifications or if LCIS involved greater than 5 TDLU. Observation with 6-month imaging and clinical follow-up was recommended for all cases of FEA and mucocele-like lesions without atypia. The 11 cases determined at the conference to lack radiologic-pathologic correlation were referred for surgical excision, resulting in a diagnosis of breast cancer in 2 patients.[17] There were no upgrades in 8 patients who elected to undergo surgery despite receiving a recommendation for surveillance. All of the patients who were observed had stable radiologic and clinical findings at the time of last follow-up (range 6.2–46.3 months).[17]

KEY CONSIDERATIONS

Radiologic-Pathologic Correlation
- Multidisciplinary
  - Radiology
  - Surgery
  - Pathology
- Regularly occurring
  - Prospective (in real time)
  - Issue recommendations for management
- Case selection
  - All core needle biopsies (CNB)
  - Nondiagnostic (CNB)
  - Benign CNB with BI-RADS 4c or 5 imaging
  - All BI-RADS 4b cases
  - Specific pathologic diagnoses
- Documentation
  - Note in the medical record
  - Addendum to radiology report
- Feasibility and cost
  - Physician time
  - Not a billable activity

RADIOLOGIC-PATHOLOGIC CORRELATION: FUTURE DIRECTIONS

The peer-reviewed literature emphasizes radiological-pathological correlation as an essential component of the multidisciplinary management of patients with nonmalignant diagnoses on image-guided breast CNB. There is an evolving consensus on the deescalation of surgery for many benign and atypical breast lesions in the setting of careful radiologic-pathologic correlation. However, multidisciplinary radiologic-pathologic correlation is not a requirement for laboratory, imaging center, or breast center accreditation. The approach to correlation is not standardized, and management recommendations for specific diagnoses may vary among physicians and institutions.[7] Participation in multidisciplinary conferences requires allocation of physician time to an activity for which there is no reimbursement.[57,58] It may be difficult to measure and improve the quality of decision-making at multidisciplinary conferences.[59] It also must be noted that adherence to standards may not necessarily lead to measurable improvement in the most important patient outcomes. Participants in the NAPBC program believe that compliance with accreditation standards leads to better oncologic outcomes,[60] but the effect of NAPBC centers on breast cancer mortality is not well documented.[61] The opportunity and the challenge in standardization of radiologic-correlation is to incorporate the best features of existing multidisciplinary programs and demonstrate meaningful improvement in patient outcomes.

CLINICS CARE POINTS

- There is an emerging consensus on limiting the role of surgery for many benign and atypical breast lesions diagnosed on core needle biopsy after careful radiologic-pathologic correlation.
- Multidisciplinary radiologic-pathologic correlation is not a requirement for laboratory, imaging center, or breast center accreditation.
- Radiological-pathological correlation is not standardized across institutions and management recommendations often vary.

DISCLOSURE

Dr B.C. Calhoun is a Member of the Oncology Advisory Board for Luminex Corp. Dr E.B. Ambinder does not have any financial relationships to disclose.

REFERENCES

1. Calhoun BC. Core needle biopsy of the breast: an evaluation of contemporary data. Surg Pathol Clin 2018;11(1):1–16.
2. Dupont WD, Page DL. Risk factors for breast cancer in women with proliferative breast disease. N Engl J Med 1985;312(3):146–51.
3. Collins LC, Baer HJ, Tamimi RM, et al. Magnitude and laterality of breast cancer risk according to histologic type of atypical hyperplasia: results from the Nurses' Health Study. Cancer 2007;109(2):180–7.
4. Hartmann LC, Sellers TA, Frost MH, et al. Benign breast disease and the risk of breast cancer. N Engl J Med 2005;353(3):229–37.

5. Morrow M, Schnitt SJ, Norton L. Current management of lesions associated with an increased risk of breast cancer. Nat Rev Clin Oncol 2015;12(4):227–38.

6. Nakhlis F. How do we approach benign proliferative lesions? Curr Oncol Rep 2018;20(4):34.

7. Georgian-Smith D, Lawton TJ. Variations in physician recommendations for surgery after diagnosis of a high-risk lesion on breast core needle biopsy. AJR Am J Roentgenol 2012;198(2):256–63.

8. Kappel C, Seely J, Watters J, et al. A survey of Canadian breast health professionals' recommendations for high-risk benign breast disease. Can J Surg 2019;62(5):358–60.

9. Nizri E, Schneebaum S, Klausner JM, et al. Current management practice of breast borderline lesions–need for further research and guidelines. Am J Surg 2012;203(6):721–5.

10. Michaels AY, Ginter PS, Dodelzon K, et al. High-risk lesions detected by MRI-guided core biopsy: upgrade rates at surgical excision and implications for management. AJR Am J Roentgenol 2021; 216(3):622–32.

11. Weinfurtner RJ, Patel B, Laronga C, et al. Magnetic resonance imaging-guided core needle breast biopsies resulting in high-risk histopathologic findings: upstage frequency and lesion characteristics. Clin Breast Cancer 2015;15(3):234–9.

12. Francis A, Thomas J, Fallowfield L, et al. Addressing overtreatment of screen detected DCIS; the LORIS trial. Eur J Cancer 2015;51(16):2296–303.

13. Elshof LE, Tryfonidis K, Slaets L, et al. Feasibility of a prospective, randomised, open-label, international multicentre, phase III, non-inferiority trial to assess the safety of active surveillance for low risk ductal carcinoma in situ – The LORD study. Eur J Cancer 2015;51(12):1497–510.

14. Hwang ES, Hyslop T, Lynch T, et al. The COMET (Comparison of Operative versus Monitoring and Endocrine Therapy) trial: a phase III randomised controlled clinical trial for low-risk ductal carcinoma in situ (DCIS). BMJ Open 2019;9(3):e026797.

15. Mercado CL. BI-RADS update. Radiol Clin North Am 2014;52(3):481–7.

16. Krishnamurthy S, Bevers T, Kuerer H, et al. Multidisciplinary considerations in the management of high-risk breast lesions. AJR Am J Roentgenol 2012; 198(2):W132–40.

17. Li X, Ma Z, Styblo TM, et al. Management of high-risk breast lesions diagnosed on core biopsies and experiences from prospective high-risk breast lesion conferences at an academic institution. Breast Cancer Res Treat 2021;185(3):573–81.

18. Middleton LP, Sneige N, Coyne R, et al. Most lobular carcinoma in situ and atypical lobular hyperplasia diagnosed on core needle biopsy can be managed clinically with radiologic follow-up in a multidisciplinary setting. Cancer Med 2014;3(3):492–9.

19. Ma Z, Arciero CA, Styblo TM, et al. Patients with benign papilloma diagnosed on core biopsies and concordant pathology-radiology findings can be followed: experiences from multi-specialty high-risk breast lesion conferences in an academic center. Breast Cancer Res Treat 2020;183(3):577–84.

20. Krishnamurthy S, Bevers T, Kuerer HM, et al. Paradigm shifts in breast care delivery: impact of imaging in a multidisciplinary environment. AJR Am J Roentgenol 2017;208(2):248–55.

21. Swapp RE, Glazebrook KN, Jones KN, et al. Management of benign intraductal solitary papilloma diagnosed on core needle biopsy. Ann Surg Oncol 2013;20(6):1900–5.

22. Bennett LE, Ghate SV, Bentley R, et al. Is surgical excision of core biopsy proven benign papillomas of the breast necessary? Acad Radiol 2010;17(5):553–7.

23. Shah-Khan MG, Geiger XJ, Reynolds C, et al. Long-term follow-up of lobular neoplasia (atypical lobular hyperplasia/lobular carcinoma in situ) diagnosed on core needle biopsy. Ann Surg Oncol 2012; 19(10):3131–8.

24. Nagi CS, O'Donnell JE, Tismenetsky M, et al. Lobular neoplasia on core needle biopsy does not require excision. Cancer 2008;112(10):2152–8.

25. Nakhlis F, Gilmore L, Gelman R, et al. Incidence of adjacent synchronous invasive carcinoma and/or ductal carcinoma in-situ in patients with lobular neoplasia on core biopsy: results from a prospective multi-institutional registry (TBCRC 020). Ann Surg Oncol 2016;23(3):722–8.

26. Nakhlis F, Baker GM, Pilewskie M, et al. The incidence of adjacent synchronous invasive carcinoma and/or ductal carcinoma in situ in patients with intraductal papilloma without atypia on core biopsy: results from a prospective multi-institutional registry (TBCRC 034). Ann Surg Oncol 2020;28(5): 2573–8.

27. Miller CL, West JA, Bettini AC, et al. Surgical excision of radial scars diagnosed by core biopsy may help predict future risk of breast cancer. Breast Cancer Res Treat 2014;145(2):331–8.

28. Phantana-Angkool A, Forster MR, Warren YE, et al. Rate of radial scars by core biopsy and upgrading to malignancy or high-risk lesions before and after introduction of digital breast tomosynthesis. Breast Cancer Res Treat 2019;173(1):23–9.

29. Ropka ME, Keim J, Philbrick JT. Patient decisions about breast cancer chemoprevention: a systematic review and meta-analysis. J Clin Oncol 2010;28(18): 3090–5.

30. Smith SG, Sestak I, Forster A, et al. Factors affecting uptake and adherence to breast cancer chemoprevention: a systematic review and meta-analysis. Ann Oncol 2016;27(4):575–90.

31. Cuzick J, Sestak I, Cawthorn S, et al. Tamoxifen for prevention of breast cancer: extended long-term

follow-up of the IBIS-I breast cancer prevention trial. Lancet Oncol 2015;16(1):67–75.

32. Farshid G, Buckley E. Meta-analysis of upgrade rates in 3163 radial scars excised after needle core biopsy diagnosis. Breast Cancer Res Treat 2019;174(1):165–77.

33. Mammography quality standards act regulations. Available at: https://www.fda.gov/radiation-emitting-products/regulations-mqsa/mammography-quality-standards-act-regulations. Accessed April 28, 2021.

34. ACR practice parameter for the performance of ultrasound-guided percutaneous breast interventional procedures. Available at: https://www.acr.org/-/media/acr/files/practice-parameters/us-guided breast.pdf. Accessed April 28, 2021.

35. D'Orsi CJ, Sickles EA, Mendelson EB, et al. ACR BI-RADS® atlas, breast imaging reporting and data system. Reston, VA: American College of Radiology; 2013.

36. Park VY, Kim EK, Moon HJ, et al. Evaluating imaging-pathology concordance and discordance after ultrasound-guided breast biopsy. Ultrasonography 2018;37(2):107–20.

37. Youk JH, Kim EK, Kim MJ, et al. Missed breast cancers at US-guided core needle biopsy: how to reduce them. Radiographics 2007;27(1):79–94.

38. Huang ML, Adrada BE, Candelaria R, et al. Stereotactic breast biopsy: pitfalls and pearls. Tech Vasc Interv Radiol 2014;17(1):32–9.

39. Ciatto S, Houssami N, Bernardi D, et al. Integration of 3D digital mammography with tomosynthesis for population breast-cancer screening (STORM): a prospective comparison study. Lancet Oncol 2013; 14(7):583–9.

40. Durand MA, Haas BM, Yao X, et al. Early clinical experience with digital breast tomosynthesis for screening mammography. Radiology 2015;274(1): 85–92.

41. Friedewald SM, Rafferty EA, Rose SL, et al. Breast cancer screening using tomosynthesis in combination with digital mammography. JAMA 2014; 311(24):2499–507.

42. Michell MJ, Iqbal A, Wasan RK, et al. A comparison of the accuracy of film-screen mammography, full-field digital mammography, and digital breast tomosynthesis. Clin Radiol 2012;67(10):976–81.

43. Bernardi D, Ciatto S, Pellegrini M, et al. Prospective study of breast tomosynthesis as a triage to assessment in screening. Breast Cancer Res Treat 2012; 133(1):267–71.

44. Andersson I, Ikeda DM, Zackrisson S, et al. Breast tomosynthesis and digital mammography: a comparison of breast cancer visibility and BIRADS classification in a population of cancers with subtle mammographic findings. Eur Radiol 2008;18(12): 2817–25.

45. Durand MA, Wang S, Hooley RJ, et al. Tomosynthesis-detected architectural distortion: management algorithm with radiologic-pathologic correlation. Radiographics 2016;36(2):311–21.

46. Taskin F, Durum Y, Soyder A, et al. Review and management of breast lesions detected with breast tomosynthesis but not visible on mammography and ultrasonography. Acta Radiol 2017;58(12):1442–7.

47. Bahl M, Lamb LR, Lehman CD. Pathologic outcomes of architectural distortion on Digital 2D versus tomosynthesis mammography. AJR Am J Roentgenol 2017;209(5):1162–7.

48. Freer PE, Niell B, Rafferty EA. Preoperative tomosynthesis-guided needle localization of mammographically and sonographically occult breast lesions. Radiology 2015;275(2):377–83.

49. Ray KM, Turner E, Sickles EA, et al. Suspicious findings at digital breast tomosynthesis occult to conventional digital mammography: imaging features and pathology findings. Breast J 2015;21(5):538–42.

50. Partyka L, Lourenco AP, Mainiero MB. Detection of mammographically occult architectural distortion on digital breast tomosynthesis screening: initial clinical experience. AJR Am J Roentgenol 2014; 203(1):216–22.

51. Skaane P, Bandos AI, Gullien R, et al. Comparison of digital mammography alone and digital mammography plus tomosynthesis in a population-based screening program. Radiology 2013;267(1):47–56.

52. Bassett LW, Mahoney MC, Apple SK. Interventional breast imaging: current procedures and assessing for concordance with pathology. Radiol Clin North Am 2007;45(5):881–94, vii.

53. Idowu MO, Hardy LB, Souers RJ, et al. Pathologic diagnostic correlation with breast imaging findings: a College of American Pathologists Q-Probes study of 48 institutions. Arch Pathol Lab Med 2012;136(1): 53–60.

54. Mihalik JE, Krupka L, Davenport R, et al. The rate of imaging-histologic discordance of benign breast disease: a multidisciplinary approach to the management of discordance at a large university-based hospital. Am J Surg 2010;199(3):319–23, [discussion 323].

55. Prakash S, Venkataraman S, Slanetz PJ, et al. Improving patient care by incorporation of multidisciplinary breast radiology-pathology correlation conference. Can Assoc Radiol J 2016;67(2):122–9.

56. Youk JH, Kim EK, Kim MJ, et al. Concordant or discordant? Imaging-pathology correlation in a sonography-guided core needle biopsy of a breast lesion. Korean J Radiol 2011;12(2):232–40.

57. Shenoy-Bhangle AS, Putta N, Adondakis M, et al. Prospective analysis of radiology resource utilization and outcomes for participation in oncology multidisciplinary conferences. Acad Radiol 2020;28(9): 1219–24.

58. Kane B, Luz S, O'Briain DS, et al. Multidisciplinary team meetings and their impact on workflow in radiology and pathology departments. BMC Med 2007;5:15.

59. Fahim C, McConnell MM, Wright FC, et al. Use of the KT-MCC strategy to improve the quality of decision making for multidisciplinary cancer conferences: a pilot study. BMC Health Serv Res 2020;20(1):579.

60. Knutson AC, McNamara EJ, McKellar DP, et al. The role of the American College of Surgeons' cancer program accreditation in influencing oncologic outcomes. J Surg Oncol 2014;110(5):611–5.

61. Pardo JA, Fan B, Valero M, et al. Impact of geographic distribution of accredited breast centers. Breast J 2020;26(11):2194–8.

Metaplastic Breast Carcinoma Revisited; Subtypes Determine Outcomes
Comprehensive Pathologic, Clinical, and Molecular Review

Thaer Khoury, MD

KEYWORDS

- Metaplastic carcinoma • Triple-negative breast cancer • Histologic subtype • Spindle cell lesion
- Immunohistochemistry • Immunotherapy • Molecular subtypes • Diagnostic algorithm

Key points

- Metaplastic breast carcinoma (MpBC) is a heterogeneous group of tumors that clinically could be divided into low risk and high risk.
- It is important to recognize the different types of MpBC, as the high-risk subtypes have worse clinical outcomes than triple-negative breast cancer.
- Spindle cell lesion of the breast has a wide range of differential diagnoses. It is important for the pathologist to be aware of the MpBC entities and use the herein proposed algorithms to assist in the diagnosis.
- Metaplastic breast carcinoma has less response rate to the traditional chemotherapy (adjuvant or neoadjuvant) than the other types of breast cancer.
- Few options of target therapies and immunotherapy are available for the patients with MpBC .

ABSTRACT

Metaplastic breast carcinoma (MpBC) is a heterogeneous group of tumors that clinically could be divided into low risk and high risk. It is important to recognize the different types of MpBC, as the high-risk subtypes have worse clinical outcomes than triple-negative breast cancer. It is important for the pathologist to be aware of the MpBC entities and use the proposed algorithms (morphology and immunohistochemistry) to assist in rendering the final diagnosis. Few pitfalls are discussed, including misinterpretation of immunohistochemistry and certain histomorphologies, particularly spindle lesions associated with complex sclerosing lesions.

OVERVIEW

The name origin of metaplasia is from the Greek verb *metaplasein*, which means "change in form." It is the transformation from one differentiated cell type to another differentiated cell type. Metaplastic breast carcinoma (MpBC) is a heterogeneous group of tumors that have only one thing in common. The tumor cells transformed from the benign mammary cell (epithelial or myoepithelial) to a cell type with malignant properties such as squamous cell, chondroid cells, and so forth. These tumors have more differences than similarities, including the morphology, the biology, and more importantly the prognosis and therefore the management.

Pathology Department, Roswell Park Comprehensive Cancer Center, Elm & Carlton Streets, Buffalo, NY 14263, USA
E-mail address: thaer.khoury@roswellpark.org
Twitter: @KhouryThaer (T.K.)

Surgical Pathology 15 (2022) 159–174
https://doi.org/10.1016/j.path.2021.11.011
1875-9181/22/© 2021 Elsevier Inc. All rights reserved.

surgpath.theclinics.com

The World Health Organization (WHO) classified these tumors into 5 subtypes: low-grade adenosquamous carcinoma (LGASC), fibromatosis-like metaplastic carcinoma (FLMC), squamous cell carcinoma (SqCC), spindle cell carcinoma (SpCC), and metaplastic carcinoma with heterologous mesenchymal differentiation (MCHMD). When a tumor has mixed components, it is designated as mixed metaplastic carcinoma (MMC).[1] In this review, the following subjects are going to be discussed: the histomorphologic features of each subtype, a proposed approach to spindle cell lesions detected in a core needle biopsy (CNB) with the differential diagnosis and the immunohistochemistry (IHC) workup, the molecular alterations, tumor microenvironment, and up-to-date target therapy and immunotherapy.

PATHOLOGY

HISTOLOGIC SUBTYPES

Low-Grade Adenosquamous Carcinoma

The LGASC is an ill-defined tumor with infiltrating borders, composed of a mixture of infiltrating neoplastic glandular and squamous structures, all present in the background of sclerotic or desmoplastic stroma with bland nuclear morphology.[2] The glandular component usually reveals well-developed glandular and tubular formations with minimal, if any, angulation, unlike tubular carcinoma. The squamous component varies from extensive epidermoid growth, syringomalike differentiation, and isolated small clusters and solid nests.[3] The overall nuclear grade is low with minimal, if any, mitotic figures. Aggregates of lymphocytes located within or at the periphery of the tumor having "Cannonball"-like configuration can also be encountered[1] (**Fig. 1**A, B). These tumors are usually negative for myoepithelial markers.[4] However, p63 stains the squamous component with nonmyoepithelial-like diffuse staining pattern. Therefore, other myoepithelial markers are required to confirm the invasive nature of the tumor (**Fig. 1**C–E). The radiologic imaging (mammography or ultrasound) of LGASC is nonspecific with the mammography usually demonstrating ill-defined infiltrating lesion (**Fig. 1**F).

Fibromatosis-Like Metaplastic Carcinoma

The FLMC, as the name implies, has similar histologic morphology to breast fibromatosis. FLMC may show epithelioid or squamous cell differentiation and may have ductal carcinoma in situ (DCIS). When these histologic features are absent, IHC staining with epithelial markers (cytokeratin [CK] and p63) can be helpful to differentiate between these 2 lesions (**Fig. 2**).[5,6] The tumor cells are spindle and bland with rare, if any, mitotic figures, arranged in a wavy, interlacing fascicle or long

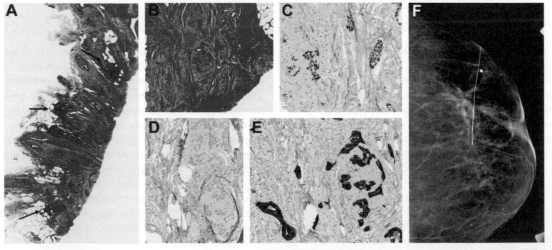

Fig. 1. Low-grade adenosquamous carcinoma. (*A*) Scanning magnification of core biopsy showing infiltrating epithelial neoplasm within a background of dense stroma; note the aggregates of lymphocytes at the periphery of the tumor (*arrows*) (H&E); (*B*) higher magnification image showing both components of infiltrating glandular and squamous clusters of cells in a background of sclerotic and desmoplastic stroma (H&E, 4x); (*C*) p63 staining showing diffuse nonmyoepithelial-like staining pattern (10x); (*D*) smooth muscle myosin image showing lack of myoepithelial cell layer in both squamous and glandular components, confirming invasion (5x); (*E*) cytokeratin 5/6 image showing diffuse staining in both the squamous and glandular components (10x); (*F*) mammography image showing ill-defined infiltrating tumor in the upper part of the breast.

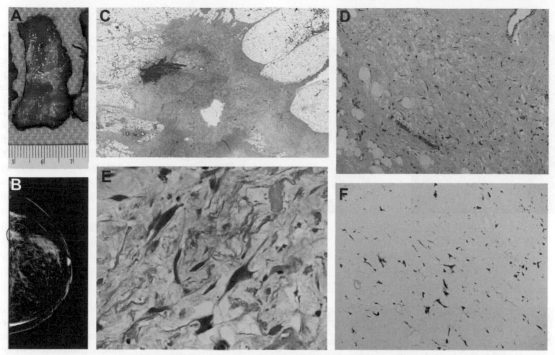

Fig. 2. Fibromatosis-like metaplastic carcinoma. (*A*) Gross image showing white fibrotic infiltrating lesion; (*B*) mammography showing irregular deeply seated lesion in the upper half of the breast; (*C*) scanning magnification of the tumor showing infiltrating fingerlike projections into the surrounding adipose tissue, corresponding to the gross image (H&E); (*D*) high power magnification showing infiltrating bland spindle cells with background of collage fibers (20x, H&E); (*E*) occasional intermediate to high atypical nuclei (60x, H&E); (*F*) pancytokeratin (AE1/3) IHC stain decorating the tumor cells (20x).

fascicle with fingerlike extensions infiltrating the adjacent breast tissue. The tumor has infiltrating borders with a background of varying degrees of collagenization.[1] FLMC and SpCC are spectrum of the spindle cell neoplasm with substantial difference in the outcomes and treatment. Some cases could pose a challenge for the pathologist to classify. The degree of nuclear atypia, the mitotic count, and percentage of spindle cell component seem to help subclassify these tumors.[7–10] In the author's opinion, when in doubt, the case should be discussed in a multidisciplinary approach.

Squamous Cell Carcinoma

Primary breast SqCC could be pure, mixed with invasive carcinoma of no special type (NST) (high-grade adenosquamous carcinoma) or metaplastic carcinoma with pseudoangiomatous acantholytic pattern. Moreover, SpCC could have a component of squamous differentiation. Pure SqCC usually presents as cystic mass lined up with squamous cells with varying degrees of differentiation. The periphery of the tumor shows infiltration into the surrounding stroma in forms of sheets, cords, or nests (**Fig. 3**). Some investigators classify this tumor separately from MpBC.[11] It is important to correlate with the clinical presentation, in order to rule out skin-based SqCC, or

more importantly metastatic SqCC, from other organs such as lung. High-grade adenosquamous carcinoma is composed of 2 components, adenocarcinoma (ductal) and carcinoma with squamous differentiation. They are usually intermingled and difficult to appreciate the morphologic difference. Therefore, this entity is underrecognized (**Fig. 4**). The squamous component varies in proportion with a spectrum of differentiation ranging from mature keratinizing epithelium to spindle cell or with pseudoangiomatous growth pattern. Metaplastic carcinoma with pseudoangiomatous acantholytic pattern has distinctive histologic architecture with closed or interconnected irregular spaces lined with atypical malignant squamous cells (**Fig. 5**). Some investigators classify this entity under SpCC.[3] It is important to recognize this entity, as the differential diagnosis includes angiosarcoma.[12] IHC staining can be helpful, as the tumor is usually positive for one of the CK stains (high-molecular-weight or CK5) and negative for CD34.[13]

Spindle Cell Carcinoma

The SpCC or carcinosarcoma is a spectrum of spindle neoplastic disease with varying degrees of nuclear atypia, growth patterns, and differentiation. As the name implies, the tumor has spindle

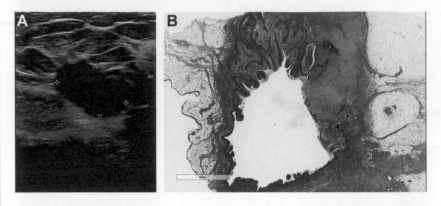

Fig. 3. Pure SqCC. (*A*) Ultrasound showing hypoechoic complex cystic and solid mass with irregular margins and some thick internal septations; (*B*) scanning magnification showing cystic formation lined up with well-differentiated SCC (H&E).

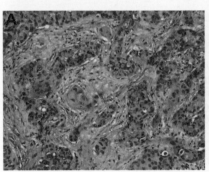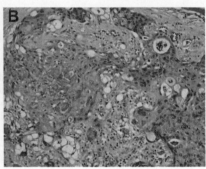

Fig. 4. Adenosquamous carcinoma. (*A*) Adenocarcinoma with intracellular mucin production intermingled with SCC (H&E, 10x); (*B*) SCC component with better differentiation (H&E, 10x).

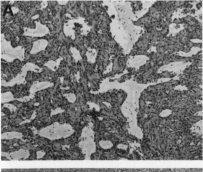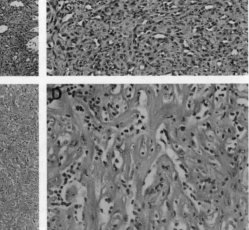

Fig. 5. SqCC acantholytic pseudoangiomatous pattern. (*A*) Dilated partially interconnected staghorn-like spaces and pseudoangiomatous growth pattern (H&E, 10x); (*B*) other areas may show only pseudoangiomatous growth pattern mimicking high-grade angiosarcoma (H&E, 20x); (*C*) another case showing collagenous background mimicking pseudoangiomatous stromal hyperplasia (H&E, 10x); (*D*) with intermediate-grade nuclear atypia (H&E, 40x).

cell morphology with epithelioid differentiation (**Fig. 6**A). The tumor could be pure spindle cell (**Fig. 6**B) or mixed with ductal (**Fig. 6**C), or squamous differentiation/metaplasia (**Fig. 6**D). To differentiate this tumor from the less aggressive tumor FLMC, the tumor must have intermediate or highly atypical nuclei, easily identifiable or brisk mitotic figures. The other differential diagnosis is primary or metastatic sarcoma (fibrosarcoma) when the tumor has a fascicular growth pattern (see **Fig. 6**B).[14,15] Sarcoma (primary or metastatic) is treated differently from SpCC, making the distinction clinically essential. SpCC also could have variable growth pattern in which the fascicles are long, herringbone, or interwoven (see **Fig. 6**B), to short and storiform (**Fig. 6**E).[10,14,16] Presence of DCIS (**Fig. 6**F),[10] epithelioid cells (see **Fig. 6**A), and/or expression of one of the epithelial markers favors SpCC (see **Fig. 6**E, inset). When spindle cell lesion of the breast is encountered in a CNB, MpBC diagnosis should be on the top of the differential diagnosis (see later discussion).

Metaplastic Carcinoma with Heterologous Mesenchymal Differentiation

The MCHMD, also known as heterologous metaplastic carcinoma,[3] are mixed epithelial/mesenchymal variants of metaplastic carcinoma with chondroid or osseous differentiation.[17] The hallmark of these tumors is having heterologous elements, including chondroid, osseous, rhabdoid, or neurologic differentiation (**Fig. 7**A, B).[1] The other component of the tumor could be glandular, tubular, or squamous (**Fig. 7**C, D).[14,18,19] These components (heterologous elements and conventional breast carcinoma) could have either an abrupt transition or intervening zones of spindle cell metaplasia (**Fig. 7**C–E). In some cases, the tumor is completely composed of the heterologous elements with no epithelial differentiation. These tumors pose a challenge differentiating it from primary or metastatic sarcoma (osteosarcoma, chondrosarcoma, rhabdomyosarcoma). The only way of making the diagnosis is the positive staining of epithelial markers favoring carcinoma. In some instances, however, the definitive diagnosis might not be possible.

Mixed Metaplastic Breast Carcinoma

The MMC is defined as a carcinoma with a mixture of different histologic elements including various metaplastic components (SqSS, SpCC, MCHMD) or any of these elements and conventional breast carcinoma such as NST and lobular, among others (see **Fig. 4**A, B, **6**C, D, **7**D, **Fig. 8**). Because MpBCs have worse clinical outcomes than conventional breast carcinoma (see later discussion), it is recommended to report it as metaplastic carcinoma and mention the distinct conventional carcinoma components.[1] In the author's opinion, a percentage of each component should be mentioned when possible.

Some investigators classify carcinoma with multinucleated giant cells resembling osteoclasts and carcinoma with choriocarcinomatous morphology as MpBC.[3] However, these tumors are currently reclassified by the WHO under invasive breast carcinoma NST with special morphologic patterns.[1]

UNUSUAL CLINICAL AND PATHOLOGIC PRESENTATION

Metaplastic Carcinoma Arising Within Complex Sclerosing Lesions

There are a few reports of complex sclerosing lesions (sclerosing papilloma and nipple adenoma) associated with metaplastic carcinoma.[20–23] In the largest series of 33 cases reported by Gobbi and colleagues, most of the cases had dominant spindle cell component with various degrees of atypia, with the majority having fibromatosis-like or low-grade morphology. Squamous metaplasia and low-grade glandular elements are common features (**Fig. 9**). DCIS and invasive mammary carcinoma could be seen but less common. Ten cases stained with IHC markers, all showing expression of at least one of the CK markers (HMW-CK, AE1/3, or CK7).[23] This entity is very important to recognize, as it can easily be overlooked when evaluating complex sclerosing lesions.

APPROACH TO SPINDLE CELL LESIONS OF THE BREAST DETECTED IN A CORE BIOPSY

Because MpBC is a major differential diagnosis for spindle cell lesions detected in a CNB, the author herein presents a short summary of the differential diagnosis and pitfalls and recommends histologic and IHC algorithmic approaches.

For histomorphology, first look for specific morphology such as epithelium (intimately admixed or separately coexisted) or vascular spaces. If the tumor is composed of pure spindle cells, evaluate the nuclear atypia. In this situation, clinical history of trauma or prior malignancy could be helpful. For imagining the borders of the tumor, well-defined versus infiltrative could narrow down the diagnosis (**Fig. 10**).

The IHC staining should be used in the context of the clinical and histologic findings; otherwise, they could be misleading. Identifying the cell

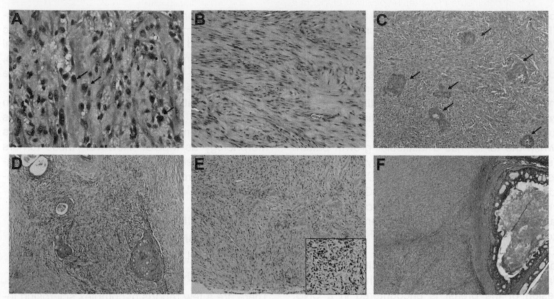

Fig. 6. SpCC. (*A*) Spindle cells with epithelioid morphology (*arrows* indicate epithelioid cells, H&E, 40x); (*B*) pure spindle cell with long sweeping fascicles (H&E, 20x); (*C*) mixed with ductal carcinoma of no special type, resembling malignant adenomyoepithelioma but lacks myoepithelial staining (*arrows* indicate ductal component, H&E, 10x); (*D*) mixed with SqCC (H&E, 10x); (*E*) pure spindle cell with short storiform fascicles (H&E, 10x; inset pancytokeratin AE1/3 staining 10x); (*F*) SpCC with DCIS (H&E, 4x).

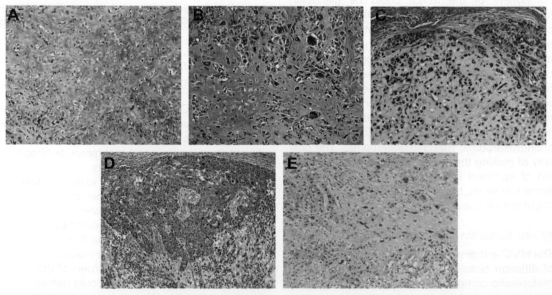

Fig. 7. MCHMD. (*A*) Matrix producing (chondroid) (H&E, 20x); (*B*) matrix producing (osteoid) (H&E, 20x); (*C*) carcinomatous (no special type) area at the periphery, note abrupt transition (H&E, 20x); (*D*) carcinomatous (squamous) area at the periphery, note abrupt transition (H&E, 20x); (*E*) zones of spindle cell metaplasia intervening between the carcinomatous and chondroid component (H&E, 20x).

Fig. 8. Mixed metaplastic carcinoma. (*A*) MCHMD-chondroid (upper half) and lobular carcinoma (lower half) (H&E, 20x); (*B*) mixed MCHMD-chondroid (left) and SqCC (right), note the squamous pearl (H&E, 20x).

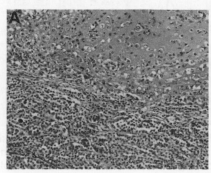 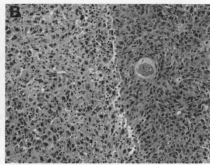

lineage is the key in the IHC approach (epithelial, vascular vs other). First and foremost, MpBC should be at the top of the differential diagnosis, and the stains should aim to rule it in or out. The most commonly used epithelial stains are AE1/3, MNF-116, HMW-CK, CK5/6, and p63.[10,24] Diffuse and strong staining patterns are usually encountered in MpBC (**Fig. 11**).

Pitfalls

- Atypical cells may be seen in benign entities such as nodular fasciitis and biopsy site, whereas some malignant entities could have bland cells such as FLMC.[1]

- It has been reported and it is in the author's experience that focal staining for keratin and p63 markers could occur in MpBC and non-MpBC tumors such as sarcoma and phyllodes tumor (PT).[25,26]

- β-catenin in PT and MpBC: Lacroix-Triki reported that all fibromatosis cases, 23% of MpBC, and 57% of PT (benign and malignant) expressed nuclear beta-catenin. However, β-catenin is usually focal when stains MpBC.[27] The author came across a case of a woman whose breast CNB had MpBC but mistakenly diagnosed as fibromatosis based on the expression of β-catenin and misinterpretation of CK stain. She presented 6 months later with double the size of the tumor. Therefore, β-catenin should be interpreted with caution in the context of the rest of the clinical and histologic findings.

MOLECULAR ALTERATIONS AND TARGET THERAPY

MpBC is usually triple-negative (estrogen receptor [ER] negative/progesterone receptor [PR] negative/HER-2/neu negative).[1,28–31] Intrinsic gene profiling classified these tumors under basal-like or claudin-low.[32,33] Further subclassification of these tumors grouped them under mesenchymal-like molecular subtype of triple-negative breast cancer (TNBC) as proposed by Lehmann and colleagues.[34] There have been many studies performed to elucidate the molecular alterations of these tumors in order to identify actionable genetic changes for potential targeted therapeutic intervention. The gene mutations are detailed in a review by González-Martínez and colleagues.[35] They reviewed 14 series with a total of 539 molecularly characterized tumors.[36–49] *TP53* was the most common mutation, followed by *PIK3CA*. *MYC* was the most amplified gene followed by *EGFR*. The most common gene loss was *CDKN2A/CDKN2B* locus (**Table 1**). There are limited data on MpBC in proper with regard to the effect of the target therapy on the actionable genes. Often, they are combined with TNBC clinical trials. However, in breast cancer in general, these monoclonal antibodies could be classified into tiers I to V and X based on the strength of the clinical evidence as explained by Condorelli and colleagues.[50] Sporadic case reports and small clinical trials have been published illustrating variety of therapeutic approaches. The author and his colleagues reported a case of a metastatic MpBC with osseous differentiation and *BRCA1* mutation who had a marked response to liposomal doxorubicin.[51] A phase I trial on 59 patients with metastatic MpBC treated with liposomal doxorubicin, bevacizumab, with either temsirolimus or everolimus, revealed an objective response rate of 21%. All 4 patients who achieved a complete response had a mutation in the *PI3K* pathway.[52] Another observation is that MpBC patients should be tested for *BRCA* germline mutations. In addition to the benefit from adding platinum agents, they are more susceptible to Poly (ADP-ribose) polymerase inhibitors.[53]

This diverse molecular profile reflects, in part, the diversity of the histologic subtypes of MpBC.

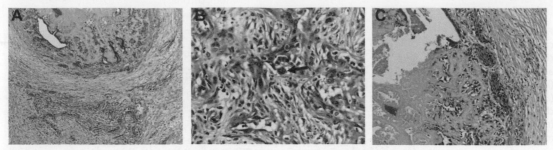

Fig. 9. Metaplastic carcinoma arising within complex sclerosing lesion. (*A*) Sclerosing lesion with infiltrative epithelioid cells (H&E, 4x); (*B*) plump fusiform and polygonal atypical tumor cells with rounded nuclei and prominent nucleoli (*arrow* indicates atypical mitotic figure) (H&E 40x); (*C*) squamous metaplasia at the periphery of the papilloma (H&E, 10x).

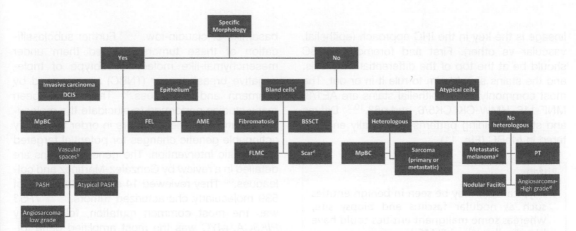

Fig. 10. Suggested algorithm of spindle cell lesion detected in core needle biopsy. [a]FEL and AME: both epithelium and stromal growths separately coexist with different proportions (AME: the spindle cells are predominantly myoepithelial). [b]IHC: CD31 positive in angiosarcoma and negative in PASH. [c]BSSCT: well-defined borders by imaging, whereas fibromatosis, FLMB, and scar: ill-defined infiltrative. [d]Scar: history of recent trauma; metastatic melanoma and metastatic sarcoma: history of the diseases; angiosarcoma: history of radiation therapy. AME, adenomamyoepithelioma; BSSCT, benign stromal spindle cell tumor (includes myofibroblastoma, spindle cell lipoma, solitary fibrous tumor); FEL, fibroepithelial lesion; FLMC, fibromatosis-like metaplastic carcinoma; MpBC, metaplastic breast carcinoma; PASH, pseudoangiomatous stromal hyperplasia; PT, phyllodes tumor.

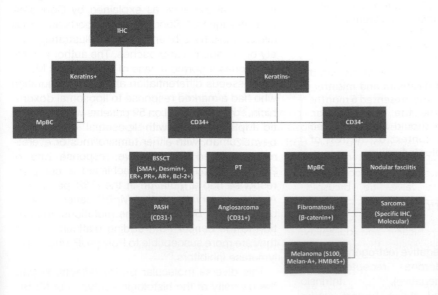

Fig. 11. Suggested IHC algorithm of spindle cell lesions detected in core needle biopsy. Keratin stains and CD34 are the major markers that can narrow down the diagnosis. Additional stains such as CD31 could be helpful. The rest of IHC should be used based on the histologic and clinical suspicion (eg, β-catenin for fibromatosis, melanoma markers, and so forth). BSSCT, benign stromal spindle cell tumor; IHC, immunohistochemistry; MpBC, metaplastic breast carcinoma; PASH, pseudoangiomatous stromal hyperplasia; PT, phyllodes tumor.

Table 1
Molecular alteration in metaplastic carcinoma

Mutation	
Gene	**Frequency (%)**
TP53	58.7 (26–70)[a]
PIK3CA	32.8 (12–48)[a]
TERT	25
PI3K/AKT Pathway	
PTEN	12.7
PIK3R1	11.2
NF1	9.8
HRAS	8.5
AKT1	—
WNT Pathway	
APC	5
FAT1	11
DNA Repair	
BRCA1	3–15
BRCA2	2–6
ATM	2–12
Chromatin Remodeling	
KMT2D	17
ARID1A	6
Copy Number Variation (CNV)	
Amplification	
MYC	17.3
EGFR	17.2
CCND1	8.4
CCNE1	5.9
CDK4	4
CCND3	15
CCND2	5
FGFR1	5
ERBB2	4.8
RAS	5
NF1	5
PIK3CA	5
SOX2	5
AKT3	5
Gene Loss	
CDKN2A/CDKN2B	19
PTEN	14.9
RB1	6.5

[a] Median (range).

Adapted from González-Martínez S, Pérez-Mies B, Carretero-Barrio I, et al. Molecular Features of Metaplastic Breast Carcinoma: An Infrequent Subtype of Triple Negative Breast Carcinoma. Cancers (Basel). 2020;12(7):1832. Published 2020 Jul 8. https://doi.org/10.3390/cancers12071832

However, when dissecting through the studies, variation could be appreciated among the MpBC subtypes (SpCC, SqCC, MCHMD). SqCC and MCHMD had more frequent TP53 mutation, whereas PIK3CA alterations were more frequent in SpCC.[36,46] TERT alteration was seen in SpCC and SqCC but not in MCHMD.[42] When MpBC was compared with non-MpBC-TNBC, the former had more PIK3CA alteration and less TP53 alteration. It is worth noting that these studies focused on high-grade tumors excluding FLMC and LGASC.

TUMOR MICROENVIRONMENT AND IMMUNOTHERAPY

With the advancement of immunotherapy, few studies investigated the immune microenvironment of MpBC. Two monoclonal antibodies have been approved by the Food and Drug Administration to treat locally advanced and metastatic TNBC expressing PD-L1 with TECENTRIQ (atezolizumab) or KEYTRUDA (pembrolizumab). The corresponding IHC assays are clone SP142 and 22C3, respectively.[54,55]

Tumor infiltrating lymphocytes (TILs) and PD-L1 have been extensively studied in TNBC. However, only a few focused on MpBC. Lien and colleagues scored TILs in 82 MpBC and found that 34.1% had intermediate (>10% to 60%) or high TILs (>60%) (SqCC [50%], MMC [34.1%], SpCC [30.8%], and MCHMD [14.3%]). Multivariate analysis showed that high/intermediate TILs correlated with better survival.[56] Chao and colleagues also found high TILs density in SqCC compared with other subtypes. Interestingly, in mixed MpBC/NST, TILs were denser in MpBC component than in INST component. Overall, TILs, high CD4, and high CD8 had borderline significance in correlating with clinical outcomes. In SqCC, TILs had stronger correlation with outcomes.[57]

Lien and colleagues investigated the expression of PD-L1 (SP142) in MpBC and found that it is expressed in 72% of 82 cases. When different metaplastic components were compared, the rate of expression was highest in SqCC (61.1%) and MMC (52.9%) and lowest in the chondroid component (14.3% in both the MCHMD and MMC). PD-L1 positivity did not correlate with the outcomes.[56] Other studies included MpBC as part of TNBC or breast carcinomas of all types.[44,58]

It would be clinically relevant to investigate the role of TILs in the response to neoadjuvant chemotherapy, particularly with the recent call of deescalating the therapy in patients with TNBC.

TREATMENT

ADJUVANT THERAPY

Classic therapeutic approaches including adjuvant chemotherapy, surgery, and radiation therapy have been previously discussed, and it is beyond the scope of this review.[59,60]

It is worth noting here in this brief review of the adjuvant treatment that as the variation in the subtypes in terms of the histopathology and the prognosis, the treatment also varies. Although high-risk MpBC is treated with surgical removal and chemotherapy, low-risk tumors (eg, LGASC and FLMC) are treated with surgical removal alone unless presented with positive lymph node.[61] Tumors that have intermediate morphology between SpCC and FLMC must be managed in a multidisciplinary approach as mentioned earlier.

NEOADJUVANT THERAPY

There is also a dearth of studies examining the role of neoadjuvant chemotherapy in MpBC. It is long thought that MpBC do not respond well due to the epithelial mesenchymal transformation that is commonly seen in these tumors.[62,63] Three studies with 1, 12, and 21 cases, respectively, reported low rate of pathology complete response (pCR).[64–66] In the author's experience 2 of 6 patients achieved pCR. However, in a recent study by Han and colleagues who studied 29 patients, 5 (17%) achieved pCR, most of whom were MCHMD type.[67] Overall, the rate of response is lower than the nonmetaplastic TNBC.[68] However, all these studies are retrospective and have small number of cases, making it difficult to draw any conclusions.

PROGNOSIS

There are many limitations to the published studies that investigated the clinical behavior of MpBC. MpBC is heterogeneous in terms of its clinical behavior. More specifically, these tumors can be grouped into 2 categories: low risk that includes LGASC and high risk that includes SqCC, SpCC, and MCHMD. FLMC is a unique entity, as it has intermediate risk and is considered as part of the SpCC spectrum (see later discussion). All published studies are retrospective. In the author's experience, defining MpBC is not always straightforward. For instance, in the author's published study, 28 of 81 (34.6%) reported MpBC were reclassified on review to carcinoma of NST.[69] Therefore, there is doubt about the studies that included large number of cases without pathologic

review and verification.[66,70–72] On the other hand, studies with small number of cases lack statistical powers.

LGASC is largely indolent but locally aggressive. Rarely, the tumor develops lymph node or distant metastasis. In the largest series of 32 cases, the clinical outcome correlated with the tumor size.[73] FLMC is locally aggressive tumor and has the potential of distant metastasis. The risk of local recurrence could reach up to 44%.[74] Few studies reported the tumor could have potential to metastasize to other organ such as the lung,[10,75,76] although this tumor seems less aggressive than the SpCC. However, the histologic distinction between the 2 entities could be challenging. More studies are required to better define this entity, in order to better manage the patient and minimize the incidence of local or distant recurrence.

Overall, MpBC is an aggressive disease that presents as advanced disease more often than the other types of breast carcinomas. About 20% present with positive lymph node and about 25% with stage III or IV.[66,72] Often SqCC, SpCC, and MCHMD are combined in one category and compared with other tumors such as nonmetaplastic TNBC,[69–71,77–80] or NST, although matched for ER and HER2.[48,81] There are sporadic studies that investigated a single diagnosis such as SpCC[8] or MCHMD.[18] Other studies investigated if these 3 subtypes differ in the outcomes.[69,80,81] Most of these studies revealed that MpBC has worse clinical outcomes than TNBC, including 2 studies with large number of cases; the hazard ratio ranged from 1.36 and 3.99.[8,69–71,77–79] Only a single study with relatively large number of cases revealed no statistical significance between MpBC versus matching NST when only stages 1 and 2 cases were included in the analysis[81] (Table 2). Some studies attempted to compare the clinical outcomes between the different MpBC subtypes but limited by the small sample size.[69,82] However, Tadros and colleagues found that MCHMD had the best outcome and SqCC had the worst.[80] Rakha and colleagues revealed that SpCC, pure or mixed with SqCC, had worse clinical outcomes than SqCC or MCHMD.[81] Downs-Kelly and colleagues found that less matrix (<40%) in MCHMD signified worse clinical outcome.[18]

COMMENTS

MpBCs are diverse group of tumors with 2 extremes, the very low risk and the very high risk. Therefore, the author recommends revising the WHO classification by proceeding the diagnoses of the least malignant tumors LGASC and FLMC

Table 2
Studies comparing the clinical outcome between metaplastic breast carcinoma and nonmetaplastic breast carcinoma (mostly triple-negative breast cancer)

Ref	Cases (No.)	Institution	Histologic Subtypes (%)	• Matching Criteria • No. Case-to-Case	DFS	OS	Multivariate Analysis	DFS (HR)	OS (HR)
Lester et al,[8] 2012	47	Single	SpCC (100)	• Age, stage, therapy (CT, RT) • One-to-one	MpBC > TNBC	Not calculated	Not calculated	Not available	Not available
Downs-Kelly et al,[18] 2009	32	Single	MCHMD (100)	• Age, stage, grade • One-to-two	MpBC > BC[a]	Not calculated	Not calculated	Not available	Not available
Jung et al,[77] 2010	35	Single	SqCC (60) MCHMD (11.4) SpCC (11.4) Mixed (14.3) LGASC (2.9)	• Grade • One-to-one	MpBC > TNBC	MpBC > TNBC	Yes	3.99	3.14
Luini et al,[78] 2007	37	Single	MCHMD (51.4) SqCC (8.1) Carcinosarcoma (24.3) SqCC (18.9) With osteoclastic giant cell (2.7)	• Grade, year of surgery, T-stage, N-stage • One-to-two	Not significant	MpBC > TNBC HR = 5.0	Not calculated	Not calculated	Not calculated
Lee et al,[79] 2012	67	Single	SqCC (52.2) SpCC (13.4) MCHMD (23.9) Mixed (7.5)[b]	• Stage • All cases	MpBC > TNBC	MpBC > TNBC	Yes	2.53	2.56
El Zein et al,[69] 2017	46	Single	MCHMD (37) SqCC (26.1) SpCC (30.4) Mixed (6.5)	• Age, stage, Nottingham grade, therapy (CT, RT) • One-to-one	MpBC > TNBC	MpBC > TNBC	Yes	1.99	Not significant
Beatty et al,[48] 2006	24	Single	SqCC (50) MCHMD (12.5) SpCC (25) Not stated (16.5)[c]	• Date of diagnosis, age, tumor size, node status, ER, PR, and HER2 (all cases TNBC) • Three-to-one	Not significant	Not significant	No	Not calculated	Not calculated

(continued on next page)

Table 2
(continued)

Ref	Cases (No.)	Institution	Histologic Subtypes (%)	• Matching Criteria • No. Case-to-Case	DFS	OS	Multivariate Analysis	DFS (HR)	OS (HR)
Rakha et al,[81] 2015	405	Multi-institutional	SpCC (31.9)[d] SqCC (21.1) Mixed SpCC/SqCC (13.5) MCHMD (28.6) FLMC (4.9)	• Age, Nottingham grade, N-stage, ER and HER2 • 405–285	Not significant[e]	Not recorded	No	Not calculated	Not calculated
Li et al,[70] 2019	586	SEER	Not recorded	• Age, race, grade, AJCC stage, therapy (CT, RT) • One-to-three	MpBC > TNBC	MpBC > TNBC	Yes	1.42	1.36
Polamraju et al,[71] 2020	5142	NCDB (2004–2013)	Not recorded	• Age, race, insurance status, T-stage, N-stage, grade, Charlson Deyo Score, year of diagnosis, income, therapy (CT, HT, RT) • All cases	Not performed	MpBC > TNBC	Yes	Not calculated	1.48
Tadros et al,[80] 2021	132	Single	SpCC (19.7) SqCC (19.7) Mixed SpCC/SqCC (22.7) MCHMD (34.1)	• Age, year of surgery, type of surgery, T-stage, N-stage, • All cases	MpBC > TNBC	MpBC > TNBC	Yes	2.3	1.9

Abbreviations: DFS, disease-free survival; MpBC, metaplastic breast carcinoma; NCDB, National Cancer Data Base, OS, overall survival; SEER, Surveillance Epidemiology End Result; TNBC, triple-negative breast carcinoma.

[a] DFS (regional and distant).

[b] Two cases were not subtyped (see **Table 2**, Lee et al[79]).

[c] Cases do not add up to 100% (Beatty et al[48]).

[d] Only 364 cases had reported subtypes.

[e] Breast cancer–specific survival was calculated.

with the term "low risk" and the most malignant tumors SqCC, SpCC, and MCHMD with "high risk." The high-risk tumors have the worst clinical outcomes, with some suggesting that MCHMD has better outcomes. The novel discoveries of tumor microenvironment and molecular alterations have led to the advancement in immunotherapies and target therapy. However, with few successful and promising therapies presented in the literature in the form of case reports and small clinical trials, unfortunately most of the patients succumb to this disease. Therefore, further discoveries are urgently needed.

CLINICS CARE POINTS

- High-risk MpBC has worse clinical outcomes than TNBC.

- Combining various histologic subtypes under one entity designated as MpBC is misleading.

- Some of the subtypes have the worst clinical outcomes among all breast carcinomas, whereas the other group has indolent clinical behavior.

- SpCC associated with complex sclerosing lesions could be challenging to diagnose, and the pathologists should be aware of this entity.

- Proper histomorphology interpretation and wise choices of immunohistochemistry staining could assist in rendering the correct diagnosis of spindle cell lesion of the breast.

- Target therapy and immunotherapy are promising ways to combat high-risk MpBC of various molecular alterations and up-to-date target therapy and immunotherapy.

DISCLOSURE

Breast Pathology Faculty Advisor for AstraZeneca on HER2 assay.

REFERENCES

1. Reis-Filho JS GH, McCart Reed AE, Rakha EA, et al. Metaplastic carcinoma. WHO classification of tumours of the breast. 5th edition. Lyon (France): International Agency for Research on Cancer (IARC); 2019. p. 134–8.

2. Rosen PP, Ernsberger D. Low-grade adenosquamous carcinoma. A variant of metaplastic mammary carcinoma. Am J Surg Pathol 1987;11(5):351–8.

3. Brogi E. Carcinoma with Metaplasia. In: Rosen PP, editor. Rosen's breast pathology. 5th edition. Mexico: Wolters Kluwer; 2021. p. 592–649.

4. Kawaguchi K, Shin SJ. Immunohistochemical staining characteristics of low-grade adenosquamous carcinoma of the breast. Am J Surg Pathol 2012; 36(7):1009–20.

5. Dwyer JB, Clark BZ. Low-grade fibromatosis-like spindle cell carcinoma of the breast. Arch Pathol Lab Med 2015;139(4):552–7.

6. Rungta S, Kloer CG. Metaplastic carcinomas of the breast: diagnostic challenges and new translational insights. Arch Pathol Lab Med 2012;136(8):896–900.

7. Davis WG, Hennessy B, Babiera G, et al. Metaplastic sarcomatoid carcinoma of the breast with absent or minimal overt invasive carcinomatous component: a misnomer. Am J Surg Pathol 2005;29(11):1456–63.

8. Lester TR, Hunt KK, Nayeemuddin KM, et al. Metaplastic sarcomatoid carcinoma of the breast appears more aggressive than other triple receptor-negative breast cancers. Breast Cancer Res Treat 2012; 131(1):41–8.

9. Zhu H, Li K, Dong DD, et al. Spindle cell metaplastic carcinoma of breast: A clinicopathological and immunohistochemical analysis. Asia-Pacific J Clin Oncol 2017;13(2):e72–8.

10. Carter MR, Hornick JL, Lester S, et al. Spindle cell (sarcomatoid) carcinoma of the breast: a clinicopathologic and immunohistochemical analysis of 29 cases. Am J Surg Pathol 2006;30(3):300–9.

11. Hoda SA. Squamous Cell Carcinoma. In: Rosen PP, editor. Rosen's breast pathology. 5th edition. Mexico: Wolters Kluwer; 2021. p. 650–64.

12. Eusebi V, Lamovec J, Cattani MG, et al. Acantholytic variant of squamous-cell carcinoma of the breast. Am J Surg Pathol 1986;10(12):855–61.

13. Aulmann S, Schnabel PA, Helmchen B, et al. Immunohistochemical and cytogenetic characterization of acantholytic squamous cell carcinoma of the breast. Virchows Arch 2005;446(3):305–9.

14. Wargotz ES, Deos PH, Norris HJ. Metaplastic carcinomas of the breast. II. Spindle cell carcinoma. Hum Pathol 1989;20(8):732–40.

15. Pitts WC, Rojas VA, Gaffey MJ, et al. Carcinomas with metaplasia and sarcomas of the breast. Am J Clin Pathol 1991;95(5):623–32.

16. Gersell DJ, Katzenstein AL. Spindle cell carcinoma of the breast. A clinocopathologic and ultrastructural study. Hum Pathol 1981;12(6):550–61.

17. Fattaneh AT. Uncommon Variants of Carcinoma. In: AFIP, editor. AFIP atlas of tumor pathology-tumors of the mammary gland, vol. 10, 4th edition. Washington, DC: Sliver Spring; 2009. p. 217–40.

18. Downs-Kelly E, Nayeemuddin KM, Albarracin C, et al. Matrix-producing carcinoma of the breast: an aggressive subtype of metaplastic carcinoma. Am J Surg Pathol 2009;33(4):534–41.

19. Oberman HA. Metaplastic carcinoma of the breast. A clinicopathologic study of 29 patients. Am J Surg Pathol 1987;11(12):918–29.

20. Pastolero GC, Bowler L, Meads GE. Intraductal papilloma associated with metaplastic carcinoma of the breast. Histopathology 1997;31(5):488–90.

21. Pitt MA, Wells S, Eyden BP. Carcinosarcoma arising in a duct papilloma. Histopathology 1995;26(1):81–4.

22. Denley H, Pinder SE, Tan PH, et al. Metaplastic carcinoma of the breast arising within complex sclerosing lesion: a report of five cases. Histopathology 2000;36(3):203–9.

23. Gobbi H, Simpson JF, Jensen RA, et al. Metaplastic spindle cell breast tumors arising within papillomas, complex sclerosing lesions, and nipple adenomas. Mod Pathol 2003;16(9):893–901.

24. Lee AH. Recent developments in the histological diagnosis of spindle cell carcinoma, fibromatosis and phyllodes tumour of the breast. Histopathology 2008;52(1):45–57.

25. Cimino-Mathews A, Sharma R, Illei PB, et al. A subset of malignant phyllodes tumors express p63 and p40: a diagnostic pitfall in breast core needle biopsies. Am J Surg Pathol 2014;38(12):1689–96.

26. Chia Y, Thike AA, Cheok PY, et al. Stromal keratin expression in phyllodes tumours of the breast: a comparison with other spindle cell breast lesions. J Clin Pathol 2012;65(4):339–47.

27. Lacroix-Triki M, Geyer FC, Lambros MB, et al. β-catenin/Wnt signalling pathway in fibromatosis, metaplastic carcinomas and phyllodes tumours of the breast. Mod Pathol 2010;23(11):1438–48.

28. Abouharb S, Moulder S. Metaplastic breast cancer: clinical overview and molecular aberrations for potential targeted therapy. Curr Oncol Rep 2015;17(3):431.

29. Reis-Filho JS, Milanezi F, Steele D, et al. Metaplastic breast carcinomas are basal-like tumours. Histopathology 2006;49(1):10–21.

30. Schroeder MC, Rastogi P, Geyer CE Jr, et al. Early and Locally Advanced Metaplastic Breast Cancer: Presentation and Survival by Receptor Status in Surveillance, Epidemiology, and End Results (SEER) 2010-2014. Oncologist 2018;23(4):481–8.

31. Rakha EA, Coimbra ND, Hodi Z, et al. Immunoprofile of metaplastic carcinomas of the breast. Histopathology 2017;70(6):975–85.

32. Prat A, Parker JS, Karginova O, et al. Phenotypic and molecular characterization of the claudin-low intrinsic subtype of breast cancer. Breast Cancer Res 2010;12(5):R68.

33. Weigelt B, Kreike B, Reis-Filho JS. Metaplastic breast carcinomas are basal-like breast cancers: a genomic profiling analysis. Breast Cancer Res Treat 2009;117(2):273–80.

34. Lehmann BD, Bauer JA, Chen X, et al. Identification of human triple-negative breast cancer subtypes and preclinical models for selection of targeted therapies. J Clin Invest 2011;121(7):2750–67.

35. González-Martínez S, Pérez-Mies B, Carretero-Barrio I, et al. Molecular features of metaplastic breast carcinoma: an infrequent subtype of triple negative breast carcinoma. Cancers 2020;12(7):1832.

36. Piscuoglio S, Ng CKY, Geyer FC, et al. Genomic and transcriptomic heterogeneity in metaplastic carcinomas of the breast. NPJ breast cancer 2017;3:48.

37. Vranic S, Stafford P, Palazzo J, et al. Molecular Profiling of the Metaplastic Spindle Cell Carcinoma of the Breast Reveals Potentially Targetable Biomarkers. Clin Breast Cancer 2020;20(4):326–31.e1.

38. McCart Reed AE, Kalaw E, Nones K, et al. Phenotypic and molecular dissection of metaplastic breast cancer and the prognostic implications. J Pathol 2019;247(2):214–27.

39. Zhai J, Giannini G, Ewalt MD, et al. Molecular characterization of metaplastic breast carcinoma via next-generation sequencing. Hum Pathol 2019;86:85–92.

40. Tray N, Taff J, Singh B, et al. Metaplastic breast cancers: Genomic profiling, mutational burden and tumor-infiltrating lymphocytes. Breast 2019;44:29–32.

41. Afkhami M, Schmolze D, Yost SE, et al. Mutation and immune profiling of metaplastic breast cancer: Correlation with survival. PLoS One 2019;14(11):e0224726.

42. Krings G, Chen YY. Genomic profiling of metaplastic breast carcinomas reveals genetic heterogeneity and relationship to ductal carcinoma. Mod Pathol 2018;31(11):1661–74.

43. Ng CKY, Piscuoglio S, Geyer FC, et al. The Landscape of Somatic Genetic Alterations in Metaplastic Breast Carcinomas. Clin Cancer Res 2017;23(14):3859–70.

44. Joneja U, Vranic S, Swensen J, et al. Comprehensive profiling of metaplastic breast carcinomas reveals frequent overexpression of programmed death-ligand 1. J Clin Pathol 2017;70(3):255–9.

45. Edenfield J, Schammel C, Collins J, et al. Metaplastic breast cancer: molecular typing and identification of potential targeted therapies at a single institution. Clin Breast Cancer 2017;17(1):e1–10.

46. Ross JS, Badve S, Wang K, et al. Genomic profiling of advanced-stage, metaplastic breast carcinoma by next-generation sequencing reveals frequent, targetable genomic abnormalities and potential new treatment options. Arch Pathol Lab Med 2015;139(5):642–9.

47. Hayes MJ, Thomas D, Emmons A, et al. Genetic changes of Wnt pathway genes are common events in metaplastic carcinomas of the breast. Clin Cancer Res 2008;14(13):4038–44.

48. Beatty JD, Atwood M, Tickman R, et al. Metaplastic breast cancer: clinical significance. Am J Surg 2006; 191(5):657–64.

49. Reis-Filho JS, Pinheiro C, Lambros MB, et al. EGFR amplification and lack of activating mutations in metaplastic breast carcinomas. J Pathol 2006; 209(4):445–53.

50. Condorelli R, Mosele F, Verret B, et al. Genomic alterations in breast cancer: level of evidence for actionability according to ESMO Scale for Clinical Actionability of molecular Targets (ESCAT). Ann Oncol 2019;30(3):365–73.

51. Hamad L, Khoury T, Vona K, et al. A case of metaplastic breast cancer with prolonged response to single agent liposomal doxorubicin. Cureus 2016;8(1):e454.

52. Basho RK, Yam C, Gilcrease M, et al. Comparative effectiveness of an mtor-based systemic therapy regimen in advanced, metaplastic and nonmetaplastic triple-negative breast cancer. Oncologist 2018;23(11):1300–9.

53. Robson M, Im SA, Senkus E, et al. Olaparib for metastatic breast cancer in patients with a germline BRCA mutation. N Engl J Med 2017;377(6):523–33.

54. Schmid P, Adams S, Rugo HS, et al. Atezolizumab and Nab-paclitaxel in advanced triple-negative breast cancer. N Engl J Med 2018;379(22):2108–21.

55. Cortes J, Cescon DW, Rugo HS, et al. KEYNOTE-355: Randomized, double-blind, phase III study of pembrolizumab + chemotherapy versus placebo + chemotherapy for previously untreated locally recurrent inoperable or metastatic triple-negative breast cancer. J Clin Oncol 2020;38(15_suppl):1000.

56. Lien HC, Lee YH, Chen IC, et al. Tumor-infiltrating lymphocyte abundance and programmed death-ligand 1 expression in metaplastic breast carcinoma: implications for distinct immune microenvironments in different metaplastic components. Virchows Arch 2020;478(4):669–78.

57. Chao X, Liu L, Sun P, et al. Immune parameters associated with survival in metaplastic breast cancer. Breast Cancer Res 2020;22(1):92.

58. Dill EA, Gru AA, Atkins KA, et al. PD-L1 Expression and Intratumoral Heterogeneity Across Breast Cancer Subtypes and Stages: An Assessment of 245 Primary and 40 Metastatic Tumors. Am J Surg Pathol 2017;41(3):334–42.

59. Drekolias D, Mamounas EP. Metaplastic breast carcinoma: Current therapeutic approaches and novel targeted therapies. Breast J 2019;25(6):1192–7.

60. Reddy TP, Rosato RR, Li X, et al. A comprehensive overview of metaplastic breast cancer: clinical features and molecular aberrations. Breast Cancer Res 2020;22(1):121.

61. Network NCC. Breast Cancer (Version 5.2021). Available at: https://www.nccn.org/guidelines/guidelines-detail?category=1&id=1419. Accessed May 4, 2021.

62. Kalluri R, Weinberg RA. The basics of epithelial-mesenchymal transition. J Clin Invest 2009;119(6): 1420–8.

63. Sarrió D, Rodriguez-Pinilla SM, Hardisson D, et al. Epithelial-mesenchymal transition in breast cancer relates to the basal-like phenotype. Cancer Res 2008;68(4):989–97.

64. Takuwa H, Ueno T, Ishiguro H, et al. A case of metaplastic breast cancer that showed a good response to platinum-based preoperative chemotherapy. Breast Cancer 2014;21(4):504–7.

65. Chen IC, Lin CH, Huang CS, et al. Lack of efficacy to systemic chemotherapy for treatment of metaplastic carcinoma of the breast in the modern era. Breast Cancer Res Treat 2011;130(1):345.

66. Hennessy BT, Giordano S, Broglio K, et al. Biphasic metaplastic sarcomatoid carcinoma of the breast. Ann Oncol 2006;17(4):605–13.

67. Han M, Salamat A, Zhu L, et al. Metaplastic breast carcinoma: a clinical-pathologic study of 97 cases with subset analysis of response to neoadjuvant chemotherapy. Mod Pathol 2019;32(6):807–16.

68. Huang M, O'Shaughnessy J, Zhao J, et al. Association of pathologic complete response with long-term survival outcomes in triple-negative breast cancer: a meta-analysis. Cancer Res 2020;80(24). 5427–34.

69. El Zein D, Hughes M, Kumar S, et al. Metaplastic carcinoma of the breast is more aggressive than triple-negative breast cancer: a study from a single institution and review of literature. Clin Breast Cancer 2017;17(5):382–91.

70. Li Y, Zhang N, Zhang H, et al. Comparative prognostic analysis for triple-negative breast cancer with metaplastic and invasive ductal carcinoma. J Clin Pathol 2019;72(6):418–24.

71. Polamraju P, Haque W, Cao K, et al. Comparison of outcomes between metaplastic and triple-negative breast cancer patients. Breast 2020;49:8–16.

72. Pezzi CM, Patel-Parekh L, Cole K, et al. Characteristics and treatment of metaplastic breast cancer: analysis of 892 cases from the National Cancer Data Base. Ann Surg Oncol 2007;14(1):166–73.

73. Van Hoeven KH, Drudis T, Cranor ML, et al. Low-grade adenosquamous carcinoma of the breast. A clinocopathologic study of 32 cases with ultrastructural analysis. Am J Surg Pathol 1993;17(3):248–58.

74. Gobbi H, Simpson JF, Borowsky A, et al. Metaplastic breast tumors with a dominant fibromatosis-like phenotype have a high risk of local recurrence. Cancer 1999;85(10):2170–82.

75. Sneige N, Yazihi H, Mandavilli SR, et al. Low-grade (fibromatosis-like) spindle cell carcinoma of the breast. Am J Surg Pathol 2001;25(8):1009–16.

76. Kurian KM, Al-Nafussi A. Sarcomatoid/metaplastic carcinoma of the breast: a clinicopathological study of 12 cases. Histopathology 2002;40(1):58–64.

77. Jung SY, Kim HY, Nam BH, et al. Worse prognosis of metaplastic breast cancer patients than other patients with triple-negative breast cancer. Breast Cancer Res Treat 2010;120(3):627–37.

78. Luini A, Aguilar M, Gatti G, et al. Metaplastic carcinoma of the breast, an unusual disease with worse prognosis: the experience of the European Institute of Oncology and review of the literature. Breast Cancer Res Treat 2007;101(3):349–53.

79. Lee H, Jung SY, Ro JY, et al. Metaplastic breast cancer: clinicopathological features and its prognosis. J Clin Pathol 2012;65(5):441–6.

80. Tadros AB, Sevilimedu V, Giri DD, et al. Survival outcomes for metaplastic breast cancer differ by histologic subtype. Ann Surg Oncol 2021;28(8): 4245–53.

81. Rakha EA, Tan PH, Varga Z, et al. Prognostic factors in metaplastic carcinoma of the breast: a multi-institutional study. Br J Cancer 2015;112(2): 283–9.

82. Leyrer CM, Berriochoa CA, Agrawal S, et al. Predictive factors on outcomes in metaplastic breast cancer. Breast Cancer Res Treat 2017;165(3): 499–504.

Moving?

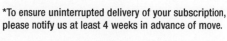

Make sure your subscription moves with you!

To notify us of your new address, find your **Clinics Account Number** (located on your mailing label above your name), and contact customer service at:

Email: journalscustomerservice-usa@elsevier.com

800-654-2452 (subscribers in the U.S. & Canada)
314-447-8871 (subscribers outside of the U.S. & Canada)

Fax number: 314-447-8029

Elsevier Health Sciences Division
Subscription Customer Service
3251 Riverport Lane
Maryland Heights, MO 63043

*To ensure uninterrupted delivery of your subscription, please notify us at least 4 weeks in advance of move.

Moving?

Make sure your subscription moves with you!

To notify us of your new address, find your Clinics Account Number (located on your mailing label above your name), and contact customer service at:

Email: journalscustomerservice-usa@elsevier.com

800-654-2452 (subscribers in the U.S. & Canada)
314-447-8871 (subscribers outside of the U.S. & Canada)

Fax number: 314-447-8029

**Elsevier Health Sciences Division
Subscription Customer Service
3251 Riverport Lane
Maryland Heights, MO 63043**

Printed and bound by CPI Group (UK) Ltd, Croydon, CR0 4YY

03/10/2024

01040372-0018